T0344431

PET/CT in Cancer

An Interdisciplinary Approach to
Individualized Imaging

PET/CT in Cancer

An Interdisciplinary Approach to Individualized Imaging

MOHSEN BEHESHTI, MD, FASNC, FEBNM
Professor of Nuclear Medicine
Head, PET-CT Center Linz
Department of Nuclear Medicine and
    Endocrinology
Ordensklinikum, St. Vincent's Hospital
Linz, Austria

WERNER LANGSTEGER, MD, FACE
Professor and Chairman
PET-CT Center Linz, Thyroid Center Linz,
    and Therapy Unit
Department of Nuclear Medicine and
    Endocrinology
Ordensklinikum, St. Vincent's Hospital
Linz, Austria

ALIREZA REZAEE, MD, ABNM
Consultant, Nuclear Medicine
Scientific Collaborator
Department of Nuclear Medicine and
    Endocrinology
Ordensklinikum, St. Vincent's Hospital
Linz, Austria

Associate Editors

MARKUS RADERER, MD
Professor of Medical Oncology
Department of Internal Medicine I
Division of Oncology
Medical University of Vienna
Vienna, Austria

NIKLAUS SCHAEFFER, MD
Professor of Nuclear Medicine and
    Medical Oncology
Department of Nuclear Medicine and
    Molecular Imaging
University of Lausanne
Lausanne, Switzerland

ELSEVIER

ELSEVIER

1600 John F. Kennedy Blvd.
Ste 1800
Philadelphia, PA 19103-2899

PET/CT IN CANCER: AN INTERDISCIPLINARY APPROACH TO
INDIVIDUALIZED IMAGING   ISBN: 978-0-323-48567-8

Notices

International Standard Book Number: 978-0-323-48567-8

Content Strategist: Robin Carter
Design Direction: Renee Duenow

Printed in United States of America

Last digit is the print number: 9 8 7 6 5 4 3 2 1

Contributors

Norbert Avril, MD
Professor and Research Scholar
Department of Radiology
Case Western Reserve University
University Hospitals Cleveland Medical Center
Cleveland, OH, USA

Mohsen Beheshti, MD, FASNC, FEBNM
Professor of Nuclear Medicine
Head, PET-CT Center Linz
Department of Nuclear Medicine and Endocrinology
Ordensklinikum, St. Vincent's Hospital
Linz, Austria

Andreas Buck, MD
Department of Nuclear Medicine
University of Würzburg
Würzburg, Germany

Martin Burian, MD
Professor and Head
Department of Otorhinolaryngology, Head and Neck
    Surgery
Ordensklinikum Linz
Linz, Austria

Alexander Drzezga, MD
Professor and Chair in Nuclear Medicine
Department of Nuclear Medicine
University Hospital of Cologne
Cologne, Germany

Norbert Galldiks, MD
Department of Neurology
University Hospital Cologne
Cologne, Germany;
Institute of Neuroscience and Medicine
Research Center Jülich
Jülich, Germany;
Center of Integrated Oncology
Universities of Cologne and Bonn
Cologne, Germany

Lukas Hefler, MD
Gynecologic Cancer Center
Ordensklinikum Linz
Linz, Austria;
Medical University of Vienna
Vienna, Austria

Ken Herrmann, MD, NBA
Ahmanson Translational Imaging Division
Department of Molecular and Medical Pharmacology
University of California, Los Angeles
Los Angeles, CA, USA;
Department of Nuclear Medicine
Universitätsklinikum Essen
Essen, Germany

Prof. Dr. Karl-Josef Langen, MD
Professor
Institute of Neuroscience and Medicine
Medical Imaging Physics
Forschungszentrum Jülich;
Department of Nuclear Medicine
Aachen University Clinic
Jülich, Germany

Werner Langsteger, MD, FACE
Professor and Chairman
PET-CT Center Linz, Thyroid Center Linz, Therapy Unit
Department of Nuclear Medicine and Endocrinology
Ordensklinikum, St. Vincent's Hospital
Linz, Austria

Markus Raderer, MD
Professor of Medical Oncology
Department of Internal Medicine I
Division of Oncology
Medical University of Vienna
Vienna, Austria

Alireza Rezaee, MD, ABNM
Consultant, Nuclear Medicine
Scientific Collaborator
Department of Nuclear Medicine and Endocrinology
Ordensklinikum, St. Vincent's Hospital
Linz, Austria

Prof. Dr. Niklaus Schaefer, MD
Professor of Nuclear Medicine and Medical Oncology
Department of Nuclear Medicine and Molecular
    Imaging
University Hospital of Lausanne
University of Lausanne
Lausanne, Switzerland

Heiko Schöder, MD
Attending Physician
Memorial Sloan Kettering Cancer Center
Professor of Radiology
Weill Cornell Medical College
New York, NY, USA

**Rathan M. Subramaniam, MD, PhD, MClinEd,
MPH, FRANZCR, FACNM**
Robert W. Parkey MD Distinguished Professor in
    Radiology
Professor and Chief, Division of Nuclear Medicine
Medical Director, Cyclotron and Molecular Imaging
    Program
Program Director, Nuclear Medicine Residency
Department of Radiology
UT Southwestern Medical Center
Dallas, TX, USA

Jochen Walz, MD
Assistant Professor
Institut Paoli-Calmettes Cancer Centre
Marseille, France

Preface

Molecular imaging with PET/CT has grown exponentially in the past decade with technical developments and the introduction of many promising and specific radiotracers. PET/CT has also become more widely available in medical centers and plays an increasingly important role in many health systems, particularly in the field of cancer diagnosis. In reality, a team of different clinical and imaging specialists, such as oncologists, radiation oncologists, oncologic surgeons, nuclear physicians, radiologists, and pathologists, is needed to prepare a road map for the best and most efficient management of a patient's cancer.

We have tried to present the appropriate indication for PET/CT imaging in different cancers, using multidisciplinary scientific data from clinical, imaging, and procedural guidelines, as well as the evidence-based literature for individualized imaging. To enable readers to quickly access pertinent information, we have organized all the chapters in the same format. The chapters are framed around important clinical information about the cancer, staging classifications, indication for PET/CT according to major clinical guidelines, evidence-based recommendations on each topic, clinical point of view from an oncologist or oncologic surgeon, PET/CT pitfalls for that malignancy, and an overview or discussion of the roles for PET/CT in staging, restaging, and evaluating the response to antineoplastic treatment, as well as its prognostic value. If indicated, the application of radiotracers beyond ^{18}F-fludeoxyglucose is discussed in some chapters. At the end of each chapter, the teaching cases section highlights the strengths and limitations of PET/CT imaging and provides clinical data, together with benign findings and pitfalls for each individual radiotracer and key points for an accurate interpretation.

In preparing this book we have had the privilege of collaborating with outstanding contributors from leading comprehensive cancer centers in Europe and North America. We believe that the authors' expertise, distinguished knowledge, and thoroughness in detailing individualized multidisciplinary approaches provide a valuable source of information and can guide decision making for physicians.

All physicians active in the field of cancer diagnosis and treatment (oncologists, oncologic surgeons, radiation oncologists, nuclear medicine physicians, and radiologists) are the target audience for this text. The book can also be used to train young specialists who are preparing for various tumor board examinations.

We dedicate this book to those who treat people with dignity and respect and to organizations and individuals committed to building a peaceful world.

Mohsen Beheshti, MD, FASNC, FEBNM
Professor of Nuclear Medicine
Head, PET-CT Center Linz
Department of Nuclear Medicine and Endocrinology
Ordensklinikum, St. Vincent's Hospital
Linz, Austria

Werner Langsteger, MD, FACE
Professor and Chairman
PET-CT Center Linz, Thyroid Center Linz, and Therapy Unit
Department of Nuclear Medicine and Endocrinology
Ordensklinikum, St. Vincent's Hospital
Linz, Austria

Alireza Rezaee, MD, ABNM
Consultant, Nuclear Medicine
Scientific Collaborator
Department of Nuclear Medicine and Endocrinology
Ordensklinikum, St. Vincent's Hospital
Linz, Austria

Contents

Abbreviations

Acetyl-CoA	Acetyl coenzyme A	**FACBC**	Anti1-amino-3-^{18}F-fluorocyclobutane-1-carboxylic acid
ACTH	Adrenocorticotropic hormone		
ALK	Anaplastic lymphoma kinase	**FAMT**	^{18}F-3-fluoro-alpha-methyl tyrosine
ASCO	American Society of Clinical Oncology	**FCH**	^{18}F-fluoromethylcholine
ATLL	Adult T-cell leukemia/lymphoma	**FDG**	2-deoxy-2-[^{18}F]-fluoro-D-glucose
ATSM	Diacetyl-bis(N(4)-methylthiosemicarbazone)	**FDOPA**	3,4-dihydroxy-6-^{18}F-fluoro-L-phenylalanine
BBB	Blood–brain barrier	**FES**	^{18}F-fluoroestradiol
BCLC	Barcelona Clinic Liver Cancer	**FET**	O-(2-^{18}F-fluoroethyl)-L-tyrosine
BCS	Breast conservation surgery	**FIGO**	Fédération Internationale de Gynécologie et d'Obstétrique (International Federation of Gynecology and Obstetrics)
BL	Burkitt lymphoma		
BPH	Benign prostatic hyperplasia		
BSO	Bilateral salpingo-oophorectomy	**FL**	Follicular lymphoma
BTV	Biologic tumor volume	**FLC**	Fibrolamellar carcinoma
CA	Cancer antigen	**FLIPI**	Follicular Lymphoma International Prognostic Index
CBD	Common bile duct		
CCRT	Chemoradiation therapy	**FLT**	^{18}F-fluorothymidine
CEA	Carcinoembryonic antigen	**FMISO**	^{18}F-fluoromisonidazole
CE-CT	Contrast-enhanced computed tomography	**FPN**	^{18}F-5-fluoropicolinamide
		G-CSF	Granulocyte-colony stimulating factor
CIM	Conventional imaging modalities	**GEP**	Gastroenteropancreatic
CLL	Chronic lymphocytic leukemia	**GGH**	Gamma-glutamyl hydrolase
CNS	Central nervous system	**GHRH**	Growth hormone releasing hormone
CRC	Colorectal cancer	**GI**	Gastrointestinal
CRF	Corticotropin-releasing factor	**GIST**	Gastrointestinal stromal tumors
CT	Computed tomography	**GLUT-1**	Glucose transporter 1
CUP	Cancers of unknown primary	**GM-CSF**	Granulocyte-macrophage colony-stimulating factor
DLBCL	Diffuse large B-cell lymphoma		
DNA	Deoxyribonucleic acid	**GS**	Gleason score
DOTA	1,4,7,10-tetraazacyclododecane-1,4,7,10-tetraacetic acid	**HBV**	Hepatitis B virus
		HCC	Hepatocellular carcinoma
DOTA-NOC	DOTA-NaI^3-Octreotide	**HCL**	Hairy cell leukemia
DOTA-TATE	DOTA-Tyr^3-Octreotate	**HCV**	Hepatitis C virus
DOTA-TOC	DOTA-Phe^1-Tyr^3-Octreotide	**HER 2**	Human epidermal growth factor receptor 2
DWI	Diffusion-weighted imaging		
EAU	European Association of Urology	**HGG**	High-grade gliomas
EBV	Epstein-Barr virus	**HGPIN**	High-grade prostatic intraepithelial neoplasia
EGFR	Epidermal growth factor receptor		
ER	Estrogen receptors	**5-HIAA**	5-hydroxyindoleacetic acid
ERCP	Endoscopic retrograde cholangiopancreatography	**HIV**	Human immunodeficiency virus
		HL	Hodgkin lymphoma
ESMO	European Society for Medical Oncology	**HNSCC**	Head and neck squamous cell carcinoma
EUS	Endoscopic ultrasound		

HPV	Human papillomavirus		PD	Programmed death
HTLV	Human T-cell lymphotropic viruses		PEM	Positron emission mammography
5-HTP	Hydroxytryptophan		PET	Positron emission tomography
IDH	Isocitrate dehydrogenase		Pg	Picograms
K-ras	Kirsten rat sarcoma viral oncogene homolog		PGL	Paraganglioma
			PID	Pelvic inflammatory disease
LAT	Large neutral amino acid transporter		P-NEN	Pancreatic neuroendocrine neoplasm
LDH	Lactate dehydrogenase		PPV	Positive predictive value
LGG	Low-grade gliomas		PRRT	Peptide receptor radionuclide therapy
LL	Lymphocytic lymphoma		PSA	Prostate-specific antigen
M	Metastasis		PSMA	Prostate-specific membrane antigen
MALT	Mucosa-associated lymphoid tissue		PTHrp	Parathyroid hormone related peptide
max	Maximum		PTLD	Post-transplant lymphoproliferative disorder
MCL	Mantle cell lymphoma			
MDCT	Multidetector computed tomography		PWI	Perfusion weighted imaging
MDP	^{99m}Tc-methylene diphosphonate		RANO	Response assessment in neuro-oncology
MEK	Mitogen-activated protein kinase kinase enzymes		RECIST	Response evaluation criteria in solid tumors
MEN	Multiple endocrine neoplasia		RGD	Arginyl-glycyl-aspartic acid
MET	^{11}C-methyl-methionine		SCC	Squamous cell carcinoma
MF	Mycosis fungoides		SCLC	Small cell lung cancer
MGMT	O6-methylguanine-DNA methyltransferase		SGO	Society of Gynecologic Oncology
			SIRT	Selective internal radionuclide therapy
MIBG	Iodine-131 metaiodobenzylguanidine			
MIPI	Mantle cell international prognostic index		SLL	Small lymphocytic lymphoma
mL	Milliliter		SLNB	Sentinel lymph node biopsy
MRCP	Magnetic resonance cholangiopancreatography		SNMMI	Society of Nuclear Medicine and Molecular Imaging
MRI	Magnetic resonance imaging		SPECT	Single-photon emission computed tomography
MTC	Medullary thyroid cancer			
MTV	Metabolic tumor volume		SPN	Solitary pulmonary nodules
MZL	Marginal zone lymphoma		SRC	Signet ring cell
N	Lymph nodes		SRS	Somatostatin receptor scintigraphy
NaF	^{18}F-sodium fluoride		SS	Sezary syndrome
NAFLD	Non-alcoholic fatty liver disease		SST-A	Somatostatin analogs
NCCN	National Comprehensive Cancer Network		SSTR	Somatostatin receptor
NEC	Neuroendocrine carcinomas		SUV	Standardized uptake value
NEN	Neuroendocrine neoplasms		TACE	Trans-arterial chemoembolization
NET	Neuroendocrine tumors		TAH	Total abdominal hysterectomy
ng	Nanogram		TB	Tuberculosis
NHL	Non-Hodgkin lymphoma		TF	Textural-features
NK	Natural killer		TKI	Tyrosine kinase inhibitors
NOPR	National Oncologic PET Registry		TLG	Total lesion glycolysis
NPV	Negative predictive value		TNM	Tumor, lymph nodes, metastasis
NSCLC	Non-small cell lung cancer		TSPO	Translocator protein
OCP	Oral contraceptive pills		UK	United Kingdom
Pap	Papanicolaou		US	United States
PCC	Pheochromocytoma		VEGF	Vascular endothelial growth factor
PCV	Procarbazine, CCNU (lomustine), and vincristine		VIP	Vasoactive intestinal polypeptide
			WHO	World Health Organization

CHAPTER 1

Head and Neck Cancers

MOHSEN BEHESHTI • RATHAN M. SUBRAMANIAM • ALIREZA REZAEE •
MARTIN BURIAN • WERNER LANGSTEGER

BACKGROUND

General

- Head and neck cancers are the sixth most common cancers among males and twice in prevalence when compared with females.[1]
- Head and neck cancers are composed of cancers arising from the paranasal sinuses, nasopharynx, oral cavity, oropharynx, hypopharynx, and larynx.[2] The cancers arising from the salivary glands and lip are not reviewed in this chapter.
- The following are the main risk factors[3–5]:
  - Tobacco and alcohol use.
  - Infection with human papillomavirus (HPV), particularly HPV-16 infection, is one of the main causes of oropharyngeal cancers.
- No screening test is available for head and neck cancers.[6]
- The hypopharyngeal, laryngeal, oropharyngeal, and nasopharyngeal cancers present with distant metastases in 19%, 16%, 13%, and 10% of cases, respectively.[7]
- Cervical lymph node metastasis is the presenting sign in about 2% to 9% of patients with head and neck squamous cell carcinoma (HNSCC) with an unknown primary site of cancer.[8]

Early Clinical Symptoms[9]

- Cervical lymphadenopathy
- Long-lasting oral cavity ulcer or sore throat
- Dysphagia
- Hoarseness
- Nasal airway obstruction

Standard Diagnostic Procedures[10]

- Clinical examination
- Panendoscopy and biopsy
- Fine-needle aspiration or core biopsy
- CT, MRI, and PET/CT (if indicated)
- HPV diagnostics

Standard Treatment[11–13]

- Surgery
- Radiation therapy
- Chemotherapy
- Targeted therapy

Prognostic Factors[13–15]

- Tumor location (worse in hypopharyngeal cancers)
- Tumor size (worse if larger)
- Lymph node status (worse if contralateral neck nodes are involved)
- Histologic grade (worse if high grade/poorly differentiated)
- Overexpression of epidermal growth factor receptor (worse prognosis)
- Tumors not associated with HPV (worse prognosis)

Five-Year Survival[16]

- Stage I: 77%
- Stage II: 61%
- Stage III: 57%
- Stage IV: 42%

TUMOR CHARACTERISTICS AND TYPICAL BEHAVIOR

Histopathology[2,17]

- Squamous cell carcinoma: >90%
- Others (adenocarcinoma, esthesioneuroblastoma, lymphoepithelioma, adenoid cystic cancer): <10%

Distribution and Localization

T-primary[2,18]

- Paranasal sinuses
- Nasopharynx
- Oral cavity
- Oropharynx
- Hypopharynx
- Larynx

N-lymph nodes[2]

The primary localization of the lymph nodes and their cervical level are provided in Table 1.1.

M-distant metastasis[2]

- Lung: 58%
- Liver: 29%
- Bone: 22%
- Distant lymph nodes: 17%
- Mediastinum: 14%
- Kidneys: 11%

TNM CLASSIFICATION[13,19]

The TNM classification system describes the stage of cancer (Table 1.2).

Guidelines

Clinical Guidelines	Initial Diagnosis (Primary Tumor)	N-staging	M-staging
ESMO[20]	• No statement	• Optional In case of doubtful findings in other imaging modalities	• Optional In case of doubtful findings in other imaging modalities
NCCN[13]	• Occult primary in cervical lymph node metastasis	• Can replace CIM in stage III-IV	• Can replace CIM in stage III-IV • Optional for nasopharyngeal cancers

CIM, conventional imaging modalities; ESMO, European Society for Medical Oncology; NCCN, National Comprehensive Cancer Network.

EVIDENCE-BASED VIEWPOINTS

- Fludeoxyglucose (FDG) PET/CT is recommended for the following[21]:
  - Staging of patients in cases in which staging is difficult clinically or there are equivocal findings on other conventional imaging modalities (because of dental artifacts in CT or movement in MRI)
  - Staging or restaging of patients (stages III and IV) with a high risk of disseminated disease
  - Identifying the primary site in patients with squamous cell carcinoma (SCC) metastatic to cervical lymph node

TABLE 1.1
N-Lymph Nodes

Primary Localization	Lymph Nodes	Cervical Levels
Nasal cavity and ethmoid sinus	• Retropharyngeal	-
Maxillary sinus	• Submandibular	I
Nasopharynx	• Retropharyngeal	-
Oropharynx	• Jugulodigastric • Superior deep cervical	II
Hypopharynx	• Mid deep cervical	III
Supraglottic region	• Jugulodigastric • Superior deep cervical • Mid deep cervical	II
Glottis	• Prelaryngeal	VI
Subglottic region	• Juguloomohyoid • Inferior deep cervical	IV
Oral cavity	• Submandibular	I
	• Jugulodigastric	II

- Evaluation of treatment response 3 to 6 months after chemoradiation therapy in patients (per NCCN guideline)
- Differentiating relapse from treatment effects
- FDG PET/CT is very accurate in restaging of HN-SCC.[22]
- FDG PET/CT shows a high diagnostic performance in detecting recurrent head and neck cancers.[23,24]
- With a very high negative predictive value (NPV), a negative posttherapy FDG PET/CT in patients with head and neck cancer is strongly suggestive of absent viable malignancy.[25]
- Pretherapy and posttherapy maximum standardized uptake values (SUV_{max}) on FDG PET/CT are predictive factors for long-term survival in patients with head and neck cancers.[26]
- Positive intratherapy or posttherapy follow-up FDG PET/CT predicts the risk of adverse events and death within a 2-year period in patients with head and neck cancers.[27]
- By determining the extent of regional nodal metastases, FDG PET/CT may dramatically change the radiation therapy target volumes, cervical dissection choices, and radiation therapy planning. It is able to detect synchronous and unknown primary tumors and metastatic disease.[24]

TABLE 1.2
Head and Neck Cancer TNM Classification

TNM[a]	N0	N1	N2	N3	M1
T1	I	III	IVA	IVB	IVC
T2	II	III	IVA	IVB	IVC
T3	III	III	IVA	IVB	IVC
T4a	IVA	IVA	IVA	IVB	IVC
T4b	IVB	IVB	IVB	IVB	IVC

TNM classification of each cancer localization in the head and neck region should be considered individually.[19]
[a]Except for nasopharyngeal cancer.

- The modality is capable of differentiating responders from nonresponders to therapy.[24]

COST-EFFECTIVENESS
- FDG PET/CT is more cost-effective and accurate than conventional anatomic imaging modalities, which is leading to better care in patients with advanced head and neck cancers and diminished costs by preventing futile surgeries of benign and nonresectable malignancies.[28]
- FDG PET/CT is cost-effective for diagnostic and therapy planning in head and neck cancers, particularly in patients with subclinical lymph nodes (N0 classification) on stand-alone CT.[29,30]

CLINICAL POINT OF VIEW
From a clinical point of view, FDG PET/CT is most valuable in cancers of unknown primary (CUPs). It provides accurate information for guiding biopsy in up to 60% of all cases, which prevents unnecessary sampling. Moreover, whole-body imaging by FDG PET/CT could prevent inessential examinations (e.g., endoscopy, bronchoscopy) for detection of primary tumors beyond the aerodigestive tract.

Currently, there is no sufficient evidence to support the utility of FDG PET/CT as a standard imaging modality for staging of head and neck cancers. Contrast-enhanced (CE)-CT and MRI are still the first imaging modalities of choice in the assessment of primary tumors mainly because they are advantageous in providing morphologic information. However, the use of hybrid imaging modalities (e.g., PET/CT, PET/MRI) may significantly improve the diagnostic accuracy. In addition, PET/CT seems to be promising in the detection of synchronous second primaries, lymph nodes, and distant metastasis or clarification of equivocal lesions on conventional imaging modalities.

Posttherapeutic imaging in head and neck cancer is still challenging. In such cases, metabolic information from PET/CT is substantial for clinical decision making. The high NPV of PET/CT helps in reducing the number of unnecessary biopsies or salvage surgeries, such as posttreatment neck dissection. However, imaging should be performed at an appropriate time frame after radiochemotherapy or surgery. Short-time posttherapeutic assessment may cause false-positive results, and long-term evaluation may lead to pronounced fibrosis and scar formation, resulting in a higher complication rate in the case of salvage surgery.

PITFALLS[31–35]
False Positive
- Benign parotid tumors (e.g., Warthin tumor, pleomorphic adenoma)
- Physiologic uptake in oculomotor, mylohyoid, laryngeal, and cervical muscles, nasopharynx, salivary glands, tonsils, and vocal cords
- Unilateral vocal cord paralysis
- Treatment of vocal cord paralysis with injectable Teflon
- Inflammatory/infectious process, including postradiation inflammation
- Reactive cervical lymph nodes
- Dental hardware streak artifact (attenuation correction artifact)
- Dental disease
- Brown fat tissue
- Benign thyroid nodules

False Negative

- Lesion proximity to structures with high FDG uptake
- Necrotic metastatic lymph nodes
- Common false-negative lesions in all cancers: early-stage malignancy, hyperglycemic state, small lesions (<8 mm)

DISCUSSION

The role of FDG PET/CT imaging in staging, therapy monitoring, and long-term follow-up evaluation of HNSCC is widely investigated.[24,31,36–38]

MRI and CE-CT are currently considered as standard imaging modalities for the assessment of the primary tumor (T-staging). However, PET/CT examinations performed with appropriate CE-CT protocols are as good as or better than standard conventional imaging for T-staging.[24,39]

In pretreatment evaluation of cervical lymph nodes of head and neck cancers, the role of FDG PET/CT is well recognized.[24,31] The average sensitivity and specificity of FDG PET/CT were reported as 87% to 90% and 80% to 93% compared with 61% to 97% and 21% to 100% for MRI or CT, respectively.[40] Also, a prospective observational study of 248 patients revealed that FDG PET/CT changed TNM-staging in 32% of cases because of accurate N-staging. The modality showed a significantly higher sensitivity and accuracy, compared with conventional work-ups.[31,41,42] Furthermore, it showed valuable impact in the detection of distant metastases with a sensitivity, specificity, positive predictive value (PPV), NPV, and overall accuracy of 89%, 97%, 85%, 98%, and 96%, respectively.[43]

In addition, FDG PET/CT seems to be the diagnostic imaging method of choice for the detection of synchronous second cancers in patients with HNSCC who are at increased risk of synchronous malignancies, specifically upper aerodigestive cancers.[24,36,38,44]

Occult primary HNSCCs are presented with cervical lymph node metastases in <10% of patients.[8] In such cases, detection of the primary tumor is of crucial significance to plan for surgery or limit the field of external beam radiation.[24] This role is well played by FDG PET/CT, with detection of about 30% of unknown primary cancers.[24,36,38,44] It is more sensitive for this purpose compared with CE-CT or MRI.[45] The target volume may change in approximately 20% of cases according to FDG PET/CT data compared with stand-alone CT data.[24] Hence, the role of FDG PET/CT has been increasingly used for radiotherapy planning in HNSCC.[24,31,44,46]

In recurrent HNSCC, FDG PET/CT is more advantageous over other conventional imaging modalities because of not only higher accuracy but also early detection of disease at the time it may not be demonstrated by other imaging methods.[23,47,48] This is mainly because of the limited value of conventional imaging modalities, such as CT or MRI, after radiation therapy and surgery, as the complex anatomy of head and neck soft tissue structures may distort after treatment.[49] A systematic review and meta-analysis of 27 studies revealed a sensitivity, specificity, PPV, and NPV of 94%, 82%, 75%, and 95% for FDG PET in detecting recurrent disease, respectively.[22] It also presents a significantly higher specificity of about 90% in differentiating residual tumor from scar tissue in the primary site compared with 59% and 41% for CT and MRI, respectively.[50]

Moreover, FDG PET/CT has an approved role in the assessment of the response to therapy in HNSCC.[14,42] The overall performance of the modality for this purpose is favorable, with a markedly high NPV (>95%). Thus, a negative posttherapy scan indicates the annihilation of viable malignancy and residual disease in most patients.[25,51–53] The time frame for performing FDG PET/CT is very important to prevent false-positive and false-negative findings resulting from intervention or treatment-induced local inflammatory changes. It is highly recommended that clinicians perform FDG PET/CT 2 weeks after needle biopsy and at least 4 and 12 weeks after surgical resection and chemo/radiotherapy respectively, to minimize false-positive results.[22,43,49,54]

The functional characteristic of FDG PET/CT could provide useful predictive information. Tumor SUV_{max} is reported as an independent predicting factor of disease-free survival in HNSCC.[55] Previous studies suggested a functional multiparametric approach for predicting the outcome of the disease.[37,56–58] A tumor $SUV_{max} > 10$, total lesion glycolysis >70, metabolic tumor volume >20 cm³, and ring-shaped pattern of uptake in the primary tumor were related to an ominous prognosis.[56] Even an $SUV_{max} \geq 4$ of metastatic cervical lymph nodes from laryngeal cancer is inversely correlated with progression-free survival rates.[59] Interestingly, some investigators discovered that the relative risks of relapse and death are higher (e.g., fourfold and sevenfold, respectively) in patients with HNSCC who have a positive FDG PET/CT.[60] In another study, the authors revealed that a positive FDG PET/CT was correlated with an over sixfold increase in risk of death in 2 years, which decreased but was still significant in the 3- to 5-year follow-up.[27] Therefore, more aggressive therapeutic approaches are suggested for primary lesions with a high FDG uptake (i.e., SUV>7).[26,61] However, prospective studies are warranted to prove the prognostic or predictive value of FDG PET/CT parameter–based cut points in the outcome of patients with HNSCC.

In conclusion, FDG PET/CT is valuable in detecting unknown primary cancer in 30% of patients after anatomic imaging failed to detect the primary cancer; has the highest accuracy for detection of neck nodal and distant metastases; is the modality of choice for therapy assessment, especially after concurrent chemoradiation therapy; and is useful for detection of suspicious recurrences in the right clinical context.

TEACHING CASES
Case 1: Staging, Laryngeal Cancer
Findings

A 67-year-old male with laryngeal SCC. FDG PET/CT shows a tracer-avid primary cancer (Fig. 1.1B, arrows) and left cervical lymph nodes (Fig. 1.1C, arrows). It also shows mildly FDG-avid bilateral paramediastinal lymph nodes (Fig. 1.1A, arrows), most likely

inflammatory in nature. A faintly FDG-avid small right cervical lymph node (Fig. 1.1D, arrows), medial to sternocleidomastoid (SCM) muscle, is reactive in nature. FDG uptake in SCM is nonspecific (Fig. 1.1D, arrowhead).

Teaching points
- The laryngeal cancer presents with distant metastases in 16% of cases.
- FDG PET/CT is an encouraging modality for N- and M-staging of head and neck cancers. However, its role in T-staging has been controversial.
- The small cervical lymph nodes that are positive on PET do not meet the criteria to be suspicious on CT. This reveals the superiority of PET/CT to stand-alone CT for this purpose.
- Use of semiquantitative parameters (e.g., SUV) and dual-time imaging helps FDG PET/CT to differentiate malignant from reactive lymph nodes.

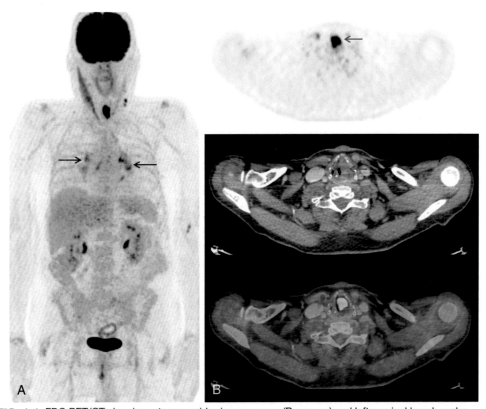

FIG. 1.1 FDG PET/CT showing a tracer-avid primary cancer (B, *arrows*) and left cervical lymph nodes (C, *arrows*). It also shows mildly FDG-avid bilateral paramediastinal lymph nodes (A, *arrows*), most likely inflammatory in nature. A faintly FDG-avid small right cervical lymph node (D, *arrows*), medial to the sternocleidomastoid (SCM) muscle, is reactive in nature. FDG uptake in SCM is nonspecific (D, *arrowhead*).

Continued

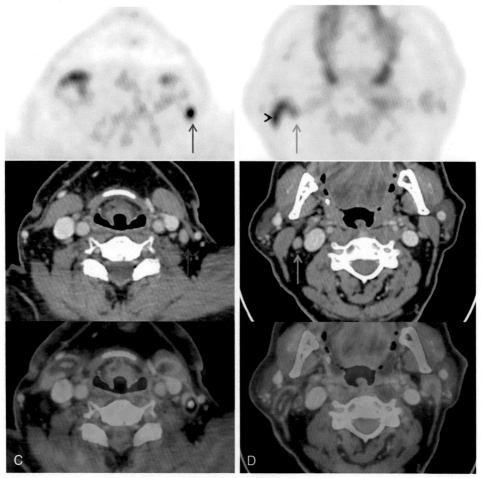

FIG. 1.1, cont'd

- An $SUV_{max} \geq 4$ of metastatic cervical lymph nodes from laryngeal cancer is inversely correlated with progression-free survival rates.

Pitfalls
- Reactive paramediastinal lymph nodes should not be interpreted as metastatic disease.

Case 2: Staging, SCC, Base of the Tongue
Findings
A 58-year-old male with SCC on the base of the tongue. FDG PET/CT shows a tracer-avid primary tumor in the base of the tongue (Fig. 1.2B, arrows) and bilateral FDG-avid cervical lymphadenopathy (Fig. 1.2A and B). There is a focal FDG uptake, corresponding to a small lytic lesion of the right ninth posterior rib on CT, consistent with metastasis (Fig. 1.2C, arrows).

Teaching points
- The role of FDG PET/CT imaging in staging, restaging, therapy monitoring, and long-term follow-up evaluation of HNSCC is widely investigated and approved.
- The small lytic lesion of the rib could be missed on stand-alone CT.
- The most common sites of distant metastasis are the lungs (~60%) and liver (~30%).
- Tumor SUV is reported as an independent predicting factor of disease-free survival in HNSCC.

Case 3: Staging, Sinus Piriform Cancer
Findings
A 69-year-old male with SCC of piriform sinus. FDG PET/CT shows a tracer-avid primary malignancy (Fig. 1.3A and B, red arrows) with right cervical lymph node metastasis (Fig. 1.3A, black arrow). There is a small FDG-avid metastatic lymph node in the prelaryngeal

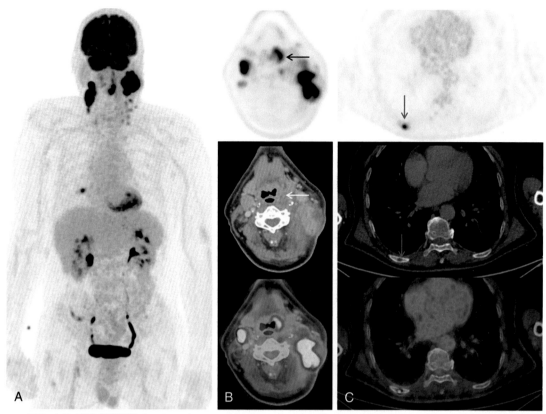

FIG. 1.2 FDG PET/CT showing a tracer-avid primary tumor in the base of the tongue (B, *arrows*) and bilateral FDG-avid cervical lymphadenopathy (A and B). There is a focal FDG uptake, corresponding to a small lytic lesion of the right ninth posterior rib on CT, consistent with metastasis (C, *arrows*).

region (Fig. 1.3C, arrows). Incidental findings are two small FDG-avid nodules within the left parotid, most likely benign in nature, such as Warthin tumor or pleomorphic adenoma (Fig. 1.3D, arrows).

Teaching points
- FDG PET/CT is an encouraging tool for the detection of small atypical metastatic lymph node metastases in HNSCC.
- FDG PET/CT examinations performed with appropriate CE-CT protocols may be as good as or better than standard conventional imaging, such as MRI and CE-CT, for T-staging of primary HNSCC.
- Lymph node involvement is a poor prognostic factor in head and neck cancers.

Pitfalls
- Benign parotid neoplasms, such as Warthin tumor and pleomorphic adenoma, may show an increased FDG uptake and are in the differential diagnosis of malignancy.

Case 4: Cancer of Unknown Primary
Findings
A 42-year-old female with CUP. FDG PET/CT shows a tracer-avid primary tumor in the right base of the tongue (Fig. 1.4B, black arrow) and known right cervical lymphadenopathy (Fig. 1.4B, red arrows). An incidental finding is symmetric vocal cord FDG uptake (arrow head), most likely inflammatory in nature. Streak artifact from dental amalgam is noted on CT (Fig. 1.4).

Teaching points
- FDG PET/CT is a promising modality to identify the primary site in patients with SCC metastatic to cervical lymph nodes and more sensitive for this purpose compared with CE-CT or MRI.
- The detection of the primary tumor is of crucial significance to plan for surgery or limit the field of external beam radiation.
- Cervical lymph node metastases are the presenting sign in about 2% to 9% of patients with HNSCC with an unknown primary cancer.

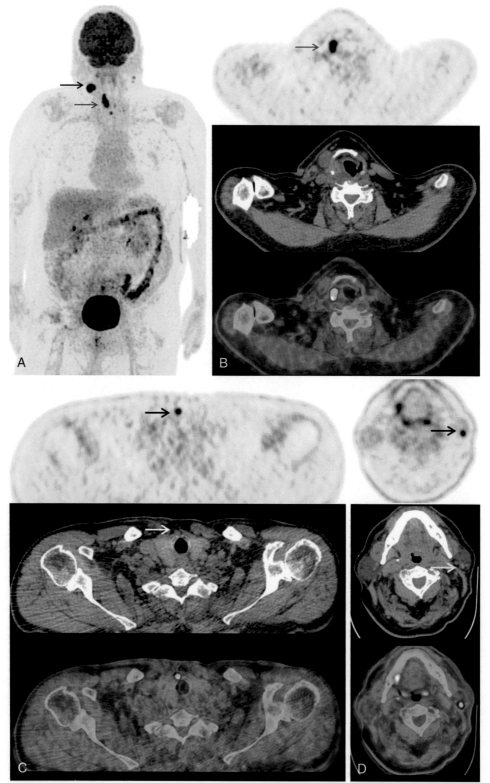

FIG. 1.3 FDG PET/CT showing a tracer-avid primary malignancy (A and B, *red arrows*) with right cervical lymph node metastasis (A, *black arrow*). There is a small FDG-avid metastatic lymph node in the prelaryngeal region (C, *arrows*). An incidental finding are two small FDG-avid nodules within the left parotid, most likely benign in nature, such as Warthin tumor or pleomorphic adenoma (D, *arrows*).

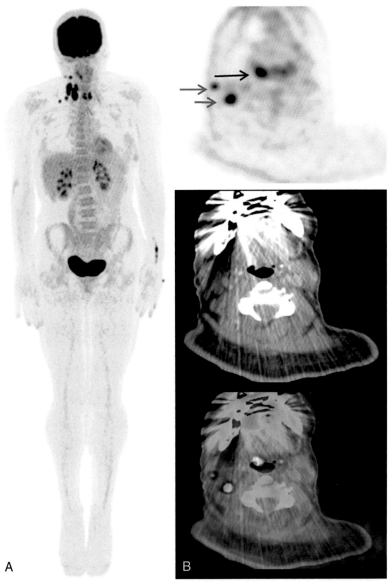

FIG. 1.4 FDG PET/CT showing a tracer-avid primary tumor in the right base of the tongue (B, *black arrow*) and known right cervical lymphadenopathy (B, *red arrows*). An incidental finding is a symmetric vocal cord FDG uptake (*arrowhead*), most likely inflammatory in nature. Streak artifact from dental amalgam is noted on CT.

- More aggressive therapeutic approaches are suggested for primary lesions with a high FDG uptake (i.e., SUV > 7).

Pitfalls
- A symmetric FDG uptake of the vocal cords can be physiologic or inflammatory in nature and should not be interpreted as malignancy.

- An asymmetric focal FDG uptake of the vocal cords may be functional because of recurrent nerve paralysis.

Case 5: Staging, Adenoid Cystic Carcinoma
Findings
A 79-year-old male with oropharyngeal adenoid cystic carcinoma. FDG PET/CT shows a primary tumor

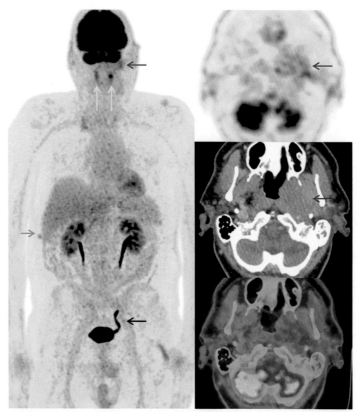

FIG. 1.5 FDG PET/CT showing a primary tumor in the nasopharyngeal and oropharyngeal region with a faint tracer uptake (*red arrows*). There is an asymmetric FDG uptake of the tonsils, more prominent on the left side (*yellow arrows*), most likely inflammatory in nature. A focal tracer uptake in the right 10th rib is posttraumatic (*green arrow*). There is atypical radioactive urine accumulation in the left distal ureter (*black arrow*).

in the nasopharyngeal and oropharyngeal region with a faint tracer uptake (red arrows). There is an asymmetric FDG uptake of the tonsils, more prominent on the left side (yellow arrows), most likely inflammatory in nature. A focal tracer uptake in the right 10th rib is posttraumatic (green arrow). There is atypical radioactive urine accumulation in the left distal ureter (black arrow) (Fig. 1.5).

Teaching point

- FDG PET/CT may show limited diagnostic accuracy in the evaluation of primary adenoid cystic carcinoma because of relatively low glucose metabolism. However, it shows higher sensitivity in the assessment of lymph node and distant metastases.

Pitfalls

- Tonsillar uptake is a common physiologic change mostly because of the inflammatory process and

should be interpreted with caution. This may limit the specificity of FDG PET/CT and may obscure the malignancy in the tonsillar region. Delayed acquisition may improve the diagnostic accuracy of this modality because malignant lesions usually show an increasing pattern on delayed scan.

Case 6: Staging, Tonsillar Cancer With Incidental Second Cancer
Findings

A 73-year-old female with left tonsillar SCC and incidental second primary gastric adenocarcinoma (intestinal type). FDG PET/CT shows a tracer-avid primary tonsillar cancer (Fig. 1.6A and B, red arrows) with left cervical lymph node metastasis (Fig. 1.6A and B, blue arrows). An incidental finding is the FDG-avid primary gastric adenocarcinoma (Fig. 1.6A and C, yellow arrows). There is a focal FDG uptake within the vagina (Fig. 1.6D, arrow), which could represent an inflammatory or a malignant process. The pathology was indeterminate in this patient (Fig. 1.6).

Teaching points
- Patients with HNSCC are more prone to second primary malignancies, most commonly of the head and neck, lung, and esophagus, which must be differentiated from either local recurrence or metastasis of the primary tumor.
- The lung is one of the most common sites for both distant metastases (particularly in patients with HPV-associated head and neck cancers) and second primary cancer in patients with HNSCC. Accurate differentiation of primary from metastatic lung malignancies is of crucial importance for patient management.
- FDG PET/CT is a promising method to detect second primary malignancy in patients with index head and neck cancers.
- Gastric cancer may be missed on stand-alone CT.

Pitfalls
- Inflammation is in the differential diagnosis of gastric cancer; however, it usually presents with a more diffuse pattern.
- Nonspecific FDG uptake in gynecologic structures is a common pitfall in PET/CT imaging. However, intensive focal versus mild to moderate diffuse increased uptake may be helpful to differentiate inflammatory from malignant disease. Nevertheless, each suspicious FDG-positive lesion should be further evaluated.

Case 7: Staging, Oropharyngeal Cancer, Myelodysplastic Syndrome
Findings
A 64-year-old male with SCC of the base of the tongue. FDG PET/CT shows a tracer-avid primary malignancy (Fig. 1.7A and B, yellow arrows). There is a diffuse FDG uptake in the axial and appendicular skeleton

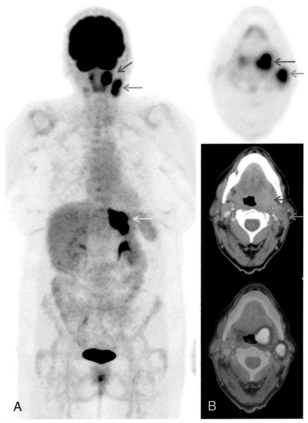

FIG. 1.6 FDG PET/CT showing a tracer-avid primary tonsillar cancer (A and B, *red arrows*) with left cervical lymph node metastasis (A and B, *blue arrows*). An incidental finding is the FDG-avid primary gastric adenocarcinoma (A and C, *yellow arrows*). There is a focal FDG uptake within the vagina (D, *arrow*), which could represent an inflammatory or a malignant process.

Continued

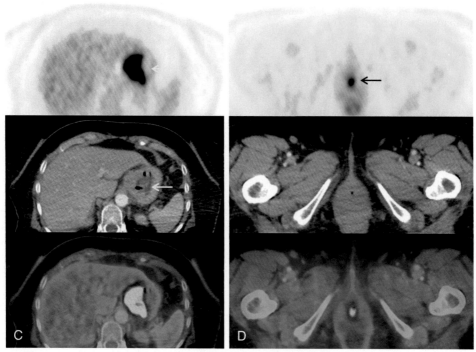

FIG. 1.6, cont'd

(Fig. 1.7A) and in bilateral mandibular condyles (Fig. 1.7A, arrowheads). Also, a moderate increased uptake is noted in the spleen (Fig. 1.7A, arrow), compared with the liver. This was confirmed to be a myelodysplastic syndrome on bone marrow biopsy (Fig. 1.7).

Teaching points
- FDG PET/CT is a promising technique to exclude second malignancy in patients with head and neck cancers.
- A diffuse homogeneous bone marrow FDG uptake is usually the result of bone marrow hyperplasia, which can happen after therapy with granulocyte colony-stimulating factor, chemotherapy, or erythropoietin or in the course of a pathologic process, such as myelodysplastic syndromes, chronic myelogenous leukemia, β-thalassemia, or severe anemia, and less likely with diffuse marrow metastases.
- The relative risks of relapse and death are higher (e.g., fourfold and sevenfold, respectively) in patients with HNSCC who have a positive FDG PET/CT.

Case 8: HNSCC, Recurrence
Findings
An 85-year-old male with right laryngeal SCC recurrence after laryngectomy. FDG PET shows a tracer-avid

local recurrent cancer with undetermined finding on CT (Fig. 1.8A and B, red arrows). There are multiple FDG-avid bilateral small lymph node metastases (Fig. 1.8C, arrows) and metastases to the oropharyngeal region (Fig. 1.8D, arrows). An incidental finding is bilateral hilar lymph nodes with a faint uptake (Fig. 1.8A, black arrows), most likely inflammatory in nature (Fig. 1.8).

Teaching points
- FDG PET/CT is a promising modality in the assessment of recurrent head and neck cancers.
- Conventional imaging methods may have limitations in postsurgical head and neck cancers because of distortion of the complex regional anatomy.

Pitfalls
- Hilar lymph nodes may present with a mild uptake, are usually reactive in nature, and should not be interpreted as metastatic disease.

Case 9: Therapy Monitoring, Nasopharyngeal Cancer
Findings
A 72-year-old male with nasopharyngeal SCC, status postradiation therapy. FDG PET/CT shows a tracer-avid

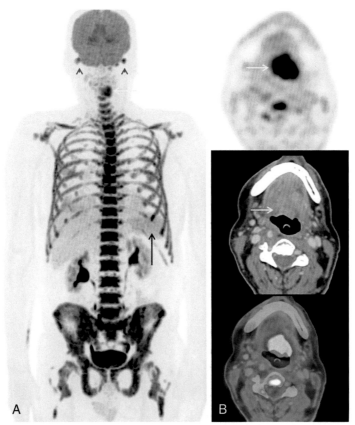

FIG. 1.7 FDG PET/CT showing a tracer-avid primary malignancy (A and B, *yellow arrows*). There is a diffuse FDG uptake in the axial and appendicular skeleton (A) and in the bilateral mandibular condyles (A, *arrowheads*). Also, a moderate increased uptake is noted in the spleen (A, *arrow*), compared with the liver.

primary malignancy (Fig. 1.9A and C, arrow). Follow-up examination demonstrates an excellent complete metabolic response to therapy (Fig. 1.9B and D, arrow).

Teaching points
- More than 90% of head and neck cancers are SCC.
- Surgery and radiotherapy are the cornerstone of treatment in head and neck cancers.
- FDG PET/CT is a promising method for therapy monitoring.
- Nasopharyngeal cancer has a high propensity for distant metastasis and is one of the main indications for FDG PET/CT to rule out distant metastases.
- The most commonly involved local lymph nodes from nasopharyngeal cancers are retropharyngeal stations. Distant lymph nodes are involved in 17% of cases.
- Determination of the extent of regional nodal metastases using FDG PET/CT may dramatically change

radiation therapy target volumes and cervical dissection choices.
- FDG PET/CT is recommended for the evaluation of treatment response 3 to 6 months after chemoradiation therapy in patients with indeterminate findings on conventional imaging.
- With a very high NPV, a negative posttherapy FDG PET/CT in patients with head and neck cancer is strongly suggestive of absent viable malignancy.

Case 10: Staging and Restaging Rhabdomyosarcoma
Findings
A 19-year-old male with rhabdomyosarcoma. FDG PET/CT shows a heterogeneous FDG uptake in the right nasoethmoidal primary malignancy (Fig. 1.10A and C, red arrows) along with bilateral cervical lymph node metastases (Fig. 1.10A, black arrows). There are disseminated FDG-avid axial and appendicular

histopathologically approved skeletal metastases (Fig. 1.10A). Follow-up examination demonstrates an excellent metabolic response to chemotherapy (Fig. 1.10B and D). A symmetric increased pharyngeal FDG uptake is seen after chemotherapy (Fig. 1.10B, arrow).

Teaching points
- The value of FDG PET/CT in the assessment of sarcoma is controversial.
- FDG PET/CT is superior to stand-alone CT in the early detection of marrow-based bone metastases.
- FDG PET/CT is a promising modality for treatment monitoring in sarcoma when malignant lesions are FDG avid on baseline examination.

- The heterogeneous pattern of marrow FDG uptake is changed to homogeneous after treatment.

Pitfalls
- A symmetric pharyngeal FDG uptake after chemotherapy is most likely inflammatory.
- A symmetric homogeneous mild to moderate bone marrow uptake after chemotherapy is reactive in nature and caused by hyperplasia.
- A focal FDG uptake in the lower abdomen on PET is caused by urinary retention.

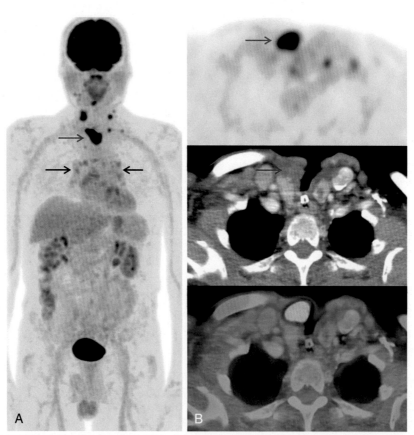

FIG. 1.8 FDG PET showing a tracer-avid local recurrent cancer with undetermined finding on CT (A and B, *red arrows*). There are multiple FDG-avid bilateral small lymph node metastases (C, *arrows*) and metastases to the oropharyngeal region (D, *arrows*). An incidental finding is bilateral hilar lymph nodes with a faint uptake (A, *black arrows*), most likely inflammatory in nature.

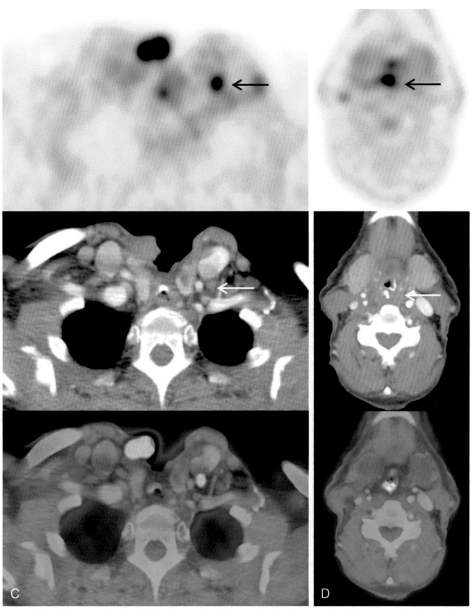

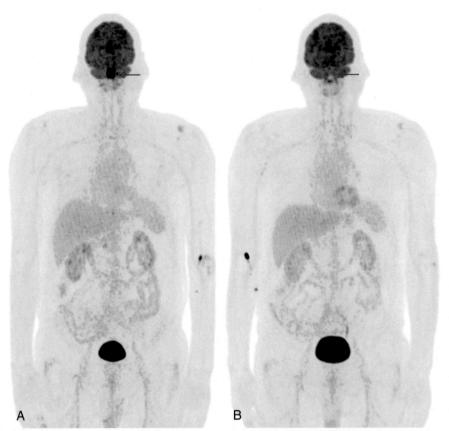

FIG. 1.9 FDG PET/CT showing a tracer-avid primary malignancy (A and C, *arrow*). Follow-up examination demonstrates an excellent complete metabolic response to therapy (B and D, *arrow*).

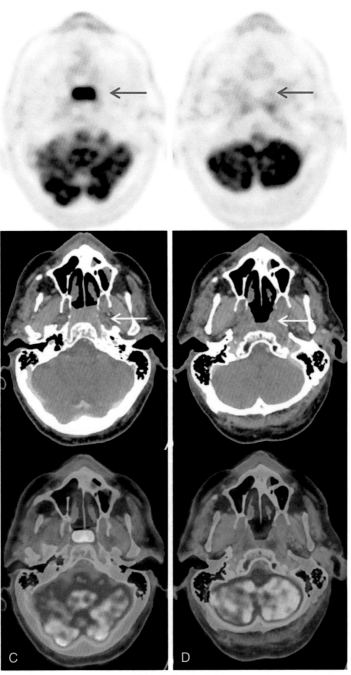

FIG. 1.9, cont'd

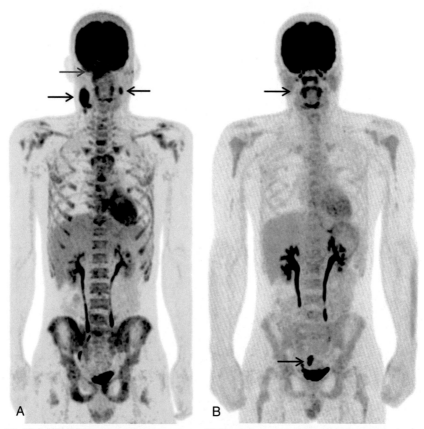

FIG. 1.10 FDG PET/CT showing a heterogeneous FDG uptake in the right nasoethmoidal primary malignancy (A and C, *red arrows*) along with bilateral cervical lymph node metastases (A, *black arrows*). There are disseminated FDG-avid axial and appendicular histopathologically approved skeletal metastases (A). Follow-up examination demonstrates an excellent metabolic response to chemotherapy (B and D). A symmetric increased pharyngeal FDG uptake is seen after chemotherapy (B, *arrow*).

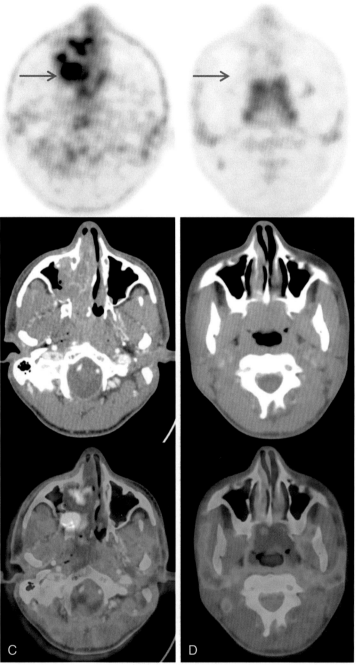

FIG. 1.10, cont'd

REFERENCES

1. Siegel RL, Miller KD, Jemal A. Cancer statistics, 2016. *CA: A Cancer Journal for Clinicians*. January-February 2016;66(1):7–30.
2. Head and Neck Primary Sites. In: Robin P, Hansen JT, eds. *TNM Staging Atlas With Oncoanatomy*. 2nd ed. Philadelphia, USA: Wolters Kluwer/LWW; 2012:1–124.
3. Chaturvedi AK, Engels EA, Pfeiffer RM, et al. Human papillomavirus and rising oropharyngeal cancer incidence in the United States. *Journal of Clinical Oncology: Official Journal of the American Society of Clinical Oncology*. November 10, 2011;29(32):4294–4301.
4. Gandini S, Botteri E, Iodice S, et al. Tobacco smoking and cancer: a meta-analysis. *International Journal of Cancer*. January 1, 2008;122(1):155–164.
5. Okami K. Clinical features and treatment strategy for HPV-related oropharyngeal cancer. *International Journal of Clinical Oncology*. July 5, 2016.
6. Screening Guidelines. https://www.mskcc.org/cancer-care/types/head-neck/screening-guidelines-head-neck.
7. Carvalho A, Nishimoto I, Califano J, Kowalski L. Trends in incidence and prognosis for head and neck cancer in the United States: a site-specific analysis of the SEER database. *International Journal of Cancer*. 2004;114(5):806–816.
8. Jereczek-Fossa BA, Jassem J, Orecchia R. Cervical lymph node metastases of squamous cell carcinoma from an unknown primary. *Cancer Treatment Reviews*. April 2004;30(2):153–164.
9. What are the Symptoms of Head and Neck Cancers? http://www.cancer.gov/types/head-and-neck/head-neck-fact-sheet#q3.
10. *Diagnosis and Management of Head and Neck Cancer - A National Clinical Guideline*. Edinburgh: Scottish Intercollegiate Guidelines Network; 2006.
11. Head and Neck Cancer - Treatment Options. http://www.cancer.net/cancer-types/head-and-neck-cancer/treatment-options.
12. Kurzweg T, Kimmeyer J, Knecht R, et al. Curative treatment of head and neck squamous cell carcinoma: organ preservation strategies in clinical routine in German-speaking countries. *HNO*. July 2016;64(7):501–507.
13. Head and Neck Cancers. Version 1. *NCCN Clinical Practice Guidelines in Oncology*. ; 2016. www.NCCN.org.
14. Cojocariu OM, Huguet F, Lefevre M, Perie S. Prognosis and predictive factors in head-and-neck cancers. *Bulletin du cancer*. April 2009;96(4):369–378.
15. Mehanna H, West CM, Nutting C, Paleri V. Head and neck cancer–part 2: treatment and prognostic factors. *BMJ*. 2010;341:c4690.
16. Winning the Battle Against Head and Neck Cancer. The Five-Year Survival Rates for Head and Neck Cancer Patients. http://www.seattlecca.org/diseases/head-neck-cancer-survival-rates.cfm.
17. Pai SI, Westra WH. Molecular pathology of head and neck cancer: implications for diagnosis, prognosis, and treatment. *Annual Review of Pathology*. 2009;4:49–70.
18. What are Cancers of the Head and Neck? http://www.cancer.gov/types/head-and-neck/head-neck-fact-sheet#r5.
19. *The AJCC Cancer Staging Manual*. 7th ed. Chicago, IL: Springer Science + Business Media, LLC (SBM); 2010.
20. Gregoire V, Lefebvre JL, Licitra L, Felip E, EHNS–ESMO–ESTRO Guidelines Working Group. Squamous cell carcinoma of the head and neck: EHNS-ESMO-ESTRO Clinical Practice Guidelines for diagnosis, treatment and follow-up. *Annals of Oncology: Official Journal of the European Society for Medical Oncology/ESMO*. May 2010;21(suppl 5):v184–v186.
21. *The Royal College of Physicians and the Royal College of Radiologists. Evidence-Based Indications for the Usage of PET-CT in the UK*. London: RCP, RCR; 2013.
22. Isles MG, McConkey C, Mehanna HM. A systematic review and meta-analysis of the role of positron emission tomography in the follow up of head and neck squamous cell carcinoma following radiotherapy or chemoradiotherapy. *Clinical Otolaryngology: Official Journal of ENT-UK; Official Journal of Netherlands Society for Oto-Rhino-Laryngology & Cervico-Facial Surgery*. June 2008;33(3):210–222.
23. Sheikhbahaei S, Taghipour M, Ahmad R, et al. Diagnostic Accuracy of Follow-Up FDG PET or PET/CT in Patients With Head and Neck Cancer After Definitive Treatment: A Systematic Review and Meta-Analysis. *AJR. American Journal of Roentgenology*. September 2015;205(3):629–639.
24. Quon A, Fischbein NJ, McDougall IR, et al. Clinical role of ^{18}F-FDG PET/CT in the management of squamous cell carcinoma of the head and neck and thyroid carcinoma. *Journal of Nuclear Medicine: Official Publication, Society of Nuclear Medicine*. January 2007;48(suppl 1):58S–67S.
25. Gupta T, Master Z, Kannan S, et al. Diagnostic performance of post-treatment FDG PET or FDG PET/CT imaging in head and neck cancer: a systematic review and meta-analysis. *European Journal of Nuclear Medicine and Molecular Imaging*. November 2011;38(11):2083–2095.
26. Xie P, Li M, Zhao H, Sun X, Fu Z, Yu J. ^{18}F-FDG PET or PET-CT to evaluate prognosis for head and neck cancer: a meta-analysis. *Journal of Cancer Research and Clinical Oncology*. July 2011;137(7):1085–1093.
27. Sheikhbahaei S, Ahn SJ, Moriarty E, Kang H, Fakhry C, Subramaniam RM. Intratherapy or Posttherapy FDG PET or FDG PET/CT for Patients With Head and Neck Cancer: A Systematic Review and Meta-analysis of Prognostic Studies. *AJR. American Journal of Roentgenology*. November 2015;205(5):1102–1113.
28. Valk PE, Pounds TR, Tesar RD, Hopkins DM, Haseman MK. Cost-effectiveness of PET imaging in clinical oncology. *Nuclear Medicine and Biology*. August 1996;23(6):737–743.
29. Hollenbeak CS, Lowe VJ, Stack Jr BC. The cost-effectiveness of fluorodeoxyglucose 18-F positron emission tomography in the N0 neck. *Cancer*. November 1, 2001;92(9):2341–2348.
30. Annunziata S, Caldarella C, Treglia G. Cost-effectiveness of Fluorine-18-Fluorodeoxyglucose positron emission

tomography in tumours other than lung cancer: a systematic review. *World Journal of Radiology*. March 28, 2014;6(3):48–55.

31. Castaldi P, Leccisotti L, Bussu F, Micciche F, Rufini V. Role of 18F-FDG PET-CT in head and neck squamous cell carcinoma. *Acta Otorhinolaryngologica Italica: organo ufficiale della Societa italiana di otorinolaringologia e chirurgia cervicofacciale*. February 2013;33(1):1–8.

32. Fukui MB, Blodgett TM, Snyderman CH, et al. Combined PET-CT in the head and neck: part 2. Diagnostic uses and pitfalls of oncologic imaging. *Radiographics: A Review Publication of the Radiological Society of North America, Inc.* July-August 2005;25(4):913–930.

33. Purohit BS, Ailianou A, Dulguerov N, Becker CD, Ratib O, Becker M. FDG-PET/CT pitfalls in oncological head and neck imaging. *Insights Into Imaging*. October 2014;5(5):585–602.

34. Sarji S. Physiological uptake in FDG PET simulating disease. *Biomedical Imaging and Intervention Journal*. 2006;2(4):e59.

35. Paquette CM, Manos DC, Psooy BJ. Unilateral vocal cord paralysis: a review of CT findings, mediastinal causes, and the course of the recurrent laryngeal nerves. *Radiographics: A Review Publication of the Radiological Society of North America, Inc.* May-June 2012;32(3):721–740.

36. Al-Ibraheem A, Buck A, Krause BJ, Scheidhauer K, Schwaiger M. Clinical applications of FDG PET and PET/CT in head and neck cancer. *Journal of Oncology*. 2009;2009:208725.

37. Paidpally V, Chirindel A, Lam S, Agrawal N, Quon H, Subramaniam RM. FDG-PET/CT imaging biomarkers in head and neck squamous cell carcinoma. *Imaging in Medicine*. December 2012;4(6):633–647.

38. Wassef HR, Hanna N, Colletti P. PET/CT in Head-neck Malignancies: The Implications for Personalized Clinical Practice. *PET Clinics*. July 2016;11(3):219–232.

39. Ha PK, Hdeib A, Goldenberg D, et al. The role of positron emission tomography and computed tomography fusion in the management of early-stage and advanced-stage primary head and neck squamous cell carcinoma. *Archives of Otolaryngology–Head & Neck Surgery*. January 2006;132(1):12–16.

40. Schoder H, Yeung HW. Positron emission imaging of head and neck cancer, including thyroid carcinoma. *Seminars in Nuclear Medicine*. July 2004;34(3):180–197.

41. Ryu IS, Roh JL, Kim JS, et al. Impact of 18F-FDG PET/CT staging on management and prognostic stratification in head and neck squamous cell carcinoma: a prospective observational study. *European Journal of Cancer*. June 8, 2016;63:88–96.

42. Tantiwongkosi B, Yu F, Kanard A, Miller FR. Role of 18F-FDG PET/CT in pre and post treatment evaluation in head and neck carcinoma. *World Journal of Radiology*. May 28, 2014;6(5):177–191.

43. Ryan WR, Fee Jr WE, Le QT, Pinto HA. Positron-emission tomography for surveillance of head and neck cancer. *The Laryngoscope*. April 2005;115(4):645–650.

44. Subramaniam RM, Truong M, Peller P, Sakai O, Mercier G. Fluorodeoxyglucose-positron-emission tomography imaging of head and neck squamous cell cancer. *AJNR. American Journal of Neuroradiology*. April 2010;31(4):598–604.

45. Lee JR, Kim JS, Roh JL, et al. Detection of occult primary tumors in patients with cervical metastases of unknown primary tumors: comparison of 18F FDG PET/CT with contrast-enhanced CT or CT/MR imaging-prospective study. *Radiology*. March 2015;274(3):764–771.

46. Deantonio L, Beldi D, Gambaro G, et al. FDG-PET/CT imaging for staging and radiotherapy treatment planning of head and neck carcinoma. *Radiation Oncology*. 2008;3:29.

47. Kim JW, Roh JL, Kim JS, et al. 18F-FDG PET/CT surveillance at 3–6 and 12 months for detection of recurrence and second primary cancer in patients with head and neck squamous cell carcinoma. *British Journal of Cancer*. December 10, 2013;109(12):2973–2979.

48. Lowe VJ, Boyd JH, Dunphy FR, et al. Surveillance for recurrent head and neck cancer using positron emission tomography. *Journal of Clinical Oncology: Official Journal of the American Society of Clinical Oncology*. February 2000;18(3):651–658.

49. Abgral R, Querellou S, Potard G, et al. Does 18F-FDG PET/CT improve the detection of posttreatment recurrence of head and neck squamous cell carcinoma in patients negative for disease on clinical follow-up? *Journal of Nuclear Medicine: Official Publication, Society of Nuclear Medicine*. January 2009;50(1):24–29.

50. Kitagawa Y, Nishizawa S, Sano K, et al. Prospective comparison of 18F-FDG PET with conventional imaging modalities (MRI, CT, and 67Ga scintigraphy) in assessment of combined intraarterial chemotherapy and radiotherapy for head and neck carcinoma. *Journal of Nuclear Medicine: Official Publication, Society of Nuclear Medicine*. February 2003;44(2):198–206.

51. McCollum AD, Burrell SC, Haddad RI, et al. Positron emission tomography with 18F-fluorodeoxyglucose to predict pathologic response after induction chemotherapy and definitive chemoradiotherapy in head and neck cancer. *Head & Neck*. October 2004;26(10):890–896.

52. Min M, Lin P, Lee M, et al. Prognostic Value of 2-[18F] Fluoro-2-deoxy-D-glucose Positron Emission Tomography-Computed Tomography Scan Carried out During and After Radiation Therapy for Head and Neck Cancer Using Visual Therapy Response Interpretation Criteria. *Clincal Oncology (The Royal College of Radiologists)*. 2016;28(6):393–401.

53. Schoder H, Fury M, Lee N, Kraus D. PET monitoring of therapy response in head and neck squamous cell carcinoma. *Journal of Nuclear Medicine: Official Publication, Society of Nuclear Medicine*. May 2009;50(suppl 1):74S–88S.

54. Lowe VJ, Stack Jr BC. Esophageal cancer and head and neck cancer. *Seminars in Roentgenology*. April 2002;37(2):140–150.

55. Dequanter D, Shahla M, Aubert C, Deniz Y, Lothaire P. Prognostic value of FDG PET/CT in head and neck squamous cell carcinomas. *OncoTargets and Therapy*. 2015;8:2279–2283.

56. Koyasu S, Nakamoto Y, Kikuchi M, et al. Prognostic value of pretreatment ^{18}F-FDG PET/CT parameters including visual evaluation in patients with head and neck squamous cell carcinoma. *AJR. American Journal of Roentgenology*. April 2014;202(4):851–858.

57. Min M, Lin P, Lee M, et al. ^{18}F-FDG PET-CT performed before and during radiation therapy of head and neck squamous cell carcinoma: are they independent or complementary to each other? *Journal of Medical Imaging and Radiation Oncology*. 2016;60(3):433–440.

58. Pak K, Cheon GJ, Nam HY, et al. Prognostic value of metabolic tumor volume and total lesion glycolysis in head and neck cancer: a systematic review and meta-analysis. *Journal of Nuclear Medicine: Official Publication, Society of Nuclear Medicine*. June 2014;55(6):884–890.

59. Kitajima K, Suenaga Y, Kanda T, et al. Prognostic value of FDG PET imaging in patients with laryngeal cancer. *PLoS One*. 2014;9(5):e96999.

60. Wong RJ, Lin DT, Schoder H, et al. Diagnostic and prognostic value of [^{18}F]fluorodeoxyglucose positron emission tomography for recurrent head and neck squamous cell carcinoma. *Journal of Clinical Oncology: Official Journal of the American Society of Clinical Oncology*. October 15, 2002;20(20):4199–4208.

61. Torizuka T, Tanizaki Y, Kanno T, et al. Prognostic value of ^{18}F-FDG PET in patients with head and neck squamous cell cancer. *AJR. American Journal of Roentgenology*. April 2009;192(4):W156–W160.

CHAPTER 2

Lung Cancer

ALIREZA REZAEE • KEN HERRMANN • MARKUS RADERER •
WERNER LANGSTEGER • MOHSEN BEHESHTI

BACKGROUND

General[1]

- Lung cancer is the second most common cancer in both genders (13% of all new cancers).
- It is the leading cause of cancer-related death in both genders.
- Two-thirds of the cases of lung cancer are diagnosed in patients 65 years or older.
- Metastatic disease is found at first presentation in 30%–40% of patients with non-small cell lung cancer (NSCLC), and even more in those with small cell lung cancer (SCLC).[2-4]
- Risk factors: Active and passive smoking, radiation therapy, environmental toxins (asbestos; radon gas; metals such as nickel, arsenic, chromium; ionizing radiation; and polycyclic aromatic hydrocarbons), human immunodeficiency virus infection, pulmonary fibrosis, and family history of lung cancer.[5]

Clinical Signs/Symptoms[6]

Cough (50%–75%), hemoptysis (25%–50%), shortness of breath (25%), chest pain (20%), and weight loss (36%) are the clinical signs found in lung cancer.

Primary Diagnostic Procedures[7-12]

The primary diagnostic procedures used are chest x-ray, contrast-enhanced chest and upper abdominal CT scan, fludeoxyglucose (FDG) PET/CT scan, and tissue diagnosis.

Standard Treatments[13-26]

Non-small cell lung cancer

Surgery and chemotherapy are the treatments of choice for early and advanced stage NSCLC, respectively.

Stages I and II: Surgical resection (sublobar resection), radiation therapy, and adjuvant chemotherapy for large tumors (i.e., stage 1B or II) as an alternative, if unable to tolerate surgery.

Stage III: Chemoradiation therapy.

Stage IV: Chemotherapy and targeted therapy (antiangiogenic therapy, epidermal growth factor receptor inhibitors, anti-abnormal anaplastic lymphoma kinase proteins therapy).

Small cell lung cancer

Chemotherapy with or without radiation therapy is the treatment of choice for SCLC.

Limited stage: Chemotherapy + hyperfractionated radiation therapy + prophylactic cranial radiation in the case of complete response to chemotherapy.

Extended stage: Chemotherapy + prophylactic cranial radiation.

Prognostic Factors[27-33]

Non-small cell lung cancer

- Stage of the disease
- Patient's performance status
- Weight loss
- Degree of tumor differentiation
- Lymphatic invasion
- Total lesion glycolysis (TLG) on ^{18}F-FDG PET

Small cell lung cancer

- Stage of the disease

Five-Year Survival[34]

Non-small cell lung cancer

- Stage IA: 50%
- Stage IB: 43%
- Stage IIA: 36%
- Stage IIB: 25%
- Stage IIIA: 19%
- Stage IIIB: 7%
- Stage IV: 2%

Small cell lung cancer

- Limited stage: 10%–13%
- Extended stage: 1%–2%

TUMOR CHARACTERISTICS AND TYPICAL BEHAVIOR

Histopathology[1]

- NSCLC: 80%–85%
  - Adenocarcinoma: 38%
  - Squamous cell carcinoma: 20%
  - Other NSCLC: 18%

(Adenosquamous, mucoepidermoid, adenoid cystic carcinoma)
- Large cell carcinoma: 5%
- SCLC: 13%
- Others: 6%

Distribution and Localization[11,12,34]
T-primary
- Central: squamous cell carcinoma, SCLC
- Peripheral: adenocarcinoma, large cell carcinoma

N-lymph nodes
- NSCLC: interlobar, hilar
- SCLC: mediastinum

M-distant metastasis
- The most common sites are adrenal gland (50%), liver (30%–50%), brain (20%), and bone (20%)

TNM CLASSIFICATION[34,35]
TNM classification is provided in Table 2.1.

Primary Tumor (T)
TX: The primary tumor cannot be assessed, or the tumor is proved by the presence of malignant cells in sputum or bronchial washing but is not visualized by imaging or bronchoscopy.

T0: There is no evidence of a primary tumor.

Tis: Carcinoma in situ.

T1: The tumor is ≤3 cm in the greatest dimension, surrounded by lung or visceral pleura; there is no bronchoscopic evidence of invasion more proximal than the lobar bronchus (not in the main bronchus); there is superficial spreading of the tumor in the central airways (confined to the bronchial wall).

T1a: The tumor is ≤2 cm in the greatest dimension.

T1b: The tumor is >2 cm but ≤3 cm in the greatest dimension.

T2: The tumor is >3 cm but ≤7 cm, or the tumor has any of the following characteristics:
- Invades visceral pleura
- Involves the main bronchus ≥2 cm distal to the carina
- Is associated with atelectasis/obstructive pneumonitis extending to the hilar region but not involving the entire lung

T2a: The tumor is >3 cm but ≤5 cm in the greatest dimension.

T2b: The tumor is >5 cm but ≤7 cm in the greatest dimension.

T3: The tumor is >7 cm or:
- The tumor directly invades any of the following: chest wall (including superior sulcus tumors), diaphragm, phrenic nerve, mediastinal pleura, or parietal pericardium; or
- The tumor is in the main bronchus <2 cm distal to the carina but without involvement of the carina; or
- There is associated atelectasis/obstructive pneumonitis of the entire lung or separate tumor nodule(s) in the same lobe.

T4: The tumor is of any size and invades any of the following: mediastinum, heart, great vessels, trachea, recurrent laryngeal nerve, esophagus, vertebral body, or carina; or there are separate tumor nodule(s) in a different ipsilateral lobe.

Regional Lymph Nodes (N)
NX: Regional lymph nodes cannot be assessed.

N0: There is no regional node metastasis.

N1: There is metastasis in the ipsilateral peribronchial and/or ipsilateral hilar lymph nodes and intrapulmonary nodes, including involvement by direct extension.

N2: There is metastasis in the ipsilateral mediastinal and/or subcarinal lymph node(s).

N3: There is metastasis in the contralateral mediastinal, contralateral hilar, ipsilateral or contralateral scalene, or supraclavicular lymph nodes.

Distant Metastasis (M)
MX: Distant metastasis cannot be assessed.

M0: There is no distant metastasis.

M1: Distant metastasis is found.

M1a: Separate tumor nodule(s) are found in a contralateral lobe; tumor has pleural nodules or malignant pleural (or pericardial) effusion.

M1b: Distant metastasis is found.

TABLE 2.1 Lung Cancer TNM Classification					
TNM	**T1**	**T2a**	**T2b**	**T3**	**T4**
N0	IA	IB	IIA	IIB	IIIA
N1	IIA	IIA	IIB	IIIA	IIIA
N2	IIIA	IIIA	IIIA	IIIA	IIIB
N3	IIIB	IIIB	IIIB	IIIB	IIIB
M1	IV	IV	IV	IV	IV

GUIDELINES
The major guidelines are provided in Table 2.2.

EVIDENCE-BASED VIEWPOINTS

- The usefulness of FDG PET/CT is well agreed on in the evidence-based medical literature. ^{18}F-FDG PET/CT is the standard in the evaluation of solitary pulmonary nodules (SPNs) and preoperative staging of lung cancers. If the findings are suggestive of benign SPN, unnecessary biopsies or thoracotomies could be prevented.[42,43]
- Whole-body FDG PET/CT reduces the cost and side effects of unnecessary invasive procedures.[44-46]
- FDG PET/CT is more accurate than CT in lymph node staging of NSCLC. It is also the standard choice to investigate response to treatment.[47-50]
- FDG PET/CT has a higher sensitivity and specificity compared with MRI or conventional whole-body bone scan to detect bone metastasis from lung cancer.[47,50]
- TLG is an independent predictive factor of survival in patients with advanced NSCLC. The higher maximum standardized uptake value (SUV_{max}) of the primary NSCLC is associated with greater tumor invasiveness and postsurgical recurrence.[51,52]
- In countries with endemic infectious granulomatous disease, the specificity of FDG PET/CT for the detection of lymph node metastasis from lung cancer is reduced.[53]

COST-EFFECTIVENESS[46,54-56]

- Although FDG PET/CT is an expensive imaging modality, its use diminishes overall expenses by:
  - Preventing futile diagnostic examinations
  - Reducing expensive futile radical therapeutic procedures
  - Early detection of occult distant metastasis

TABLE 2.2
Lung Cancer ESMO and NCCN Guidelines[36-41]

Clinical Guidelines	Initial Diagnosis (Primary Tumor)	Metastatic Disease
ESMO	**Recommended** in patients with potentially curative treatment	**Recommended**
NCCN	**Recommended in NSCLC** limited stage of SCLC. Supplemental in neuroendocrine tumors	**Recommended** in case of inconclusive findings on CT or MRI, if PET/CT data make changes in management

ESMO, European Society for Medical Oncology; *NCCN*, National Comprehensive Cancer Network.

CLINICAL POINT OF VIEW

Suspected Disease

Solitary pulmonary nodules: The likelihood of malignancy is ascertained to determine the optimal approach (wait and watch versus biopsy or upfront surgery for lesions with a high likelihood of malignancy).

Initial Diagnosis

- Extent of disease
- Local spread/resectability
- Lymph node involvement
- Presence/absence of distant metastases

Non-small Cell Lung Cancer

Differentiation between patients with stage I/II (upfront surgery), stage III (induction chemotherapy or radio/chemotherapy), and stage IV (palliative systemic therapy) is of critical importance for determining the treatment approach in newly diagnosed NSCLC. Accurate lymph node staging is of great clinical relevance to prevent unnecessary surgical procedures, particularly in the detection of small/subclinical metastases that might be missed by conventional imaging.

Small Cell Lung Cancer

Determination of limited versus extended stage is pivotal, especially in view of additional radiotherapy in the limited—versus systemic chemotherapy in the extended—stage. Also, it may play an important role for defining patients with limited-stage cancer who may benefit from potential prophylactic cranial irradiation with complete remission after initial therapy.

Suspected Recurrence After Potentially Curative Therapy

- Likelihood of malignancy versus inflammation/nonmalignant process
- Extent of suspected recurrence (localized versus disseminated)

Metastatic Disease

- Extent of metastases/localization: in the case of cerebral deposits, gamma-knife or whole-brain radiotherapy will be considered.
- The intensity of radiotracer uptake by means of SUV may correlate with patients' prognosis; however, it will not change the treatment of choice.

Response to Therapy

- Considering the side effects of chemotherapies, early identification of nonresponders may protect them from unnecessary toxicities. In addition, use of targeted agents will rarely result in pronounced measurable regression on stand-alone CT. Hence, determination of an early metabolic response to treatment may be helpful in guiding the duration of therapy in case of toxicities.

PITFALLS[57–59]

False Positive

- Infection, including tuberculosis (TB; including tuberculoma and TB lymphadenopathy), histoplasmosis, aspergillosis, cryptococcosis, paragonimiasis, pneumocystis infection
- Postsurgical changes
- Radiation therapy-induced changes
- Talc pleurodesis
- Flare phenomenon
- Rib fractures
- Inflammatory process, such as sarcoidosis, rheumatoid nodules, Wegener granulomatosis, amyloidosis, and pneumoconiosis
- Sclerosing hemangioma

False Negative

- Bronchioloalveolar carcinoma or adenocarcinoma in situ
- Carcinoid tumor
- Lung metastasis of mucinous origin
- Lung metastases from prostate cancer, renal cell carcinoma, testicular malignancy, and some invasive lobular breast cancers
- Common in all cancers: early-stage malignancy, hyperglycemic state, small lesions (<8 mm)

DISCUSSION

Solitary Pulmonary Nodules

The role of FDG PET/CT in investigating SPNs as the standard diagnostic imaging modality is well documented in the medical literature. FDG PET is superior to contrast-enhanced CT (ceCT) in the assessment of SPN. A comparative study of PET and ceCT performed by Christensen and colleagues on the assessment of 42 SPNs resulted for ceCT in a sensitivity, specificity, positive predictive value (PPV), and negative predictive value (NPV) of 100%, 29%, 68%, and 100%, respectively. Corresponding values for FDG PET were 96%, 76%, 86%, and 93%, respectively. The authors concluded that FDG PET is superior based on its markedly better specificity and PPV with just unremarkably lower sensitivity and NPV. The latter two are most likely a result of inclusion of lesions smaller than 8 mm, which are beyond the resolution of FDG PET.

However, the nodule-enhancement CT might still be helpful because of its excellent NPV and lower cost. In a meta-analysis the authors calculated a pooled sensitivity and specificity of 96.8% and 77.8%, respectively, for FDG PET to detect SPN. By the introduction of combined PET/CT scanners in the late 1990s, the overall accuracy increased even more. Reviewing published studies resulted for combined FDG PET/CT in sensitivities ranging from 88% to 97% and corresponding specificities of 83%–89% for malignancy differentiation of SPN. These studies demonstrate the superiority of combined FDG PET/CT in the noninvasive diagnosis of SPN. Importantly, the negative predictive value for all these studies is consistently greater than 90%, which significantly reduces futile thoracotomies or biopsies in the case of a benign nodule, preventing unnecessary side effects and reducing costs.[39,40,43]

Nevertheless, given that FDG is not a specific radiotracer for malignancy and can also be taken up by inflammatory and infectious lesions, the FDG PET/CT readers have to take into account this limitation, especially in geographic regions with endemic infectious pulmonary diseases. It is reported that the average adjusted specificity of FDG PET is 16% lower in the endemic infectious area.[53]

Staging Lung Cancer

With a higher sensitivity and specificity compared with CT, FDG PET/CT is a useful modality for staging and restaging of SCLC and NSCLC, as well as for the evaluation of corresponding lymph node metastases. This is well documented and incorporated in major clinical guidelines. In addition, FDG PET/CT is recommended by the National Comprehensive Cancer Network as a supplemental diagnostic modality in pulmonary neuroendocrine tumors.[39,40]

A prospective study compared the accuracy of FDG PET/CT with that of stand-alone CT for the preoperative assessment of 106 patients with NSCLC. The accuracy of primary tumor detection was 79% for CT versus 86% for FDG PET/CT. Corresponding sensitivity, specificity, and accuracy for lymph node staging were 70%, 69%, and 69% for CT and 85%, 84%, and 84% for FDG PET/CT, respectively. In summary, the authors concluded that FDG PET/CT is superior to stand-alone CT for T- and N-staging of NSCLC.[60]

Wu and colleagues evaluated the value of FDG PET/CT for the diagnosis of metastases from NSCLC in a meta-analysis. A total of 56 studies including 8699 patients were analyzed. FDG PET/CT was found to be significantly more sensitive and specific than ceCT alone. Li and colleagues performed a meta-analysis including nine studies and a total of 780 patients evaluating the accuracy of FDG PET/

CT for M-staging. Pooled sensitivity and specificity were 93% and 96%, respectively. FDG PET/CT correctly identified metastases of the adrenal gland, a common site of metastases, and correctly differentiated benign adenoma from metastatic disease in about 99% of cases. Moreover, previous studies reported a higher sensitivity and accuracy of FDG PET/CT (91% and 94%, respectively) for the detection of bone metastases when compared with conventional methylene diphosphonate (MDP) whole-body bone scintigraphy (75% and 85%, respectively).[47,61,62]

However, for the detection of cerebral metastases, dedicated brain MRI is recommended as the imaging of choice because of the high physiologic cerebral FDG uptake and the subsequent limited sensitivity.[61]

In addition, FDG PET/CT may have an impact on the management of patients with lung cancer. In a prospective study of 24 patients with NSCLC, FDG PET/CT led to upstaging, downstaging, and change of management in 29%, 13%, and 21% of patients, respectively.[63] In a retrospective study of 55 patients with SCLC, FDG PET/CT upstaged 11% of patients.[64] Hence, accurate staging with FDG PET/CT may prevent unnecessary surgeries because of change in patients' stage, which reduces the healthcare cost and shows the cost-effectiveness of this modality as well.

Moreover, FDG PET/CT plays an important role in the assessment of recurrent lung cancer. Systematic reviews reported a higher efficiency of FDG PET than CT in the evaluation of recurrent lung cancer. FDG PET was found to be a sensitive and specific modality, providing a high NPV for exclusion of disease recurrence.[65]

Prognostic Value

FDG PET/CT showed a high prognostic value in lung cancer and is recommended for treatment monitoring after chemotherapy or radiation therapy because the patient with a better response to therapy often has better outcomes. TLG, which is calculated based on FDG PET, is an independent prognostic factor for survival in patients with advanced NSCLC. In a retrospective study including 63 patients with metastatic stage IV NSCLC, TLG and metabolic tumor volume (MTV) were measured on both primary and posttreatment FDG PET/CT. The authors found pretreatment and posttreatment TLG and MTV to be independent prognostic factors for overall and progression-free survival.[66] The same concept was confirmed in patients with SCLC in another study. In addition, the higher SUV_{max} of the primary tumor is associated with greater tumor invasiveness and recurrence; thus, median survival is reduced with an increased SUV_{max}.[64]

A review of a database of 315 patients with NSCLC showed that the SUV_{max} is an independent predictive factor for tumor pathologic nature and stage. In this study, the SUV_{max} of most poorly differentiated tumors with advanced stage was >10. The authors also suggested SUV_{max} as the best prognostic factor for disease-free survival.[67] In a meta-analysis by Berghmans and colleagues investigating the prognostic value of the pretreatment SUV_{max} in patients with NSCLC involving 13 studies with a total of 1474 patients, the SUV_{max} was found to be a reliable prognostic marker.[68] In another study with 136 patients with stage I NSCLC, the patients were separated into two groups depending on whether the SUV_{max} of the primary tumor was above or below the cutoff point of 5.5 for a median SUV_{max} of the primary tumor. The recurrence rates were 37% and 14% for the initial SUV_{max} above or below the median, respectively. Accordingly, the authors concluded that an initial $SUV_{max} \geq 5.5$ is an independent prognostic factor for recurrence and cancer-related death in patients with stage I NSCLC.[69] Antoniou and colleagues retrospectively studied 261 patients with biopsy-proven lung cancer and demonstrated that FDG PET/CT has a prognostic value for overall survival, particularly if the age is less than 70 years.[70] Also, systematic reviews reported the FDG uptake of newly diagnosed NSCLC as an independent prognostic factor for these patients.[65]

Tixier and colleagues developed a textural-features (TF) automated quantification system for comparison of FDG heterogeneity and visual evaluation in patients with NSCLC. The SUV, metabolic volume of the tumor, and high tumor heterogeneity (based on TF-automated quantification findings) were identified as independent factors of prognosis and overall survival among these patients.[71]

Therapy Monitoring

FDG PET/CT is the imaging modality of choice for assessing response to treatment. A reduction in tumor FDG uptake, early after initiation of therapy, is prognostic for improved survival and guides the oncologists in determining the most effective chemotherapy regimen. In a study assessing response to neoadjuvant chemoradiation therapy in patients with stage III NSCLC, the authors demonstrated that a visually negative FDG PET/CT scan or a minimum reduction of 80% in the posttherapy SUV is the best prognosticator for outcome.[72] In a retrospective study of 17 patients, Kremer and colleagues reviewed preneoadjuvant and postneoadjuvant FDG PET/CT. A patient-based visual investigation of the metastatic N2 lymph node response to therapy revealed accuracy, sensitivity, specificity, NPV, and PPV of 94%, 100%, 93%, 100%, and 75%, respectively.[73] There is a clinically relevant correlation between the response to therapy detected on follow-up FDG PET/

CT and improved survival of patients with NSCLC and SCLC.[74,75] Weber and colleagues studied 57 patients with stage IIIB or IV NSCLC and revealed that a >20% diminished SUV of the primary tumor after one cycle of chemotherapy is significantly associated with a better final outcome.[76] In conclusion, a reduced FDG uptake of the primary tumor after therapy is significantly associated with a pathologic tumor response and better overall survival.[77–80]

Detection of Tumor Burden and Planning for Radiation Therapy

FDG PET/CT seems to be superior to conventional imaging modalities for guiding tumor biopsies. It is shown that necrosis within the lung cancerous lesion or resultant atelectasis at the vicinity of the tumor may obscure the real borders of the mass or nodule on CT. In contrast, FDG PET/CT allows the delineation of the actual vital tumor territory for optimal tissue sampling. Guiding the biopsy to the most FDG-avid part of the malignancy improves the sampling success rate and prevents false-negative pathology results.[81]

Furthermore, FDG PET/CT is very helpful for treatment planning of external beam radiation and sparing radiation to normal pulmonary parenchyma. FDG PET/CT-guided radiation therapy planning based on the maximum FDG uptake within the tumor provides an improved radiation dose escalation and results in the reduction of the radiation dose to organs at risk.[82] Bradley and colleagues evaluated 26 patients with NSCLC and revealed that using FDG PET/CT instead of stand-alone CT changed the radiation therapy planning in more than 50% of the patients.[83]

Comparison With Other Modalities

Because of technical restrictions, such as the weak signal of the air-filled lung parenchyma and the low proton density of the lungs, MRI is inferior to FDG PET/CT in evaluating pulmonary pathologies. Even in the assessment of osseous metastasis from lung cancer, FDG PET/CT is more sensitive and specific compared with MRI or conventional bone scan.[42,60]

Radiopharmaceuticals Beyond FDG

FDG PET/CT is a promising imaging method to evaluate different aspects of lung cancer. However, scientists are working to identify new radiotracers with a higher sensitivity and specificity than FDG to potentially overcome its shortcomings and to assess metabolic pathways other than glucose metabolism. ^{18}F-fluorothymidine (FLT) visualizes cell proliferation

and may therefore be valuable for evaluating response to therapy; however, it is less sensitive for N-staging and primary tumors than FDG PET/CT. Wang and colleagues performed a meta-analysis of 17 studies and a total of 548 patients. The comparison expectedly showed that FLT PET is significantly less sensitive (80% vs. 89%) but more specific (82% vs. 66%) than FDG PET/CT in the evaluation of lung malignancies. For assessing benign inflammatory lesions, however, FLT PET was significantly more accurate than FDG PET/CT (57% vs. 32%).[84] Other PET tracers that have been investigated for the detection of lung nodules are ^{11}C-methionine and ^{18}F-fluoromisonidazole (^{18}F-FMISO). ^{11}C-methionine shows a higher sensitivity and specificity in the detection of pulmonary nodules, compared with FDG PET/CT.[85] ^{18}F-FMISO is a PET tracer that represents hypoxia. It has been previously reported that there is a significant correlation between the tumor oxygen content and response to treatment, particularly radiation therapy. The tumor hypoxia itself triggers tumor angiogenesis.[86,87] $\alpha V\beta 3$ is an integrin protein that is highly expressed on activated endothelial cells and associated with tumor angiogenesis. Therefore, $\alpha V\beta 3$ expression is relevant not only for diagnostic imaging but also for therapy. Other helpful PET tracers are peptide ligands visualizing the expression of the somatostatin 2 receptor, which is often expressed in well-differentiated neuroendocrine tumors. ^{68}Ga-DOTA-peptides are superior to FDG in well-differentiated neuroendocrine tumors and serve not only for diagnostic imaging but also for confirmation of somatostatin 2 receptor target expression for potential somatostatin 2 receptor–directed therapy.[85]

In addition, the utility of ^{18}F-NaF PET/CT is gaining increasing recognition for the evaluation of osseous metastases from various cancers, especially in tumor entities with a high prevalence of bone involvement, such as lung, breast, and prostate. Hillner and colleagues evaluated the impact of ^{18}F-NaF PET/CT on the management of patients with osseous metastases from different cancers based on the National Oncologic PET Registry database. They reported a change of treatment based on the ^{18}F-NaF PET/CT findings in 36% of patients with lung cancer.[88]

CONCLUSION

The evidence-based recommendations are consistent with the content of the most recent clinical guidelines. FDG PET/CT is indicated as the "imaging modality of choice" for staging and restaging of SCLC and NSCLC, as well as for the detection of distant metastasis and for response assessment. FDG PET/CT has also a prognostic role in lung cancer. In addition, FDG PET/CT is recommended for the evaluation of solitary pulmonary nodules. FDG PET/CT is also useful in further evaluation of equivocal or suspicious lesions incidentally detected by conventional imaging.

TEACHING CASES
Case 1: Staging at SCLC
Findings

A 71-year-old male with SCLC. FDG PET/CT shows an FDG-avid right lung lesion (Fig. 2.1B, arrow). In spite of the small size of the primary tumor, extensive mediastinal, supraclavicular, cervical, and axillary lymph node involvement is noted (Fig. 2.1C, arrows).

Teaching points
- The extended stage of SCLC has a poor prognosis, with a 5-year survival of 1%–2%.
- Mediastinal lymph nodes are the most common site of metastases in SCLC.
- Although SCLC and squamous cell carcinoma are usually central, they may originate from the peripheral part of the lungs.
- Differentiation of limited from extended stage has significant clinical relevance for determining the treatment approach.

Pitfalls
- A non-FDG-avid pulmonary lesion in the left upper lobe represents a subsegmental atelectasis and should not be interpreted as metastasis.

Case 2: Staging NSCLC—Early Detection of Distant Metastases
Findings

A 72-year-old male with NSCLC. FDG PET/CT shows a primary tumor and lymph node involvement on the left hilum. FDG-avid contralateral small-sized mediastinal lymph node metastasis (N3) is evident (Fig. 2.2B, arrow). Of note is an FDG-avid lesion in the right iliac bone with no significant morphologic changes on CT scan (Fig. 2.2C, arrow).

Teaching points
- FDG PET/CT showed a higher sensitivity than CT scan alone in the detection of involved lymph nodes metastases (80%–85% vs. 66%–70%).
- FDG PET/CT is superior to conventional imaging modalities in the early detection of bone marrow metastases.

Pitfalls
- A metabolically active lesion within the left lung represents postobstructive atelectasis/pneumonia caused by central bronchial involvement, which may cause false-positive FDG PET/CT interpretation.

Case 3: Staging NSCLC—Atypical Distant Metastases
Findings

An 82-year-old male with centrally necrotic poorly differentiated adenocarcinoma of the right lung. FDG PET/CT scan shows the lung malignancy with invasion to the chest wall (Fig. 2.3B, arrow). In addition, bilateral pulmonary and mediastinal lymph node metastases are evident. The left adrenal gland, as a common site of distant metastases in lung cancer, is involved (Fig. 2.3C, arrow). There is a focal FDG-avid soft tissue nodule in the ascending colon wall (Fig. 2.3D, arrow) with local lymph node involvement, which was shown to be metastases from lung cancer in pathology.

Teaching points
- The interlobar and hilar regions are the most common sites of metastases in NSCLC.
- FDG PET/CT is superior to stand-alone CT in differentiating adrenal adenoma from primary adrenal cancer or metastasis.
- The adrenal gland is the most common site of distant metastases (50%) in lung cancer.

Pitfalls
- Although FDG uptake of intestinal wall could be physiologic, close attention and follow-up are needed for the intense focal FDG uptake of the gastrointestinal (GI) tract to exclude malignancy or metastases.

Case 4: Staging NSCLC—Atypical Distant Metastases
Findings

A 52-year-old male with poorly differentiated lung adenocarcinoma. FDG PET/CT shows an extended FDG-avid central right lung malignancy with metastases to the right hilar and mediastinal lymph nodes. Although the adrenal gland, liver, and bone were spared, FDG-avid peritoneal soft tissue metastasis is noticed on the left lower abdomen (arrow) (Fig. 2.4).

Teaching points
- FDG PET/CT may lead to upstaging in 29% of NSCLC.
- The peritoneum is a very rare site of distant metastases in lung cancer and could be affected even in the case of intact adrenal and liver.

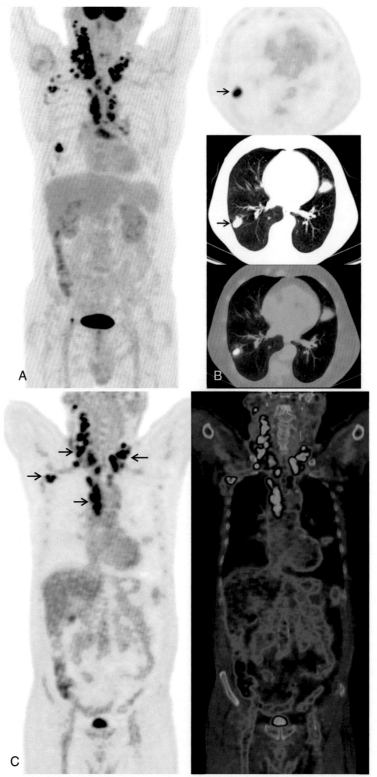

FIG. 2.1 A, MIP image. B, FDG PET/CT showing an FDG-avid right lung lesion (*arrow*). In spite of the small size of the primary tumor, extensive mediastinal, supraclavicular, cervical, and axillary lymph node involvement is noted (C, *arrows*).

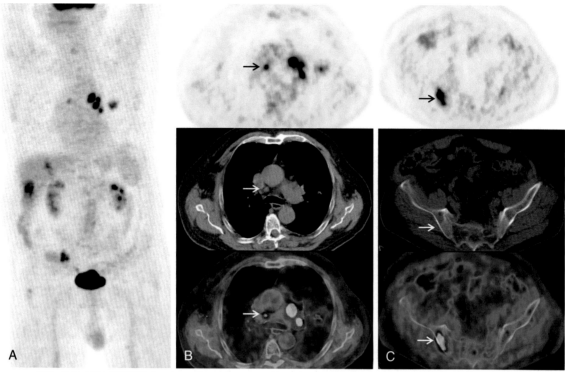

FIG. 2.2 FDG PET/CT showing primary tumor and lymph node involvement on the left hilum (A). FDG-avid contralateral small mediastinal lymph node metastasis (N3) is evident (B, *arrow*). Of note is an FDG-avid lesion in the right iliac bone with no significant morphologic changes on CT scan (C, *arrow*).

Case 5: Staging Lung Cancer—Guiding Biopsy and Radiotherapy
Findings
A 76-year-old female with bronchial carcinoma. FDG PET/CT shows a large right upper lobe lung mass with central necrosis and peripheral FDG-avid viable tumor tissues (Fig. 2.5).

Teaching points
- FDG PET/CT has an important role in guiding tumor biopsy and external radiation therapy. Tissue sampling from the central necrotic part will cause a false-negative result. Radiation should be directed to the parts with the most FDG uptake, which a representative of viable tumor cells.
- FDG PET/CT is able to rule out locoregional lymph node metastases and distant metastases in lung cancers with an advanced primary tumor.

Case 6: Staging SCLC—Differentiation of Limited From Extended Stage
Findings
A 58-year-old female with SCLC. FDG PET/CT shows an intensely FDG-avid left hilar pulmonary mass with

involved paratracheal lymph node. Of incidental note is an FDG-avid metastasis in normal-appearing spinal cord on CT (Fig. 2.6).

Teaching points
- FDG PET/CT may lead to upstaging in about 11% of SCLC cases.
- A higher FDG uptake in malignant lung lesions is related to poorer prognosis.
- This case shows superiority of FDG PET/CT to stand-alone CT in the detection of distant metastasis in the spinal cord.

Case 7: NSCLC—Recurrence
Findings
A 69-year-old male with recurrent pulmonary adenocarcinoma. FDG PET shows a focal FDG uptake in the right hilum (Fig. 2.7B, arrow), suggestive of local recurrence on the primary tumor surgical bed, with no remarkable findings on CT. There is also evidence of FDG-avid metastases to the right internal mammary and celiac lymph nodes (Fig. 2.7C and D, arrow), as well as right posterior pleura (Fig. 2.7E, arrow).

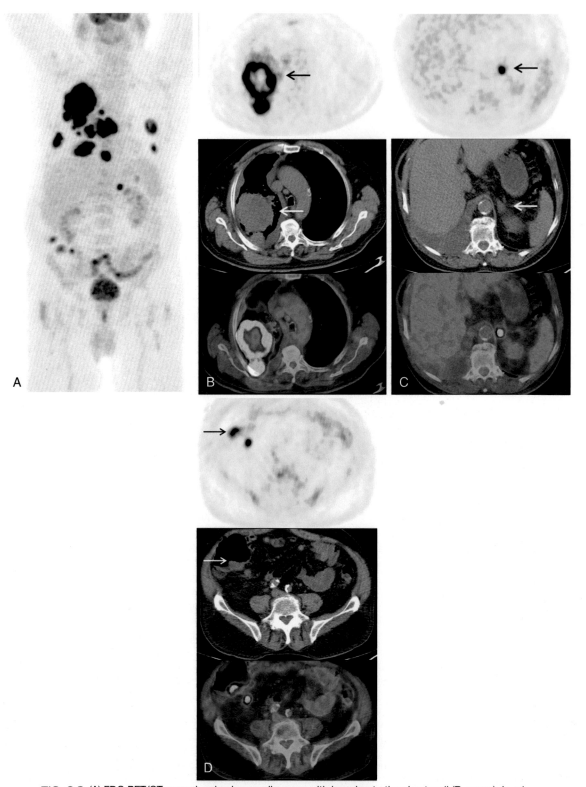

FIG. 2.3 (A) FDG PET/CT scan showing lung malignancy with invasion to the chest wall (B, *arrow*). In addition, bilateral pulmonary and mediastinal lymph node metastases are evident. The left adrenal gland, as a common site of distant metastases in lung cancer, is involved (C, *arrow*). There is a focal FDG-avid soft tissue nodule in the ascending colon wall (D, *arrow*) with local lymph node involvement, which was shown to be metastases from lung cancer in pathology.

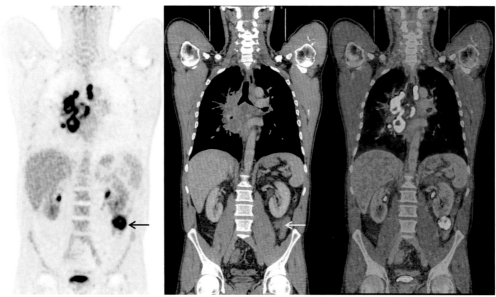

FIG. 2.4 FDG PET/CT showing an extended FDG-avid central right lung malignancy with metastases to the right hilar and mediastinal lymph nodes. Although the adrenal gland, liver, and bone are spared, FDG-avid peritoneal soft tissue metastasis is noticed on the left lower abdomen (*arrow*).

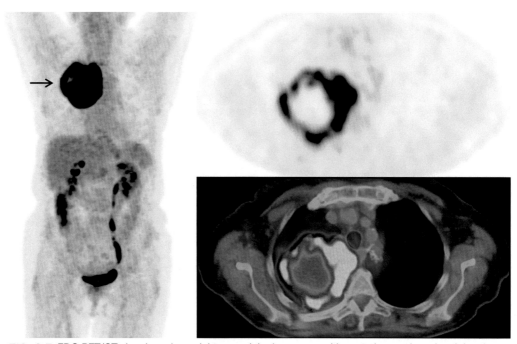

FIG. 2.5 FDG PET/CT showing a large right upper lobe lung mass with central necrosis and peripheral FDG-avid viable tumor tissues.

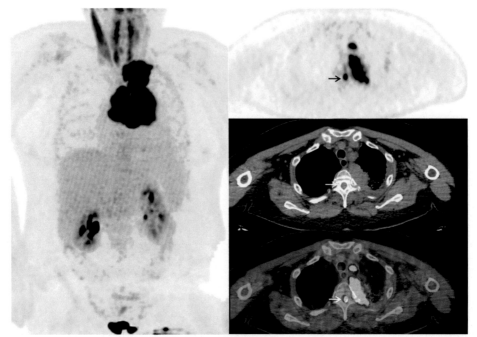

FIG. 2.6 FDG PET/CT showing an intensely FDG-avid left hilar pulmonary mass with involved paratracheal lymph node. Of incidental note is an FDG-avid metastasis in a normal-appearing spinal cord on CT.

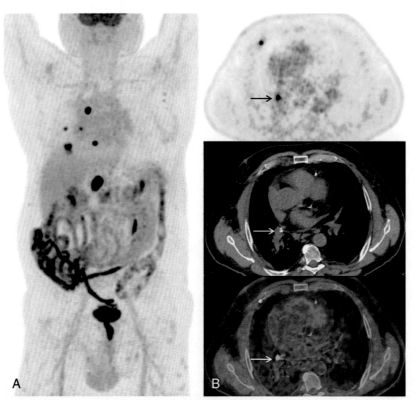

FIG. 2.7 (A) FDG PET showing a focal FDG uptake in the right hilum (B, *arrow*), suggestive of local recurrence on the primary tumor surgical bed with no remarkable findings on CT. There is also evidence of FDG-avid metastases to the right internal mammary and celiac lymph nodes (C and D, *arrow*), as well as right posterior pleura (E, *arrow*).

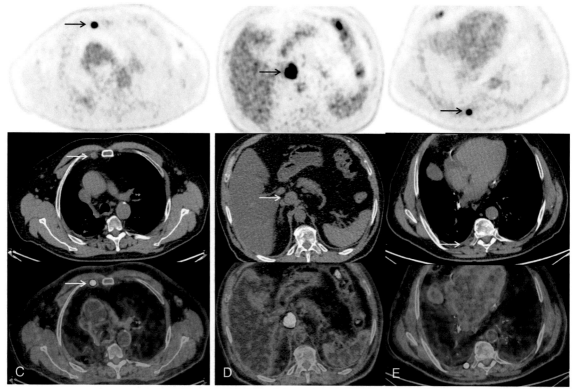

FIG. 2.7, cont'd

Teaching point
- Owing to postsurgical changes and scar tissue formation, FDG PET/CT is superior to stand-alone CT in detecting recurrent lung cancer.

Pitfalls
- Diffuse tracer uptake in the GI tract could be physiologic or drug induced (metformin) or because of a diffuse inflammatory process.

Case 8: Mesothelioma—Treatment Monitoring
Findings
A 62-year-old male with mesothelioma. FDG PET/CT before (Fig. 2.8A) and after (Fig. 2.8B) chemotherapy shows diffuse FDG-avid malignancy with favorable response to therapy (arrows).

Teaching point
- FDG PET/CT is a valuable modality to assess response to therapy earlier than conventional imaging methods. In this patient, the metabolic response is much more noticeable than anatomic changes of the tumor.

Pitfalls
- Talc pleurodesis, postsurgical changes, and radiation therapy–induced changes are the most common causes of false-positive interpretation in treatment monitoring of the lung and pleural malignancies.

Case 9: Talc Pleurodesis
Findings
A 55-year-old female with history of breast cancer and metastases to the left pleura, status post–talc pleurodesis. FDG PET/CT demonstrates pleural calcification with corresponding intense FDG uptake (Fig. 2.9).

Pitfalls
- Talc pleurodesis causes an inflammatory process, which leads to an intense FDG uptake on FDG PET and should not be interpreted as metastasis. The uptake may persist for 5 years or even longer.

Case 10: Carcinoid Tumor—Very Low FDG-Avid Malignancies
Findings
A 69-year-old female with pulmonary carcinoid tumor, which is non-FDG avid on PET (Fig. 2.10).

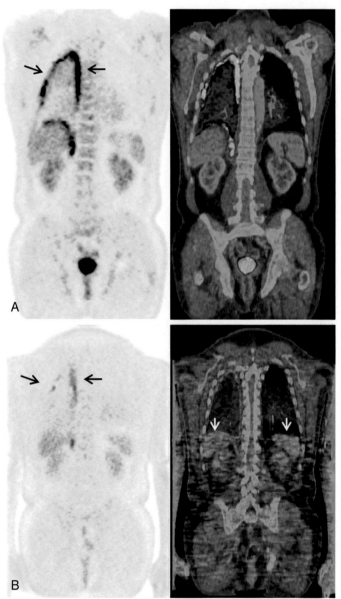

FIG. 2.8 FDG PET/CT before (A) and after (B) chemotherapy shows diffuse FDG-avid malignancy with a favorable response to therapy (*arrows*).

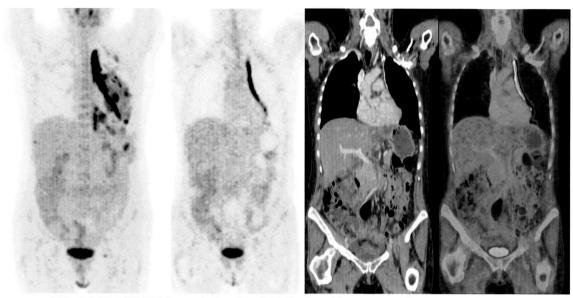

FIG. 2.9 FDG PET/CT demonstrating pleural calcification with a corresponding intense FDG uptake.

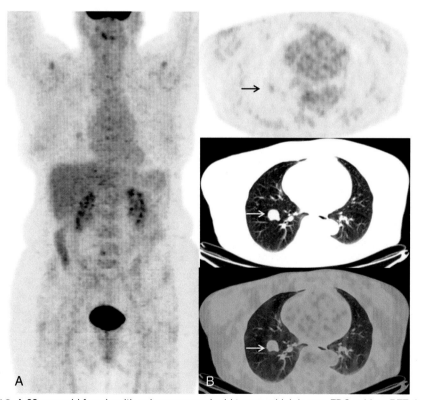

FIG. 2.10 A 69-year-old female with pulmonary carcinoid tumor, which is non–FDG avid on PET. A, MIP image; B, axial PET, CT, and fused images.

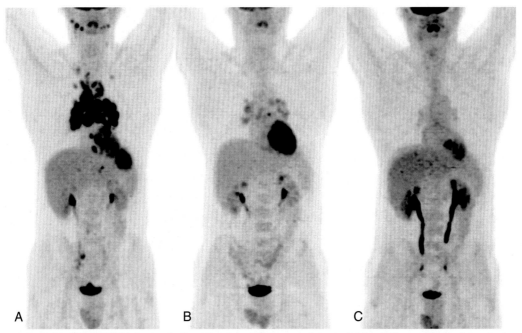

FIG. 2.11 FDG PET/CT demonstrating intensive radiotracer uptake on bilateral hilar, mediastinal, cervical, and abdominal lymph nodes. A, B, and C, MIP images. B and C, Serial posttreatment images.

Teaching points
- Some lung malignancies, such as bronchioloalveolar carcinoma (in situ pulmonary adenocarcinoma) and carcinoid tumors, although malignant, present with very low FDG uptake and should be mentioned in the differential diagnosis of non-FDG-avid lung lesions.
- ^{18}F-DOPA and ^{68}Ga-DOTA-peptide are specific tracers for staging of patients with carcinoid tumors (see Chapter 6).

Case 11: Sarcoidosis
Findings
A 39-year-old male underwent FDG PET/CT because of hilar and mediastinal masses and lymphadenopathies. FDG PET/CT demonstrates intensive radiotracer uptake on bilateral hilar, mediastinal, cervical, and abdominal lymph nodes. Histopathologic examination revealed sarcoidosis, which significantly regressed after therapy (Fig. 2.11).

Teaching points
- Inflammatory/infectious lesions, such as sarcoidosis and TB, can mimic lung cancers with lymph node metastases.
- Intensive FDG uptake on bilateral hilar and mediastinal lymph nodes is a typical pattern for sarcoidosis.

REFERENCES
1. Travis W, Colby T, Corrin B, Shimosato Y, Brambilla E. *WHO Histological Classification of Tumors: Histological Typing of Lung and Pleural Tumours*. 3rd ed. Berlin: Springer-Verlag; 1999.
2. Matsuda A, Matsuda T, Shibata A, et al. Cancer incidence and incidence rates in Japan in 2008: a study of 25 population-based cancer registries for the Monitoring of Cancer Incidence in Japan (MCIJ) project. *Japanese Journal of Clinical Oncology*. 2014;44(4):388–396.
3. Little AG, Gay EG, Gaspar LE, Stewart AK. National survey of non-small cell lung cancer in the United States: epidemiology, pathology and patterns of care. *Lung Cancer*. 2007;57(3):253–260.
4. Nakazawa K, Kurishima K, Tamura T, et al. Specific organ metastases and survival in small cell lung cancer. *Oncology Letters*. 2012;4(4):617–620.
5. Alberg AJ, Samet JM. Epidemiology of lung cancer. *Chest*. 2003;123(suppl 1):21S–49S.
6. Kocher F, Hilbe W, Seeber A, et al. Longitudinal analysis of 2293 NSCLC patients: a comprehensive study from the TYROL registry. *Lung Cancer*. 2015;87(2):193–200.
7. Silvestri GA, Gonzalez AV, Jantz MA, et al. Methods for staging non-small cell lung cancer: diagnosis and management of lung cancer. 3rd ed.: American College of Chest Physicians Evidence-Based Clinical Practice Guidelines *Chest*. 2013;143(suppl 5):e211S–e250S.

8. De Leyn P, Lardinois D, Van Schil P, et al. European trends in preoperative and intraoperative nodal staging: ESTS guidelines. *Journal of Thoracic Oncology: Official Publication of the International Association for the Study of Lung Cancer.* 2007;2(4):357–361.

9. De Wever W. Role of integrated PET/CT in the staging of non-small cell lung cancer. *JBR-BTR: organe de la Societe royale belge de radiologie.* 2009;92(2):124–126.

10. Fischer B, Lassen U, Mortensen J, et al. Preoperative staging of lung cancer with combined PET-CT. *The New England Journal of Medicine.* 2009;361(1):32–39.

11. Pieterman RM, van Putten JW, Meuzelaar JJ, et al. Preoperative staging of non-small-cell lung cancer with positron-emission tomography. *The New England Journal of Medicine.* 2000;343(4):254–261.

12. Ung YC, Maziak DE, Vanderveen JA, et al. ^{18}Fluorodeoxyglucose positron emission tomography in the diagnosis and staging of lung cancer: a systematic review. *Journal of the National Cancer Institute.* 2007;99(23):1753–1767.

13. Ginsberg RJ, Rubinstein LV. Randomized trial of lobectomy versus limited resection for T1 N0 non-small cell lung cancer. Lung Cancer Study Group. *The Annals of Thoracic Surgery.* 1995;60(3):615–622. discussion 622–613.

14. Narsule CK, Ebright MI, Fernando HC. Sublobar versus lobar resection: current status. *Cancer Journal.* 2011;17(1):23–27.

15. Mentzer SJ, DeCamp MM, Harpole Jr DH, Sugarbaker DJ. Thoracoscopy and video-assisted thoracic surgery in the treatment of lung cancer. *Chest.* 1995;107(suppl 6):298S–301S.

16. Farjah F, Wood DE, Mulligan MS, et al. Safety and efficacy of video-assisted versus conventional lung resection for lung cancer. *The Journal of Thoracic and Cardiovascular Surgery.* 2009;137(6):1415–1421.

17. Louie BE, Farivar AS, Aye RW, Vallieres E. Early experience with robotic lung resection results in similar operative outcomes and morbidity when compared with matched video-assisted thoracoscopic surgery cases. *The Annals of Thoracic Surgery.* 2012;93(5):1598–1604. discussion 1604–1595.

18. Song DY, Kavanagh BD, Benedict SH, Schefter T. Stereotactic body radiation therapy. Rationale, techniques, applications, and optimization. *Oncology.* 2004;18(11):1419–1430. discussion 1430, 1432, 1435–1416.

19. Timmerman R, Paulus R, Galvin J, et al. Stereotactic body radiation therapy for inoperable early stage lung cancer. *JAMA.* 2010;303(11):1070–1076.

20. Vansteenkiste J, De Ruysscher D, Eberhardt WE, et al. Early and locally advanced non-small-cell lung cancer (NSCLC): ESMO clinical practice guidelines for diagnosis, treatment and follow-up. *Annals of Oncology: Official Journal of the European Society for Medical Oncology.* 2013;24(suppl 6):vi89–vi98.

21. Pignon JP, Tribodet H, Scagliotti GV, et al. Lung adjuvant cisplatin evaluation: a pooled analysis by the LACE Collaborative Group. *Journal of Clinical Oncology: Official Journal of the American Society of Clinical Oncology.* 2008;26(21):3552–3559.

22. Rami-Porta R, Ball D, Crowley J, et al. The IASLC Lung Cancer Staging Project: proposals for the revision of the T descriptors in the forthcoming (seventh) edition of the TNM classification for lung cancer. *Journal of Thoracic Oncology: Official Publication of the International Association for the Study of Lung Cancer.* 2007;2(7):593–602.

23. Georgoulias V, Papadakis E, Alexopoulos A, et al. Platinum-based and non-platinum-based chemotherapy in advanced non-small-cell lung cancer: a randomised multicentre trial. *Lancet.* 2001;357(9267):1478–1484.

24. Ciuleanu T, Brodowicz T, Zielinski C, et al. Maintenance pemetrexed plus best supportive care versus placebo plus best supportive care for non-small-cell lung cancer: a randomised, double-blind, phase 3 study. *Lancet.* 2009;374(9699):1432–1440.

25. Spira A, Ettinger DS. Multidisciplinary management of lung cancer. *The New England Journal of Medicine.* 2004;350(4):379–392.

26. Auperin A, Arriagada R, Pignon JP, et al. Prophylactic cranial irradiation for patients with small-cell lung cancer in complete remission. Prophylactic Cranial Irradiation Overview Collaborative Group. *The New England Journal of Medicine.* 1999;341(7):476–484.

27. Groome PA, Bolejack V, Crowley JJ, et al. The IASLC Lung Cancer Staging Project: validation of the proposals for revision of the T, N, and M descriptors and consequent stage groupings in the forthcoming (seventh) edition of the TNM classification of malignant tumours. *Journal of Thoracic Oncology: Official Publication of the International Association for the Study of Lung Cancer.* 2007;2(8):694–705.

28. Hoang T, Xu R, Schiller JH, Bonomi P, Johnson DH. Clinical model to predict survival in chemonaive patients with advanced non-small-cell lung cancer treated with third-generation chemotherapy regimens based on eastern cooperative oncology group data. *Journal of Clinical Oncology: Official Journal of the American Society of Clinical Oncology.* 2005;23(1):175–183.

29. Blackstock AW, Herndon 2nd JE, Paskett ED, et al. Outcomes among African-American/non-African-American patients with advanced non-small-cell lung carcinoma: report from the Cancer and Leukemia Group B. *Journal of the National Cancer Institute.* 2002;94(4):284–290.

30. Stanley KE. Prognostic factors for survival in patients with inoperable lung cancer. *Journal of the National Cancer Institute.* 1980;65(1):25–32.

31. Feinstein AR. Symptomatic patterns, biologic behavior, and prognosis in cancer of the lung. Practical application of boolean algebra and clinical taxonomy. *Annals of Internal Medicine.* 1964;61:27–43.

32. Kawaguchi T, Takada M, Kubo A, et al. Performance status and smoking status are independent favorable prognostic factors for survival in non-small cell lung cancer: a comprehensive analysis of 26,957 patients with NSCLC. *Journal of Thoracic Oncology: Official Publication of the International Association for the Study of Lung Cancer.* 2010;5(5):620–630.

33. Sculier JP, Chansky K, Crowley JJ, et al. The impact of additional prognostic factors on survival and their relationship with the anatomical extent of disease expressed by the 6th edition of the TNM classification of malignant tumors and the proposals for the 7th edition. *Journal of Thoracic Oncology: Official Publication of the International Association for the Study of Lung Cancer.* 2008;3(5):457–466.

34. Goldstraw P, Crowley J, Chansky K, et al. The IASLC Lung Cancer Staging Project: proposals for the revision of the TNM stage groupings in the forthcoming (seventh) edition of the TNM classification of malignant tumours. *Journal of Thoracic Oncology: Official Publication of the International Association for the Study of Lung Cancer.* 2007;2(8):706–714.

35. Detterbeck FC, Boffa DJ, Tanoue LT. The new lung cancer staging system. *Chest.* 2009;136(1):260–271.

36. Rudin CM, Ismaila N, Hann CL, et al. Treatment of small-cell lung cancer: American Society of Clinical Oncology Endorsement of the American College of Chest Physicians Guideline. *Journal of Clinical Oncology: Official Journal of the American Society of Clinical Oncology.* 2015;33(34):4106–4111.

37. Vansteenkiste J, Crino L, Dooms C, et al. 2nd ESMO consensus conference on lung cancer: early-stage non-small-cell lung cancer consensus on diagnosis, treatment and follow-up. *Annals of Oncology: Official Journal of the European Society for Medical Oncology.* 2014;25(8):1462–1474.

38. Fruh M, De Ruysscher D, Popat S, et al. Small-cell lung cancer (SCLC): ESMO clinical practice guidelines for diagnosis, treatment and follow-up. *Annals of Oncology: Official Journal of the European Society for Medical Oncology.* 2013;24(suppl 6):vi99–vi105.

39. Non-small Cell Lung Cancer *NCCN.org.*Version 4. *NCCN Clinical Practice Guidelines in Oncology.* 2016.

40. Small Cell Lung Cancer *NCCN.org.*Version 1. *NCCN Clinical Practice Guidelines in Oncology.* 2016.

41. Masters GA, Temin S, Azzoli CG, et al. Systemic therapy for stage IV non-small-cell lung cancer: American Society of Clinical Oncology Clinical Practice Guideline Update. *Journal of Clinical Oncology: Official Journal of the American Society of Clinical Oncology.* 2015;33(30):3488–3515.

42. Sim YT, Poon FW. Imaging of solitary pulmonary nodule-a clinical review. *Quantitative Imaging in Medicine and Surgery.* 2013;3(6):316–326.

43. Christensen JA, Nathan MA, Mullan BP, Hartman TE, Swensen SJ, Lowe VJ. Characterization of the solitary pulmonary nodule: ^{18}F-FDG PET versus nodule-enhancement CT. *American Journal of Roentgenology.* 2006;187(5):1361–1367.

44. Flechsig P, Mehndiratta A, Haberkorn U, Kratochwil C, Giesel FL. PET/MRI and PET/CT in lung lesions and thoracic malignancies. *Seminars in Nuclear Medicine.* 2015;45(4):268–281.

45. Shimizu K, Okita R, Saisho S, et al. Clinical significance of dual-time-point ^{18}F-FDG PET imaging in resectable non-small cell lung cancer. *Annals of Nuclear Medicine.* 2015;29(10):854–860.

46. Mac Manus MP, Hicks RJ, Matthews JP, et al. Positron emission tomography is superior to computed tomography scanning for response-assessment after radical radiotherapy or chemoradiotherapy in patients with non-small-cell lung cancer. *Journal of Clinical Oncology: Official Journal of the American Society of Clinical Oncology.* 2003;21(7):1285–1292.

47. Qu X, Huang X, Yan W, Wu L, Dai K. A meta-analysis of ^{18}FDG-PET-CT, ^{18}FDG-PET, MRI and bone scintigraphy for diagnosis of bone metastases in patients with lung cancer. *European Journal of Radiology.* 2012;81(5):1007–1015.

48. Vansteenkiste JF, Stroobants SG, De Leyn PR, et al. Lymph node staging in non-small-cell lung cancer with FDG-PET scan: a prospective study on 690 lymph node stations from 68 patients. *Journal of Clinical Oncology: Official Journal of the American Society of Clinical Oncology.* 1998;16(6):2142–2149.

49. Pak K, Park S, Cheon GJ, et al. Update on nodal staging in non-small cell lung cancer with integrated positron emission tomography/computed tomography: a meta-analysis. *Annals of Nuclear Medicine.* 2015;29(5):409–419.

50. Petersen H, Holdgaard PC, Madsen PH, et al. FDG PET/CT in cancer: comparison of actual use with literature-based recommendations. *European Journal of Nuclear Medicine and Molecular Imaging.* 2016;43(4):695–706.

51. Im HJ, Pak K, Cheon GJ, et al. Prognostic value of volumetric parameters of ^{18}F-FDG PET in non-small-cell lung cancer: a meta-analysis. *European Journal of Nuclear Medicine and Molecular Imaging.* 2015;42(2):241–251.

52. Yildirim F, Yurdakul AS, Ozkaya S, Akdemir UO, Ozturk C. Total lesion glycolysis by ^{18}F-FDG PET/CT is independent prognostic factor in patients with advanced non-small cell lung cancer. *The Clinical Respiratory Journal.* 2015.

53. Deppen SA, Blume JD, Kensinger CD, et al. Accuracy of FDG-PET to diagnose lung cancer in areas with infectious lung disease: a meta-analysis. *JAMA.* 2014;312(12):1227–1236.

54. Dietlein M, Weber K, Gandjour A, et al. Cost-effectiveness of FDG-PET for the management of solitary pulmonary nodules: a decision analysis based on cost reimbursement in Germany. *European Journal of Nuclear Medicine.* 2000;27(10):1441–1456.

55. Verboom P, van Tinteren H, Hoekstra OS, et al. Cost-effectiveness of FDG-PET in staging non-small cell lung cancer: the PLUS study. *European Journal of Nuclear Medicine and Molecular Imaging.* 2003;30(11):1444–1449.

56. Salminen E, Mac Manus M. FDG-PET imaging in the management of non-small-cell lung cancer. *Annals of Oncology: Official Journal of the European Society for Medical Oncology.* 2002;13(3):357–360.

57. Long NM, Smith CS. Causes and imaging features of false positives and false negatives on F-PET/CT in oncologic imaging. *Insights Into Imaging.* 2011;2(6):679–698.

58. Cheran SK, Nielsen ND, Patz Jr EF. False-negative findings for primary lung tumors on FDG positron emission tomography: staging and prognostic implications. *American Journal of Roentgenology.* 2004;182(5):1129–1132.

59. Chang JM, Lee HJ, Goo JM, et al. False positive and false negative FDG-PET scans in various thoracic diseases. *Korean Journal of Radiology.* 2006;7(1):57–69.

60. Shim SS, Lee KS, Kim BT, et al. Non-small cell lung cancer: prospective comparison of integrated FDG PET/CT and CT alone for preoperative staging. *Radiology.* 2005;236(3):1011–1019.

61. Wu Y, Li P, Zhang H, et al. Diagnostic value of fluorine 18 fluorodeoxyglucose positron emission tomography/computed tomography for the detection of metastases in non-small-cell lung cancer patients. *International Journal of Cancer.* 2013;132(2):E37–E47.

62. Li J, Xu W, Kong F, Sun X, Zuo X. Meta-analysis: accuracy of ^{18}FDG PET-CT for distant metastasis staging in lung cancer patients. *Surgical Oncology.* 2013;22(3):151–155.

63. Promteangtrong C, Kunawudhi A, Phadungrerk R, Iamsa-art C, Chotipanich C. ^{18}F-FDG PET/contrast-enhanced CT for initial staging and strategic treatment of non-small cell lung cancer: a prospective study. *Journal of the Medical Association of Thailand=Chotmaihet thangphaet.* 2015;98(10):1010–1018.

64. Zer A, Domachevsky L, Rapson Y, et al. The role of ^{18}F-FDG PET/CT on staging and prognosis in patients with small cell lung cancer. *European Radiology.* 2015.

65. Vansteenkiste J, Fischer BM, Dooms C, Mortensen J. Positron-emission tomography in prognostic and therapeutic assessment of lung cancer: systematic review. *The Lancet. Oncology.* 2004;5(9):531–540.

66. Lee JW, Lee SM, Yun M, Cho A. Prognostic value of volumetric parameters on staging and posttreatment FDG PET/CT in patients with stage IV non-small cell lung cancer. *Clinical Nuclear Medicine.* 2016;41(5):347–353.

67. Cerfolio RJ, Bryant AS, Ohja B, Bartolucci AA. The maximum standardized uptake values on positron emission tomography of a non-small cell lung cancer predict stage, recurrence, and survival. *The Journal of Thoracic and Cardiovascular Surgery.* 2005;130(1):151–159.

68. Berghmans T, Dusart M, Paesmans M, et al. Primary tumor standardized uptake value (SUV_{max}) measured on fluorodeoxyglucose positron emission tomography (FDG-PET) is of prognostic value for survival in non-small cell lung cancer (NSCLC): a systematic review and meta-analysis (MA) by the European Lung Cancer Working Party for the IASLC Lung Cancer Staging Project. *Journal of Thoracic Oncology: Official Publication of the International Association for the Study of Lung Cancer.* 2008;3(1):6–12.

69. Goodgame B, Pillot GA, Yang Z, et al. Prognostic value of preoperative positron emission tomography in resected stage I non-small cell lung cancer. *Journal of Thoracic Oncology: Official Publication of the International Association for the Study of Lung Cancer.* 2008;3(2):130–134.

70. Antoniou AJ, Marcus C, Tahari AK, Wahl RL, Subramaniam RM. Follow-up or surveillance ^{18}F-FDG PET/CT and survival outcome in lung cancer patients. *Journal of Nuclear Medicine: Official Publication, Society of Nuclear Medicine.* 2014;55(7):1062–1068.

71. Tixier F, Hatt M, Valla C, et al. Visual versus quantitative assessment of intratumor ^{18}F-FDG PET uptake heterogeneity: prognostic value in non-small cell lung cancer. *Journal of Nuclear Medicine: Official Publication, Society of Nuclear Medicine.* 2014;55(8):1235–1241.

72. Eschmann SM, Friedel G, Paulsen F, et al. ^{18}F-FDG PET for assessment of therapy response and preoperative re-evaluation after neoadjuvant radiochemotherapy in stage III non-small cell lung cancer. *European Journal of Nuclear Medicine and Molecular Imaging.* 2007;34(4):463–471.

73. Kremer R, Peysakhovich Y, Dan LF, et al. FDG PET/CT for assessing the resectability of NSCLC patients with N2 disease after neoadjuvant therapy. *Annals of Nuclear Medicine.* 2016;30(2):114–121.

74. Cuaron J, Dunphy M, Rimner A. Role of FDG-PET scans in staging, response assessment, and follow-up care for non-small cell lung cancer. *Frontiers in Oncology.* 2012;2:208.

75. Ziai D, Wagner T, El Badaoui A, et al. Therapy response evaluation with FDG-PET/CT in small cell lung cancer: a prognostic and comparison study of the PERCIST and EORTC criteria. *Cancer Imaging: the Official Publication of the International Cancer Imaging Society.* 2013;13: 73–80.

76. Weber WA, Petersen V, Schmidt B, et al. Positron emission tomography in non-small-cell lung cancer: prediction of response to chemotherapy by quantitative assessment of glucose use. *Journal of Clinical Oncology: Official Journal of the American Society of Clinical Oncology.* 2003;21(14):2651–2657.

77. de Geus-Oei LF, van der Heijden HF, Visser EP, et al. Chemotherapy response evaluation with ^{18}F-FDG PET in patients with non-small cell lung cancer. *Journal of Nuclear Medicine: Official Publication, Society of Nuclear Medicine.* 2007;48(10):1592–1598.

78. Hicks RJ. Role of ^{18}F-FDG PET in assessment of response in non-small cell lung cancer. *Journal of Nuclear Medicine: Official Publication, Society of Nuclear Medicine.* 2009;50(suppl 1):31S–42S.

79. Nishino M, Hatabu H, Johnson BE, McLoud TC. State of the art: response assessment in lung cancer in the era of genomic medicine. *Radiology.* 2014;271(1):6–27.

80. Aukema TS, Kappers I, Olmos RA, et al. Is ^{18}F-FDG PET/CT useful for the early prediction of histopathologic response to neoadjuvant erlotinib in patients with non-small cell lung cancer? *Journal of Nuclear Medicine: Official Publication, Society of Nuclear Medicine.* 2010;51(9):1344–1348.

81. De Ruysscher D. PET-CT in radiotherapy for lung cancer. *Methods in Molecular Biology.* 2011;727:53–58.

82. Lee P, Kupelian P, Czernin J, Ghosh P. Current concepts in F18 FDG PET/CT-based radiation therapy planning for lung cancer. *Frontiers in Oncology.* 2012;2:71.

83. Bradley J, Thorstad WL, Mutic S, et al. Impact of FDG-PET on radiation therapy volume delineation in non-small-cell lung cancer. *International Journal of Radiation Oncology, Biology, Physics.* 2004;59(1):78–86.

84. Wang Z, Wang Y, Sui X, et al. Performance of FLT-PET for pulmonary lesion diagnosis compared with traditional FDG-PET: a meta-analysis. *European Journal of Radiology.* 2015;84(7):1371–1377.

85. Szyszko TA, Yip C, Szlosarek P, Goh V, Cook GJ. The role of new PET tracers for lung cancer. *Lung Cancer*. 2016;94:7–14.

86. Rockwell S, Dobrucki IT, Kim EY, Marrison ST, Vu VT. Hypoxia and radiation therapy: past history, ongoing research, and future promise. *Current Molecular Medicine*. 2009;9(4):442–458.

87. Brown JM. Tumor hypoxia in cancer therapy. *Methods in Enzymology*. 2007;435:297–321.

88. Hillner BE, Siegel BA, Hanna L, et al. Impact of ^{18}F-Fluoride PET on Intended Management of Patients with Cancers Other Than Prostate Cancer: Results from the National Oncologic PET Registry. *Journal of Nuclear Medicine: Official Publication, Society of Nuclear Medicine*. 2014;55(7):1054–1061.

CHAPTER 3

Breast Cancer

ALIREZA REZAEE • ANDREAS BUCK • MARKUS RADERER •
WERNER LANGSTEGER • MOHSEN BEHESHTI

BACKGROUND

General[1,2]

- Breast cancer is the most common type of invasive cancer (one-third of all cancers in women) and the second leading cause of cancer death (14%) in females after lung cancer in the United States.
- The main risk factors are:
  - Gender (100 times more among women than men)
  - Age (two-thirds of invasive cancers after the age of 55 years)
  - Race (more often within Caucasian women)
  - Personal or family history of breast cancer (10-fold more risk if positive personal history of invasive ductal carcinoma)
  - History of lobular or ductal carcinoma in situ
  - First delivery at an older age (>30 years) or nulliparity
  - Genetic mutations such as BRCA1 or BRCA2
  - History of radiation therapy
  - Long-term use of hormone replacement therapy
- Mammography is the recommended screening modality and has been shown to benefit women in the age group between 50 and 69 years. Magnetic resonance imaging (MRI) is recommended for subgroups of women at risk (e.g., familial BRCA history). There is no consensus for the use of ultrasound in the screening setting.
- At initial presentation, 5%–10% of patients already have metastatic disease.

Early Clinical Symptoms[1,3]

- Painless breast mass or lump (most common)
- Erythema, thickening, irritation, scaling, and dimpling of the skin overlying the breast
- Nipple distortion or discharge
- Axillary lymphadenopathy

Primary Diagnostic Procedures[1,4]

- Physical examination
- Mammography (bilateral)
- Ultrasound of the breasts including local lymph nodes
- MRI is not routinely recommended (considered in BRCA history, suspicion of multifocal disease)
- Pathologic examination of the primary and axillary lymph nodes if involvement is suspected

Standard Treatment[5]

All treatment decisions have to be taken by a multidisciplinary team:

- **Early stage I–IIB (T2N1):** Tumor resection (lumpectomy/mastectomy, breast conservation surgery [BCS] whenever possible), regional lymph node dissection if suspected as positive in the clinical setting or proved using ultrasound/biopsy (if negative, sentinel node biopsy) ± radiation therapy (especially in the case of BCS) ± adjuvant chemotherapy (based on the surrogate intrinsic phenotype).
- **Locally advanced IIB (T3N0)–IIIC:** Neoadjuvant chemotherapy (locally advanced and large "operable" cancers) + tumor resection if possible (lumpectomy/mastectomy, breast conservation surgery [BCS] whenever possible), regional lymph node dissection if suspected as positive in the clinical setting or proved using ultrasound/biopsy (if negative, sentinel node biopsy) ± radiation therapy (especially in the case of BCS) ± adjuvant chemotherapy (based on the surrogate intrinsic phenotype).
- **Metastatic disease stage IV:** Tumor surgery/radiation for palliative reasons, and lymph node dissection, radiation therapy, systemic therapy, e.g., chemotherapy, biologic, and/or endocrine therapy according to the biology of the disease.

A minor deviation in treatment approaches may be considered by various clinical guidelines.

Prognostic Factors[6]

- Age <35 years or ≥65 years (worse prognosis)
- Race (worse prognosis in blacks)
- Tumor stage and size (worse prognosis in stage III–IV)
- Hormone receptors (worse prognosis if triple hormone receptors are negative)
- HER2 overexpression (worse prognosis)

- Marker of proliferation (Ki67) (worse prognosis with higher levels)
- Axillary nodal involvement (worse prognosis)
- Lymphovascular invasion (worse prognosis)
- Gene expression studies showing positive harmful BRCA1 or BRCA2 mutation (worse prognosis)
- Circulating tumor cells (worse prognosis)

Five-Year Survival[7]

- Stage I: 100%
- Stage II: 93%
- Stage III: 72%
- Stage IV: 22%

TUMOR CHARACTERISTICS AND TYPICAL BEHAVIOR

Histopathology[8]

Invasive carcinoma

- Infiltrating ductal carcinoma: 75%
- Infiltrating lobular carcinoma: 8%
- Mixed ductal/lobular carcinoma: 7%
- Others such as mucinous, tubular, medullary, papillary, metaplastic carcinoma, lymphoma, sarcoma: 10%

Distribution and Localization[9–11]

T-primary

- Upper outer quadrant: 50%
- Areola/nipple: 18%
- Upper inner quadrant: 15%
- Lower outer quadrant: 11%
- Lower inner quadrant: 6%

N-lymph nodes

Tumor size and nodal positivity are provided in Table 3.1.

M-distant metastasis

- Bone: 20%
- Lung: 12%
- Liver: 12%
- Skin: 5%
- Brain: 2%

TNM CLASSIFICATION[12]

Primary Tumor (T) Categories

The TNM classification is provided in Table 3.2.

TO: no evidence of primary tumor

Tis: carcinoma in situ (or Paget disease of the nipple with no associated tumor mass)

TABLE 3.1
N-Lymph Nodes

Lymph Node Station	Tumor Size	Nodal Positivity (%)
Axillary	<2 cm	18
	2–5 cm	35
	>5 cm	56
Internal mammary	<5 cm	19
	>5 cm	37

TABLE 3.2
Breast Cancer TNM Classification

TNM	T1	T2	T3	T4
N0	I	IIA	IIB	IIIB
N1	IIA	IIB	IIIA	IIIB
N2	IIIA	IIIA	IIIA	IIIB
N3	IIIC	IIIC	IIIC	IIIC
M1	IV	IV	IV	IV

T1: ≤2 cm
- T1mi: tumor ≤1 mm
- T1a: 1 < tumor ≤5 mm
- T1b: 5 < tumor ≤10 mm
- T1c: 10 < Tumor ≤20 mm

T2: 2 to ≤5 cm

T3: > 5 cm

T4: any size growing into the chest wall or skin, including inflammatory breast cancer
- T4a: extension to chest wall, not including only pectoralis muscle adherence/invasion
- T4b: ipsilateral satellite nodules and/or ulceration and/or edema (including peau d'orange) of the skin, which do not meet the criteria for inflammatory carcinoma
- T4c: both T4a and T4b
- T4d: inflammatory carcinoma

Regional Lymph Nodes (N; Based on Looking at Them Under a Microscope)

N0: no regional lymph node metastases

N1: metastases to movable ipsilateral axillary lymph nodes

N2:

Metastases to be fixed or matted ipsilateral axillary lymph nodes

Or

Clinically apparent metastases to ipsilateral internal mammary lymph nodes without axillary lymph node involvement

- N2a: metastases in ipsilateral level I, II axillary lymph nodes fixed to one another (matted) or to other structures
- N2b: metastases only in clinically detected ipsilateral internal mammary nodes and in the absence of clinically evident level I, II axillary lymph node metastases

N3:

Metastases to ipsilateral infraclavicular lymph nodes ± axillary lymph node involvement

Or

Clinically apparent metastases to ipsilateral internal mammary lymph nodes with axillary lymph node involvement

Or

Metastases to ipsilateral supraclavicular lymph nodes ± axillary or internal mammary lymph node involvement

- N3a: metastasis in ipsilateral infraclavicular lymph node(s)
- N3b: metastasis in ipsilateral internal mammary and axillary lymph node(s)
- N3c: metastasis in ipsilateral supraclavicular lymph node(s)

Distant Metastasis (M)

M0: No distant spread is found on clinical and/or imaging examinations

M1: Cancer has spread to distant organs

EVIDENCE-BASED VIEWPOINTS[5,12,14,15]

- Fludeoxyglucose positron emission tomography/computed tomography (FDG PET/CT) can potentially replace conventional imaging modalities in staging of locally advanced breast cancer.
- It is a supplemental modality in case of equivocal or suspicious findings on conventional imaging.
- FDG PET/CT is recommended for evaluation of response to chemotherapy or radiation therapy.
- The role of FDG PET/CT is controversially discussed in the assessment of primary breast cancer or regional lymph node status and, generally, is not recommended in the screening of primary breast cancer and posttreatment disease surveillance; nevertheless:
  - It provides a sensitivity, specificity, and accuracy of 90%, 92%, and 93% for the diagnosis of pri-

mary invasive breast carcinoma and a sensitivity and specificity of 80% and 90%, respectively, for the detection of metastatic axillary lymph nodes.
- FDG uptake is higher in patients with triple-negative or HER2-positive malignant lesions and inversely correlates with prognosis.
- FDG PET/CT caused upstaging and downstaging in approximately 20%–30% of patients based on different studies.

COST-EFFECTIVENESS

No large studies have been performed to evaluate the cost-effectiveness of using FDG PET in breast cancer. However, retrospective studies show a change in management in patients with primary breast cancer (>T1 stage). There was change of management in about 40% of patients, based on FDG PET/CT data. In stage III patients the percentage of change in management was even higher (>50%).[16]

CLINICAL POINT OF VIEW

- Among many other factors, the correct staging in breast cancer remains essential. At present, CT, abdominal ultrasound, and even bone scintigraphy are still seen as the standard.
- The role of FDG PET/CT in patients with breast cancer is still controversial. In particular, prospective outcome studies showing the benefit of functional (and nonfunctional) imaging as CT on overall survival are lacking.
- Patients with inconclusive findings or high risk for metastasis benefit from FDG PET/CT scanning. The European Society for Medical Oncology therefore mentions the usefulness of FDG PET/CT in patients with locally advanced cancer or in patients with inflammatory disease, because these patients have a high risk for further previously unknown metastases.
- The current National Comprehensive Cancer Network guidelines recommend FDG PET/CT for staging in locally advanced, recurrent, or stage IV diseases. However, there is no recommendation for the earlier stages (Table 3.3).
- Because the sensitivity of FDG PET depends on the size of the tumor, best results are achieved in patients with tumors > 2 cm (>T1) with a sensitivity over 90%. In patients with T1 tumors the sensitivity drops below 70%, and FDG PET has no role in "in situ" carcinomas.

TABLE 3.3
Breast Cancer ESMO and NCCN Guidelines[5,12,13]

Clinical Guidelines	Initial Diagnosis (Primary Tumor)	N-Staging	M-Staging
ESMO	Can replace CIM in: • locally advanced or inflammatory disease (e.g., T3-4)	Can replace CIM in: • high-risk patients as candidates for neo-adjuvant chemotherapy • locally advanced (e.g., N2-3)	Can replace CIM in: • high-risk patients as candidates for neoadjuvant chemotherapy • inoperable cancer before starting therapy
NCCN	Optional for locally advanced cancer (e.g., T3-4)	Optional for locally advanced cancer (e.g., N2-3)	Optional for • stages III and IV with equivocal or suspicious conventional imaging • after primary tumor surgery if >4 axillary lymph nodes • evaluation of response to therapy

ESMO, European Society for Medical Oncology; *NCCN*, National Comprehensive Cancer Network.

- Because glucose metabolism is non–cancer specific, false-positive findings might occur in patients with dysplasia, fibroadenomas, silicone leakage, and fat necrosis, among other inflammatory and infectious etiologies.
- A negative FDG PET/CT, for example, in local lymph nodes does not exclude micrometastases, and the sentinel node procedure still remains the standard to assess lymph node involvement.
- There is broad consensus that FDG PET/CT is useful in patients with inflammatory breast cancer because these patients have a high risk of distant metastasis and the inflammatory component can be well visualized by the FDG PET component.
- FDG PET/CT outperforms bone scintigraphy in patients with osteolytic or mixed osteolytic/osteoblastic bone lesions.
- FDG PET/CT is highly useful to monitor the response to cytotoxic treatment in malignant disease, and it has been shown that early or midtreatment FDG PET is highly predictive for further response to treatment. However, the absence of FDG does not ultimately predict the absence of viable tumor cells.
- Because the uptake of FDG is dependent on the tumor metabolism, low-grade tumors might not be FDG avid. On the other hand, very aggressive subtypes, such as the triple negative breast cancer subtype, do have high FDG uptakes.
- FDG PET/CT is highly valuable in the setting of recurrence because conventional imaging might not be able to differentiate between postsurgical and postradiation scars, and functional imaging using FDG PET outperforms classical methods of restaging such as CT.
- In asymptomatic patients, there are currently no data to perform surveillance imaging either with CT or with FDG PET/CT, because no survival benefits have been proved.

PITFALLS[17]
False Positive
- Acute and chronic inflammation
- Benign breast masses (silicone granuloma, fat necrosis, fibroadenoma, fibrocystic change)
- Postsurgical and postradiation changes
- Gynecomastia in men
- Postchemotherapy bone marrow stimulation
- Physiologically avid brown fat tissue
- Traumatic bony lesions
- Vertebral compression fracture with vertebroplasty
- Flare phenomenon in antiestrogen or chemotherapy
- Image misregistration (breathing artifacts)
- Lactating breast

False Negative
- Low-grade and well-differentiated tumors
- Histologic tumor type (tubular carcinoma, lobular carcinoma, in situ carcinoma)
- Lactating breasts and high breast density may obscure tumor visualization

Common false-negative lesions in all cancers: Early-stage malignancy, hyperglycemic patients, and small-sized lesions (<8 mm).

DISCUSSION
Primary Staging-Restaging
The number of diagnosed cases of breast cancer is increasing because of widespread screening tests such as physical examination and mammography. MRI is an alternative for younger patients with dense breast tissue.

In the case of a palpable mass in the breast, however, the conventional imaging modalities including mammography, ultrasound, and MRI are recommended to detect primary breast cancer.

As another helpful examination, FDG PET/CT is now widely used to image oncology patients. It shows promising staging modality for staging of patients with primary breast tumors larger than 3 cm, with a sensitivity and specificity of 93% and 91% for the diagnosis of primary tumor as well as 80% and 90% for the detection of metastatic locoregional lymph nodes, respectively. However, the sensitivity of FDG PET/CT scan is not high enough for smaller lesions measuring <1 cm or tumor types with low FDG uptake such as lobular and in situ carcinoma.

In addition, FDG PET/CT is not able to rule out micrometastases in the axillary lymph nodes. Therefore, it could not replace sentinel lymph node biopsy or axillary lymph node dissection.[18]

Clinical guidelines generally recommend FDG PET/CT as an optional modality for locally advanced breast cancer or for high-risk patients who are candidates for neoadjuvant treatment. It is also recommended in recurrent disease or when the other conventional studies are equivocal or suspicious.[12,13,19]

Conversely, there is a group of studies that emphasize the role of FDG PET/CT staging in stage II or III breast cancers, especially in young patients, which may lead to change of patients' management. In addition, a vast majority of the studies in the medical literature highly recommend evaluation of extraaxillary lymph nodes and distant organ metastasis of breast cancer with FDG PET/CT with a sensitivity and specificity of 71%–99% and 66%–68%, respectively.[20–28]

Furthermore, initial reports noted a sensitivity of 57%–100% and specificity of 96%–100% for FDG PET/CT scan in localizing osseous metastases in patients with breast cancer.[29] In addition to its higher sensitivity compared with conventional imaging modalities, particularly in locally advanced or inflammatory breast cancers, FDG PET/CT is able to offer a whole-body examination in one session, early detection of disease before morphologic changes appear, and accurate information regarding intrathoracic lymph nodes status, as well as distant metastases.[20,30]

Moreover, FDG PET/CT is an invaluable modality for detecting breast cancer recurrence with a median sensitivity and specificity of 93% and 82%, respectively. It is much more sensitive and specific for the assessment of recurrent breast cancers compared with stand-alone CT and provides additional information that could alter patients' management.[27,31,32]

Treatment Monitoring
FDG PET/CT is an encouraging imaging biomarker for the effectiveness of breast cancer treatment, and decreased FDG uptake of metastatic lesions is associated with favorable response to therapy. When compared with conventional imaging modalities such as CT scan and MRI, FDG PET/CT has the unique ability to recognize nonresponder patients to chemotherapy even after the first or second cycle of treatment. This group of patients may therefore be referred for second-line chemotherapy before trying more cycles of the same regimen. A change in SUV_{max} has a good predictive value for monitoring pathologic response and survival in patients with inflammatory breast cancer after neoadjuvant chemotherapy. Also, available data support the role of FDG PET/CT in therapy monitoring of recurrent breast cancer.[23,29,33–35]

Prognostic Value
The prognostic value of FDG PET/CT scan is well investigated. The avidity of primary breast tumors is significantly correlated with clinicopathologic factors, which propounds the prognostic feature of the modality. For instance, FDG avidity was considerably higher in estrogen receptor (ER)-negative than in ER-positive, as well as triple negative, breast tumors. In addition, there is a good correlation between FDG uptake (SUV_{max}) and Ki-67 proliferation index, as well as tumor size in triple negative breast cancers. Furthermore, a greater FDG uptake in primary tumor is associated with lymphatic invasion and axillary lymph node metastasis. To sum up, a high FDG uptake in malignant lesions seems to be an ominous prognostic factor in primary breast cancer.[31,36–40]

PET/MRI and Positron Emission Mammography
One of the imaging modalities that is used in breast cancer evaluation is MRI. Specific breast MRI is used for local breast cancer staging with a high accuracy. Moreover,

whole-body MRI can be performed for the evaluation of distant metastases, particularly when completed with organ-specific imaging protocols. Hence, PET/MRI is an encouraging technology to evaluate breast cancer and provides excellent functional findings of PET with high-resolution anatomic details of MRI in one acquisition. On the other hand, FDG PET/MRI has better sensitivity (96% versus 85%) in detecting skeletal metastases from breast cancer when compared with FDG PET/CT. The disadvantages of FDG PET/MRI are its higher cost and long imaging time, which currently limit its usage.[41,42]

As an alternative imaging method, positron emission mammography could be a promising tool with fewer limitations in local staging and recurrence of breast cancer, as well as evaluation of response to therapy when compared with other whole-body imaging modalities. However, further investigations are needed to evaluate its value in breast cancer diagnostic guidelines.[43] However, some investigators found the technique comparable with whole-body FDG PET/CT in the detection of primary breast cancer.[44]

FDG PET/CT and Breast-Feeding

Although FDG is excreted in the milk of mothers who undergo an FDG PET/CT examination, the amount is within the allowed range for breast-fed infants, and it is the favorable method for cancer imaging in lactating mothers.[45–48] Most of the authorities do not recommend breast-feeding withdrawal after PET imaging.[46–48] However, controversial approaches are noticed in this concern. Some groups consider the lactating breast, with dramatic accumulation of radiotracer, as a source of external radiation to the baby during breast-feeding.[45,49–51] They recommend that breast-feeding be stopped for 4–12 h or for one breast-feeding and that the baby be bottle fed with pumped breast milk.[45,49] The maximum radioactivity in breast milk will be achieved approximately 3 h after injection of the FDG dose.[45]

Radiotracers Beyond FDG

Several other radiotracers are currently being investigated, which may greatly influence breast cancer management in the future. Most of these tracers target the cellular processes that are more specific than glucose metabolism. Among those are the thymidine analogues, targeting DNA replication, which represents cell proliferation; annexin V derivatives that appraise apoptosis; ER tracers; agents detecting angiogenesis; and engineered antibody fragments that bind to HER2/neu receptors. For instance, ^{18}F-fluorothymidine uptake is strongly correlated with cell proliferation in untreated patients with breast cancer and is basically

used to evaluate response to chemotherapy, particularly with taxanes anticancer medications, as early as 1 week after chemotherapy. ^{18}F-fluoroestradiol measures ER expression of the breast malignancy, as well as delivery and binding of estrogen to ER, and thus predicts response to hormone therapy (e.g., tamoxifen and aromatase inhibitors) in these patients. αVβ3 is an integrin receptor for vitronectin, which presents on angiogenic endothelial cells, and could be detected by ^{18}F-galacto-RGD PET, with a promising role in detecting primary breast cancers but not nodal or distant metastases. ^{18}F-fluoromisonidazole accumulates in viable hypoxic cancerous cells with functional nitroreductase enzyme rather than in nonviable necrotic cells.[14] By performing pretreatment HER2 PET/CT with ^{89}Zr-trastuzumab, clinicians may identify patients who are most likely to respond to trastuzumab emtansine (T-DM1) therapy. The combination of HER2 and FDG PET/CT could correctly predict morphologic response with a positive predictive value and negative predictive value of 100%.[52]

As a bone-seeking agent, ^{18}F-NaF is used as a PET radiotracer for the evaluation of skeletal metastases from breast cancer. Although whole-body MDP bone scintigraphy is still the method of choice for this purpose, ^{18}F-NaF PET/CT is a more sensitive and specific modality.[53] Considering the increasing availability of PET scanners, the authors believe that conventional bone scintigraphy will be replaced by ^{18}F-NaF PET/CT in the near future for the detection of bone metastases from breast cancer.[54]

CONCLUSION

In contrast to clinical guidelines that consider an optional role for FDG PET/CT in the staging of primary breast cancer or axillary lymph node involvement, evidence-based data show a promising role for FDG PET/CT in routine clinical practice in the staging of locally advanced or high-risk breast cancer. It changed patients' management in approximately 20%–30% of patients. FDG PET/CT is highly recommended in the evaluation of extraaxillary lymph nodes and distant metastases. It also shows superior diagnostic performance compared with conventional imaging modalities in recurrent breast cancer and therapy monitoring.

TEACHING CASES
Case 1: Staging Breast Cancer
Findings

A 40-year-old female with invasive ductal carcinoma (grade 3, ER/progesterone receptor negative) of the left breast. FDG PET/CT shows an FDG-avid left breast soft

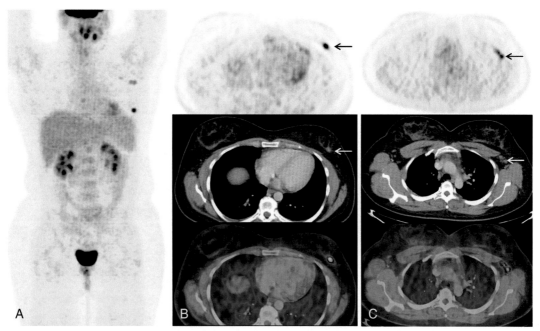

FIG. 3.1 Fludeoxyglucose (FDG) positron emission tomography/computed tomography showing an FDG-avid left breast soft tissue nodule (B, *arrow*) as the primary tumor with ipsilateral FDG-avid axillary lymph nodes (C, *arrow*) suspicious for metastatic disease. A, MIP image.

tissue nodule (Fig. 3.1B, arrow) as the primary tumor with ipsilateral FDG-avid axillary lymph nodes (Fig. 3.1C, arrow) suspicious for metastatic disease.

Teaching points
- Patients with axillary lymph node involvement have poorer prognosis.
- FDG PET/CT provides a sensitivity, specificity, and accuracy of 90%, 92%, and 93% for the diagnosis of primary invasive breast carcinoma and a sensitivity and specificity of 80% and 90% for the detection of metastatic axillary lymph nodes, respectively.

Pitfalls
- Sinus histiocytosis, reactive process, and paravenous injection of radiotracer are common pitfalls for FDG-avid lymph nodes in the axillary region.
- Increased FDG uptake on additional delayed acquisition may be suggestive of malignancy.

Case 2: Assessment of Lymph Node Metastases
Findings
A 43-year-old female with multifocal invasive ductal carcinoma, status post bilateral radical mastectomy, radiochemotherapy, and hormonal and bisphosphonate treatment, admitted for follow-up imaging. FDG PET/CT shows multiple lymph node metastases in the right axillary region (Fig. 3.2B, arrow) and in internal mammary groups (Fig. 3.2C, arrow). A solitary bone metastasis in the right ischium is also noted (Fig. 3.2D, arrow) without morphologic changes on correlated CT.

Teaching points
- The internal mammary lymph nodes do not meet CT scan criteria for metastases. FDG PET/CT is superior to stand-alone CT in the assessment of lymph node metastases.
- FDG PET/CT has the potential for whole-body imaging and is able to detect distant metastases earlier than conventional imaging modalities before morphologic changes are apparent.

Case 3: Extensive Distant Metastases
Findings
A 79-year-old female with lobular breast cancer. FDG PET/CT shows disseminated osseous metastases (Fig. 3.3A and C) without suspicious morphologic changes on CT (e.g., bone marrow infiltration). A focal FDG uptake is noted within the myocardium (Fig. 3.3B, arrow), which could be a metastatic lesion.

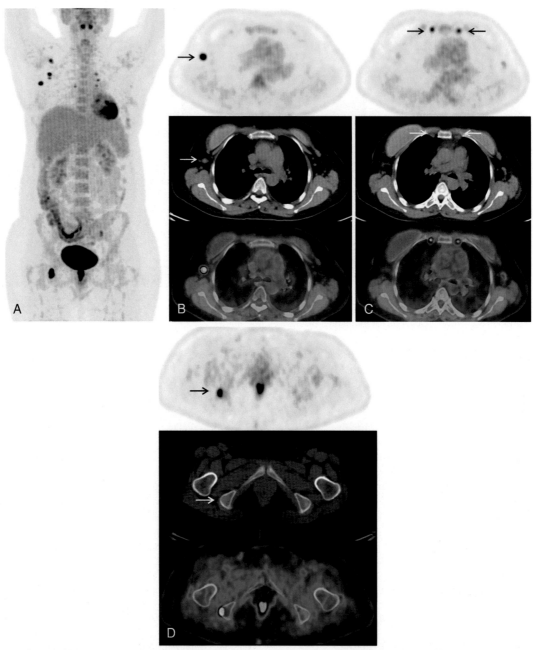

FIG. 3.2 Fludeoxyglucose (FDG) positron emission tomography/computed tomography (CT) showing multiple lymph node metastases in right axillary region (B, *arrow*), as well as in internal mammary groups (C, *arrow*). A solitary bone metastasis in right ischium is also noted (D, *arrow*) without morphologic changes on correlated CT. A, MIP image.

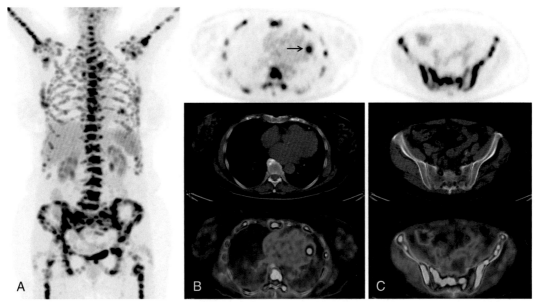

FIG. 3.3 Fludeoxyglucose (FDG) positron emission tomography/computed tomography (CT) showing disseminated osseous metastases (A, C) without suspicious morphologic changes on CT (e.g., bone marrow infiltration). A focal FDG uptake is noted within myocardium (B, *arrow*), which could be a metastatic lesion.

Teaching points
- Approximately 5%–10% of patients with breast cancer present with distant metastases.
- Bone is the most common site of distant metastasis from breast cancer (20% of cases).
- Although it is extremely rare for breast cancer to metastasize to the heart, a focal intense FDG uptake of myocardium may represent a metastatic lesion or tumor thrombosis.
- It is important to suppress myocardial FDG uptake as much as possible in oncologic patients who undergo FDG PET/CT.

Pitfalls
- Myocardial FDG uptake may obscure distant metastasis to the heart.

Case 4: Inflammatory Breast Cancer
Findings
A 71-year-old female with right inflammatory breast cancer. FDG PET/CT shows intensive FDG-avid primary tumor with bilateral axillary (Fig. 3.4B, arrow) and mediastinal lymph node as well as left adrenal (Fig. 3.4C, arrow) and thoracic vertebral metastases (Fig. 3.4E, arrow). An FDG-avid right colon soft tissue

nodule was a tubular adenomatous polyp on pathology (Fig. 3.4D, arrow).

Teaching points
- Inflammatory breast cancer is an invasive malignancy with very poor prognosis.
- Distant metastasis is usually noted at presentation.
- There is broad consensus that FDG PET/CT is useful in patients with inflammatory breast cancer because these patients have a high risk of distant metastasis.

Pitfalls
- FDG-avid benign lesions in the gastrointestinal tract could be a false-positive pitfall in PET interpretation.

Case 5: Staging, FDG Versus ^{18}F-NaF PET/CT
Findings
A 43-year-old female with right breast cancer who underwent both FDG (Fig. 3.5A) and NaF PET/CT in two consecutive days. FDG PET/CT shows a large tracer-avid right breast cancer with multiple axillary lymph nodes as well as osseous metastases. FDG PET/CT is able to detect more skeletal metastases most likely because of bone marrow involvement and osteolytic metastases. The lytic lesion in left iliac bone is merely

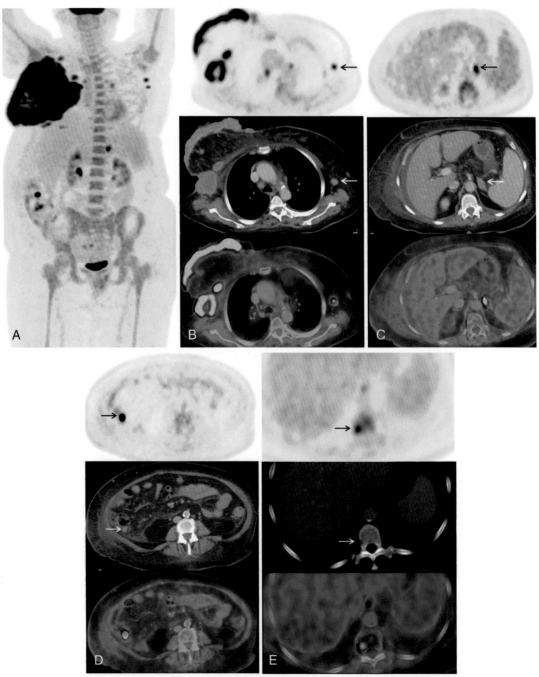

FIG. 3.4 Fludeoxyglucose (FDG) positron emission tomography/computed tomography showing intensive FDG-avid primary tumor with bilateral axillary (B, *arrow*) and mediastinal lymph node as well as left adrenal (C, *arrow*) and thoracic vertebral metastases (E, *arrow*). FDG-avid right colon soft tissue nodule was a tubular adenomatous polyp on pathology (D, *arrow*). A, MIP image.

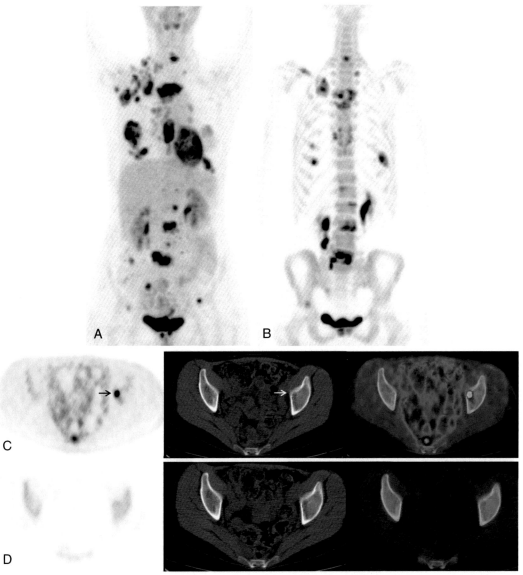

FIG. 3.5 Fludeoxyglucose (FDG) positron emission tomography/computed tomography showing a large tracer-avid right breast cancer with multiple axillary lymph nodes as well as osseous metastases. FDG PET/CT is able to detect more skeletal metastases most likely because of bone marrow involvement and osteolytic metastases. The lytic lesion in left iliac bone is merely positive on FDG (C, *arrow*) but not on NaF PET images (D). A and B, MIP images.

positive on FDG (Fig. 3.5C, arrow) but not on NaF PET images (Fig. 3.5D).

Teaching points
- FDG PET/CT is a useful modality in the assessment of primary tumor, as well as soft tissue and early bone marrow metastases from breast cancer. It also

shows higher sensitivity in the detection of malignant lytic bony lesions.
- FDG PET/CT has, however, limited sensitivity in the detection of densely sclerotic lesions mainly after treatment because of lower perfusion and fewer tumor cells in the osteoblastic metastases. In such cases, PET/CT using bone-seeking

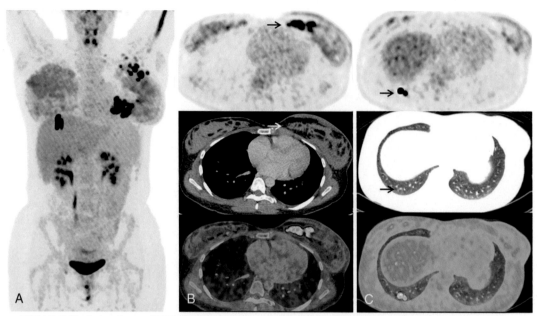

FIG. 3.6 Fludeoxyglucose (FDG) positron emission tomography/computed tomography showing multifocal tracer-avid lesions in the left breast with ipsilateral axillary, internal mammary, subpectoral, and infraclavicular lymph node metastases. A, MIP image. B and C, Axial PET, CT, and fused images.

agents (i.e., NaF) may provide more useful information.

Case 6: Breast Cancer During Breast-feeding
Findings
A 30-year-old female with multifocal triple negative invasive ductal left breast cancer, which was initially diagnosed after her delivery and during breast-feeding. FDG PET/CT shows multifocal tracer-avid lesions in the left breast with ipsilateral axillary, internal mammary, subpectoral, and infraclavicular lymph node metastases (Fig. 3.6).

Teaching points
- Triple hormone receptors negative breast cancer is related to poor prognosis.
- Breast cancer is often diagnosed at a later stage than it would be if the women were not pregnant or breast-feeding. It is also more likely to have spread to the lymph nodes. The use of FDG PET/CT may be preferable to other types of scans during breast-feeding because of the low levels and rapid disappearance of radiation.
- The amount of FDG excreted in breast milk after PET/CT is below the level of concern for the breast-fed infant, and numerous international radiation safety organizations state that no interruption of

breast-feeding is necessary. However, some groups consider the lactating breast as a source of external radiation to infant and recommend withdrawal of breast-feeding for 4–12 h.
- FDG PET/CT is superior to stand-alone CT in the detection of small nonaxillary lymph node metastases.

Pitfalls
- Diffused FDG uptake in bilateral breast parenchyma, representing physiologic accumulation of radiotracer in the lactating breast tissue, could obscure malignant lesions with low FDG uptake.
- Of incidental note are foci of FDG uptake in the right lung with no corresponding morphologic lesions on CT, most likely because of radioactive clot, representing a common pitfall of FDG PET/CT.

Case 7: Contralateral Axillary Lymph Node Involvement
Findings
A 73-year-old female with multifocal ductal carcinoma of the right breast (pT1a pN1a M0 R0 Grad III), status post lumpectomy and axillary lymph node dissection. FDG PET/CT shows primary cancer in the right breast (Fig. 3.7B, arrow) and an FDG-avid lymph node on the contralateral axillary region (Fig. 3.7C, arrow) highly suspicious for malignancy. Follow-up

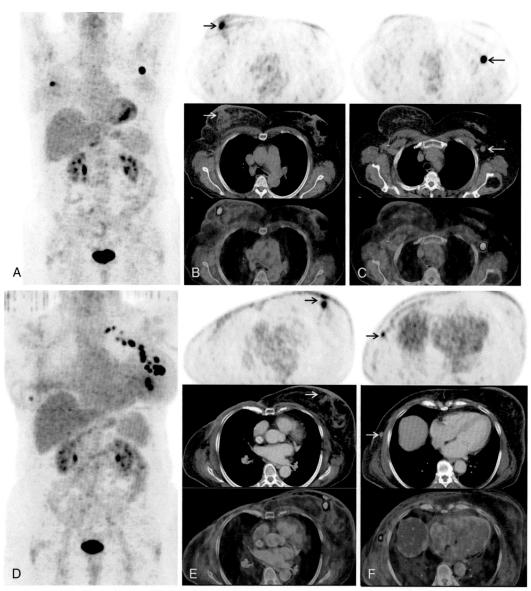

FIG. 3.7 Fludeoxyglucose (FDG) positron emission tomography/computed tomography showing primary cancer in the right breast (B, *arrow*) and an FDG-avid lymph node on the contralateral axillary region (C, *arrow*) highly suspicious for malignancy. Follow-up examination after right radical mastectomy confirmed the previous findings of left axillary lymph node involvement to be most likely because of occult primary left breast cancer (E, *arrow*) rather than a metastatic disease from right side. FDG-avid small recurrent disease is also evident on the right thoracic wall (F, *arrow*). A and D, MIP images.

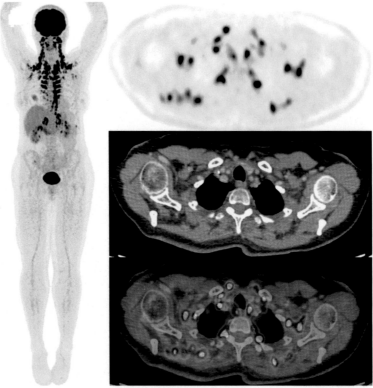

FIG. 3.8 Fludeoxyglucose (FDG) positron emission tomography/computed tomography (CT) showing numerous foci of FDG uptake in bilateral cervical, supraclavicular, paramediastinal, and paravertebral regions, corresponding to the fat tissue on CT, representing physiologic FDG-avid brown fat tissue.

examination after right radical mastectomy confirmed the previous findings of left axillary lymph node involvement to be most likely because of occult primary left breast cancer (Fig. 3.7E, arrow) rather than a metastatic disease from the right side. FDG-avid small recurrent disease is also evident on the right thoracic wall (Fig. 3.7F, arrow).

Teaching points
- Metastases to the contralateral axillary lymph nodes are uncommon. Involvement of the contralateral axilla is a manifestation of systemic disease (stage IV) or a regional metastasis from a new occult primary malignancy (T0N1, stage II).
- The most common site of primary breast cancer is the upper outer quadrant (50%), followed by the areolar region (18%).
- Axillary lymph node involvement is a poor prognostic factor in breast cancer.
- Infiltrating ductal carcinoma is the most common type of breast cancer (75%).

Case 8: Breast Cancer—Pitfall
Findings
A 59-year-old female with suspicious breast cancer. FDG PET/CT shows numerous foci of FDG uptake in bilateral cervical, supraclavicular, paramediastinal, and paravertebral regions, corresponding to the fat tissue on CT, representing physiologic FDG-avid brown fat tissue (BFT) (Fig. 3.8).

Teaching points
- FDG uptake of BFT is physiologic and should not be interpreted as metastatic disease.
- Common distribution of BFT: supraclavicular, axillae, neck, mediastinum, paravertebral, paraaortic, parahepatic, paracolic, suprarenal, and perinephric areas.
- BFT uptake can be reduced with warm temperature and pharmacologically (propranolol, reserpine, fentanyl). Warm clothing, no exposure to cold, temperature-controlled room (24°C), and 20 mg oral propranolol 1 h before FDG injection are all helpful.

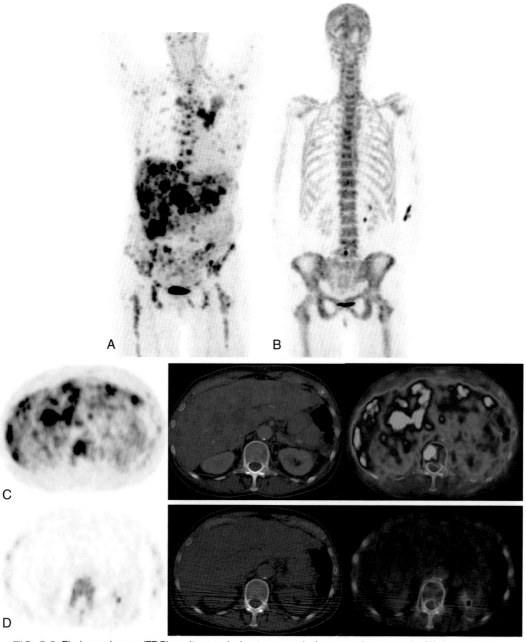

FIG. 3.9 Fludeoxyglucose (FDG) positron emission tomography/computed tomography (A) demonstrating extensive FDG-avid liver and bone marrow metastases. NaF PET/CT scan (B) shows nonhomogeneous tracer uptake but without the typical pattern of bone metastases. There is a focal increased uptake within the lower thoracic vertebral body, positive on FDG but negative on NaF PET, with no corresponding morphologic lesion on CT, most consistent with bone marrow metastasis. A and B, MIP images. C and D, Axial PET, CT, and fused images.

Pitfalls
- FDG uptake of BFT causes false-positive results on FDG PET. The pattern of tracer distribution and correlation with CT is very helpful for interpretation.

Case 9: Staging—FDG Versus NaF PET/CT
Findings
A 69-year-old female with history of multicentric lobular carcinoma of the right breast, status post mastectomy and adjuvant chemoradiation therapy. FDG PET/CT demonstrates (Fig. 3.9A) extensive FDG-avid liver and bone marrow metastases. NaF PET/CT scan shows nonhomogeneous tracer uptake but without the typical pattern of bone metastases. There is a focal increased uptake within the lower thoracic vertebral body, positive on FDG but negative on NaF PET, with no corresponding morphologic lesion on CT, most consistent with bone marrow metastasis.

Teaching points
- FDG PET/CT is superior to NaF PET/CT in the evaluation of early bone marrow metastases and is also able to assess soft tissue malignancies.
- Skeleton is the most common site for breast cancer metastases (20%), followed by liver (12%) and lung (12%).
- Age ≥65 years at diagnosis is a poor prognostic factor in patients with breast cancer.
- Patients with extensive distant metastases (stage IV disease) have poor prognosis with 5-year survival of about 22%.

Case 10: Therapy Monitoring
Findings
A 45-year-old female with left breast cancer, status post chemotherapy with Avastin/Navelbine. Primary FDG PET/CT (Fig. 3.10A) shows FDG-avid left breast primary tumor with extensive osteolytic bone metastases. The follow-up FDG PET/CT (Fig. 3.10B) revealed excellent response to therapy without any morphologic changes on CT.

Teaching points
- Although no significant changes are noted in osteolytic bone metastatic lesions, the FDG uptake is completely resolved (D, arrow), which demonstrates the incremental value of FDG PET/CT over stand-alone CT in the evaluation of response to therapy.
- Major clinical guidelines and evidence-based data support the value of FDG PET/CT for evaluation of response to chemotherapy or radiation therapy.

Case 11: Staging—Bone Seeking Agents (NaF PET/CT Versus Conventional 99mTc-MDP Bone Scan)
Findings
An 80-year-old female with history of breast cancer, admitted for assessment of skeletal metastases. 99mTc-MDP whole-body bone scintigraphy (Fig. 3.11A) shows symmetric age-adjusted distribution of radiotracer with no evidence of osseous metastasis. NaF PET/CT (Fig. 3.11B) shows a focal NaF-avid tumor in a thoracic vertebral body, suggestive of osteolytic bone metastasis (Fig. 3.11B and C; arrow).

Teaching points
- NaF PET/CT is more sensitive and specific than conventional whole-body bone scan in the detection of osseous metastases. Some investigators calculated sensitivity and specificity of 100% for this modality in the detection of bone metastases in breast and prostate cancers.
- The NaF uptake in osteolytic metastases is most likely due to reactive bone remodeling on the rim of the lesions or occult microsclerosis. Therefore, NaF PET may depict lytic lesions regarding its high tumor/background ratio.

Case 12: Breast Cancer and Silicone Implant
Findings
A 38-year-old female with left breast poorly differentiated invasive ductal carcinoma. Staging FDG PET/CT (A) shows an FDG-avid primary left breast cancer before surgery (arrow). The patient underwent bilateral (curative left and prophylactic right) mastectomy with silicone implantation. Follow-up FDG PET/CT (Fig. 3.12B) after 1 year demonstrates recurrent malignancy on the left thoracic wall (arrow). Of incidental note is the FDG uptake at the posterior wall of the right implant (arrowhead) (Fig. 3.12).

Teaching points
- FDG PET/CT is a valuable modality for the detection of breast cancer recurrence.
- Siliconoma is probably caused by the transfer of silicone particles from implants to lymph nodes by macrophages.
- Approximately 15% of modern implants may leak or rupture in 3–10 years after implantation.

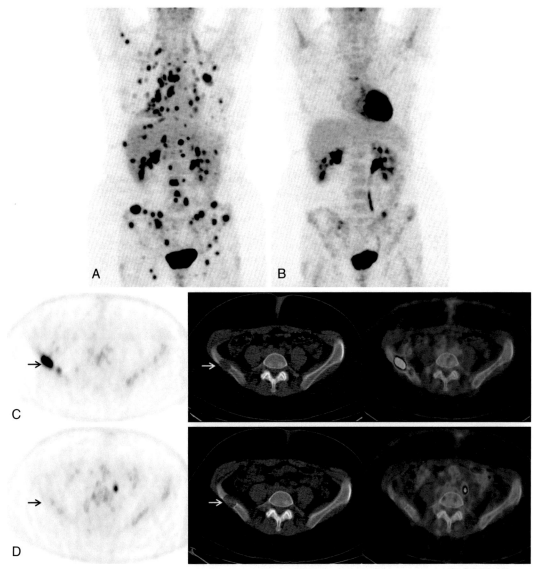

FIG. 3.10 Primary fludeoxyglucose positron emission tomography/computed tomography (FDG PET/CT) (A) shows FDG-avid left breast primary tumor with extensive osteolytic bone metastases. The follow-up FDG PET/CT (B) revealed excellent response to therapy without any morphologic changes on CT. C and D, Axial PET, CT, and fused images.

Pitfalls

- Siliconoma can cause false-positive results on FDG PET/CT and is a differential diagnosis for lymph node metastasis.

- Silicone leaks through the microscopic pores of the implant shell, without any discernible tear via a mechanism known as silicone gel bleeding, and can cause false-positive results on FDG PET/CT.

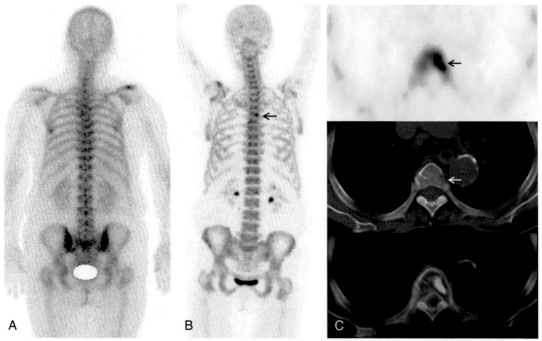

FIG. 3.11 99mTc-MDP whole-body bone scintigraphy (A) shows symmetric age-adjusted distribution of radiotracer with no evidence of osseous metastasis. NaF PET/CT (B) shows a focal NaF-avid tumor in a thoracic vertebral body, suggestive of osteolytic bone metastasis (B, C; *arrow*).

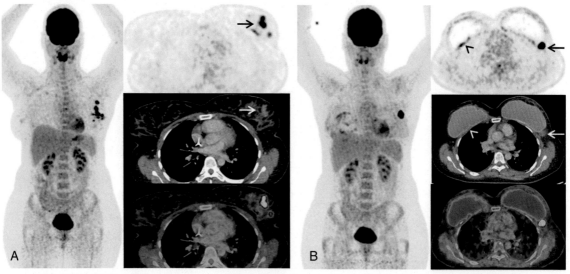

FIG. 3.12 Staging fludeoxyglucose positron emission tomography/computed tomography (FDG PET/CT) (A) shows an FDG-avid primary left breast cancer before surgery (*arrow*). The patient underwent bilateral (curative left and prophylactic right) mastectomy with silicone implantation. Follow-up FDG PET/CT (B) after 1 year demonstrates recurrent malignancy on the left thoracic wall (*arrow*). Of incidental note is the FDG uptake at the posterior wall of the right implant (*arrowhead*).

REFERENCES

1. *Cancer Facts & Figures*. Atlanta: American Cancer Society; 2016.
2. Clemons M, Goss P. Estrogen and the risk of breast cancer. *The New England Journal of Medicine*. January 25, 2001;344(4):276–285.
3. Esserman LJ, Shieh Y, Rutgers EJ, et al. Impact of mammographic screening on the detection of good and poor prognosis breast cancers. *Breast Cancer Research and Treatment*. December 2011;130(3):725–734.
4. Dizon D, Tejada-Berges T, Steinhoff M. Breast Cancer. In: Barakat RR, Markman M, Randall ME, eds. *Principles and Practice of Gynecologic Oncology*. Baltimore: Lippincott, Williams, & Wilkins; 2009:910.
5. Cardoso F, Costa A, Norton L, et al. ESO-ESMO 2nd international consensus guidelines for advanced breast cancer (ABC2)dagger. *Annals of Oncology: Official Journal of the European Society for Medical Oncology/ESMO*. October 2014;25(10):1871–1888.
6. Cristofanilli M, Budd GT, Ellis MJ, et al. Circulating tumor cells, disease progression, and survival in metastatic breast cancer. *The New England Journal of Medicine*. August 19, 2004;351(8):781–791.
7. *SEER Cancer Statistics Review 1975-2013*. Bethesda: National Cancer Institute; 2016.
8. Schnitt SJ. Classification and prognosis of invasive breast cancer: from morphology to molecular taxonomy. *Modern Pathology: An Official Journal of the United States and Canadian Academy of Pathology, Inc*. May 2010;23(suppl 2):S60–S64.
9. Darbre PD. Recorded quadrant incidence of female breast cancer in Great Britain suggests a disproportionate increase in the upper outer quadrant of the breast. *Anticancer Research*. May–June 2005;25(3c):2543–2550.
10. Beaumont T, Leadbeater M. Treatment and care of patients with metastatic breast cancer. *Nursing Standard*. June 8–14, 2011;25(40):49–56.
11. *Atlas of Clinical Positron Emission Tomography*. 2nd ed. Hodder Arnold; 2006.
12. NCCN Clinical Practice Guidelines in Oncology. *Breast Cancer*. 2016;2. National Comprehensive Cancer Network.
13. Senkus E, Kyriakides S, Ohno S, et al. Primary breast cancer: ESMO Clinical Practice Guidelines for diagnosis, treatment and follow-up. *Annals of Oncology: Official Journal of the European Society for Medical Oncology/ESMO*. September 2015;26(suppl 5):v8–30.
14. Quon A, Gambhir SS. FDG-PET and beyond: molecular breast cancer imaging. *Journal of Clinical Oncology: Official Journal of the American Society of Clinical Oncology*. March 10, 2005;23(8):1664–1673.
15. Carr C, Conant E, Rosen M, Schnall M, Davidson R. The impact of FDG PET in the staging of breast cancer. *Journal of Clinical Oncology (Meeting Abstracts)*. June 2006;24(18):530.
16. Gunalp B, Erdogan M, Ince S, Alagoz E, Arslan N. Investigation of patient selection criteria and cost-effectiveness of 18F FDG-PET/CT in primary staging of patients with breast carcinoma. *Journal of Nuclear Medicine: Official Publication, Society of Nuclear Medicine*. 2015;56(suppl 3):1308.
17. Kumar R, Rani N, Patel C, Basu S, Alavi A. False-negative and false-positive results in FDG-PET and PET/CT in breast cancer. *PET Clinics*. July 2009;4(3):289–298.
18. Liu Y. Role of FDG PET-CT in evaluation of locoregional nodal disease for initial staging of breast cancer. *World Journal of Clinical Oncology*. December 10, 2014;5(5):982–989.
19. Khatcheressian JL, Hurley P, Bantug E, et al. Breast cancer follow-up and management after primary treatment: American Society of Clinical Oncology clinical practice guideline update. *Journal of Clinical Oncology: Official Journal of the American Society of Clinical Oncology*. March 1, 2013;31(7):961–965.
20. Groheux D, Giacchetti S, Delord M, et al. 18F-FDG PET/CT in staging patients with locally advanced or inflammatory breast cancer: comparison to conventional staging. *Journal of Nuclear Medicine: Official Publication, Society of Nuclear Medicine*. January 2013;54(1):5–11.
21. Riedl CC, Slobod E, Jochelson M, et al. Retrospective analysis of 18F-FDG PET/CT for staging asymptomatic breast cancer patients younger than 40 years. *Journal of Nuclear Medicine: Official Publication, Society of Nuclear Medicine*. October 2014;55(10):1578–1583.
22. Krammer J, Schnitzer A, Kaiser CG, et al. (18) F-FDG PET/CT for initial staging in breast cancer patients – is there a relevant impact on treatment planning compared to conventional staging modalities? *European Radiology*. August 2015;25(8):2460–2469.
23. Koolen BB, Valdes Olmos RA, Elkhuizen PH, et al. Locoregional lymph node involvement on 18F-FDG PET/CT in breast cancer patients scheduled for neoadjuvant chemotherapy. *Breast Cancer Research and Treatment*. August 2012;135(1):231–240.
24. Vercher-Conejero JL, Pelegri-Martinez L, Lopez-Aznar D, Cozar-Santiago MP. Positron emission tomography in breast cancer. *Diagnostics*. 2015;5(1):61–83.
25. Gemignani ML. PET imaging and breast cancer. *Oncology*. May 2014;28(5):430, 432, 434.
26. Rosen EL, Eubank WB, Mankoff DA. FDG PET, PET/CT, and breast cancer imaging. *Radiographics: A Review Publication of the Radiological Society of North America, Inc*. October 2007;27(suppl 1):S215–S229.
27. Isasi CR, Moadel RM, Blaufox MD. A meta-analysis of FDG-PET for the evaluation of breast cancer recurrence and metastases. *Breast Cancer Research and Treatment*. March 2005;90(2):105–112.
28. Sachelarie I, Kerr K, Ghesani M, Blum RH. Integrated PET-CT: evidence-based review of oncology indications. *Oncology*. April 2005;19(4):481–490. discussion 490–482, 495–486.

29. Gaeta CM, Vercher-Conejero JL, Sher AC, Kohan A, Rubbert C, Avril N. Recurrent and metastatic breast cancer PET, PET/CT, PET/MRI: FDG and new biomarkers. *The Quarterly Journal of Nuclear Medicine and Molecular Imaging: Official Publication of the Italian Association of Nuclear Medicine.* December 2013;57(4):352–366.

30. Eubank WB, Mankoff DA, Takasugi J, et al. 18Fluorodeoxyglucose positron emission tomography to detect mediastinal or internal mammary metastases in breast cancer. *Journal of Clinical Oncology: Official Journal of the American Society of Clinical Oncology.* August 1, 2001;19(15):3516–3523.

31. Cochet A, David S, Moodie K, et al. The utility of 18 F-FDG PET/CT for suspected recurrent breast cancer: impact and prognostic stratification. *Cancer Imaging: The Official Publication of the International Cancer Imaging Society.* 2014;14:13.

32. Manohar K, Mittal BR, Senthil R, Kashyap R, Bhattacharya A, Singh G. Clinical utility of F-18 FDG PET/CT in recurrent breast carcinoma. *Nuclear Medicine Communications.* June 2012;33(6):591–596.

33. Gennari A, Donati S, Salvadori B, et al. Role of 2-[18F]-fluorodeoxyglucose (FDG) positron emission tomography (PET) in the early assessment of response to chemotherapy in metastatic breast cancer patients. *Clinical Breast Cancer.* July 2000;1(2):156–161. discussion 162–153.

34. Humbert O, Cochet A, Coudert B, et al. Role of positron emission tomography for the monitoring of response to therapy in breast cancer. *The Oncologist.* February 2015;20(2):94–104.

35. Champion L, Lerebours F, Alberini JL, et al. 18F-FDG PET/CT to predict response to neoadjuvant chemotherapy and prognosis in inflammatory breast cancer. *Journal of Nuclear Medicine: Official Publication, Society of Nuclear Medicine.* September 2015;56(9):1315–1321.

36. Jo I, Zeon SK, Kim SH, et al. Correlation of primary tumor FDG uptake with clinicopathologic prognostic factors in invasive ductal carcinoma of the breast. *Nuclear Medicine and Molecular Imaging.* March 2015;49(1):19–25.

37. Osborne JR, Port E, Gonen M, et al. 18F-FDG PET of locally invasive breast cancer and association of estrogen receptor status with standardized uptake value: microarray and immunohistochemical analysis. *Journal of Nuclear Medicine: Official Publication, Society of Nuclear Medicine.* April 2010;51(4):543–550.

38. Koo HR, Park JS, Kang KW, Han W, Park IA, Moon WK. Correlation between (18)F-FDG uptake on PET/CT and prognostic factors in triple-negative breast cancer. *European Radiology.* November 2015;25(11):3314–3321.

39. Jung NY, Kim SH, Kang BJ, Park SY, Chung MH. https://www.ncbi.nlm.nih.gov/pubmed/26219608 The value of primary tumor (18)F-FDG uptake on preoperative PET/CT for predicting intratumoral lymphatic invasion and axillary nodal metastasis. *Breast Cancer.* September 2016;23(5):712–717.

40. Evangelista L, Cervino AR, Ghiotto C, et al. Could semiquantitative FDG analysis add information to the prognosis in patients with stage II/III breast cancer undergoing neoadjuvant treatment? *European Journal of Nuclear Medicine and Molecular Imaging.* October 2015;42(11):1648–1655.

41. Kong E, Chun KA, Bae YK, Cho IH. Integrated PET/MR mammography for quantitative analysis and correlation to prognostic factors of invasive ductal carcinoma. *The Quarterly Journal of Nuclear Medicine and Molecular Imaging: Official Publication of the Italian Association of Nuclear Medicine.* January 19, 2016.

42. Catalano OA, Nicolai E, Rosen BR, et al. Comparison of CE-FDG-PET/CT with CE-FDG-PET/MR in the evaluation of osseous metastases in breast cancer patients. *British Journal of Cancer.* April 28, 2015;112(9):1452–1460.

43. Koolen BB, Vogel WV, Vrancken Peeters MJ, Loo CE, Rutgers EJ, Valdes Olmos RA. Molecular imaging in breast cancer: from whole-body PET/CT to dedicated breast PET. *Journal of Oncology.* 2012;2012:438647.

44. Teixeira SC, Rebolleda JF, Koolen BB, et al. Evaluation of a hanging-breast PET system for primary tumor visualization in patients with Stage I-III breast cancer: comparison with standard PET/CT. *American Journal of Roentgenology.* June 2016;206(6):1307–1314.

45. Hicks RJ, Binns D, Stabin MG. Pattern of uptake and excretion of (18)F-FDG in the lactating breast. *Journal of Nuclear Medicine: Official Publication, Society of Nuclear Medicine.* August 2001;42(8):1238–1242.

46. Dorbala S, Di Carli MF, Delbeke D, et al. SNMMI/ASNC/SCCT guideline for cardiac SPECT/CT and PET/CT 1.0. *Journal of Nuclear Medicine: Official Publication, Society of Nuclear Medicine.* August 2013;54(8):1485–1507.

47. Mattsson S, Johansson L, Leide Svegborn S, et al. Radiation dose to patients from radiopharmaceuticals: a compendium of current information related to frequently used substances. *Annals of the ICRP.* July 2015;44(2 suppl):7–321.

48. Leide-Svegborn S, Ahlgren L, Johansson L, Mattsson S. Excretion of radionuclides in human breast milk after nuclear medicine examinations. Biokinetic and dosimetric data and recommendations on breastfeeding interruption. *European Journal of Nuclear Medicine and Molecular Imaging.* May 2016;43(5):808–821.

49. Leide-Svegborn S. Radiation exposure of patients and personnel from a PET/CT procedure with 18F-FDG. *Radiation Protection Dosimetry.* April–May 2010;139(1–3):208–213.

50. Devine CE, Mawlawi O. Radiation safety with positron emission tomography and computed tomography. *Seminars in Ultrasound, CT, and MR.* February 2010;31(1):39–45.

51. Hendler D, Stemmer SM. Uncommon reason for high fluorodeoxyglucose positron emission tomography uptake. *Journal of Clinical Oncology: Official Journal of the American Society of Clinical Oncology.* November 10, 2010;28(32):e659–660.

52. Gebhart G, Lamberts LE, Wimana Z, et al. Molecular imaging as a tool to investigate heterogeneity of advanced HER2-positive breast cancer and to predict patient outcome under trastuzumab emtansine (T-DM1): the ZEPHIR trial. *Annals of Oncology: Official Journal of the European Society for Medical Oncology/ESMO.* April 2016;27(4):619–624.

53. Even-Sapir E, Metser U, Mishani E, Lievshitz G, Lerman H, Leibovitch I. The detection of bone metastases in patients with high-risk prostate cancer: 99mTc-MDP Planar bone scintigraphy, single- and multi-field-of-view SPECT, 18F-fluoride PET, and 18F-fluoride PET/CT. *Journal of Nuclear Medicine: Official Publication, Society of Nuclear Medicine.* February 2006;47(2):287–297.

54. Langsteger W, Heinisch M, Fogelman I. The role of fluoro-deoxyglucose, 18F-dihydroxyphenylalanine, 18F-choline, and 18F-fluoride in bone imaging with emphasis on prostate and breast. *Seminars in Nuclear Medicine.* January 2006;36(1):73–92.

CHAPTER 4

Gastroesophageal Cancer

ALIREZA REZAEE • ANDREAS BUCK • MARKUS RADERER •
WERNER LANGSTEGER • MOHSEN BEHESHTI

GASTRIC CANCER
Background
General[1,2]
- Gastric cancer is the fifth most common cancer worldwide.
- Gastric cancer incidence is higher among men.
- It is more common in developing countries, especially in Asian compared with European populations.

Early clinical symptoms[2,3]
- Epigastric pain, nausea, anorexia.

Primary diagnostic procedures[4,5]
- Upper gastrointestinal (GI) endoscopy (including endosonography for local and regional lymph node assessment) and biopsy is the diagnostic procedure of choice.
- A double-contrast barium study provides a comparable sensitivity to endoscopy, approximately 90%–95% for gastric cancer detection.

Standard treatment[6]
- The standard treatment is surgery with or without chemoradiation and/or targeted therapy:
  - Stage 0: Surgery
  - Stage I: Surgery ± chemoradiation therapy
  - Stage II: Neoadjuvant chemotherapy + surgery ± chemotherapy (or chemoradiation in selective patients with suboptimal lymph node dissection)
  - Stage III: Neoadjuvant chemotherapy + surgery + chemotherapy (or chemoradiation) therapy
  - Stage IV: Palliative chemotherapy (radiation therapy only for preventing or treating complications of metastases) ± targeted therapy (in the small percentage of patients with Her2-neu-positive cancers) + palliative care

Five-Year Survival[7]
- Stage I   57%–71%
- Stage II   33%–46%
- Stage III   9%–20%
- Stage IV   4%

Prognostic factors[2]
- Tumor stage
- Tumor grade
- Size of the primary tumor
- Location of the primary tumor (poor prognosis if the tumor is in the proximal third of the stomach)
- Lymphatic and vascular invasion

Tumor Characteristics and Typical Behavior
Histopathology[2]
- Adenocarcinoma   95%
- Others (lymphoma,   5%
  leiomyosarcoma,
  neuroendocrine
  neoplasms, squamous cell
  cancers, stromal tumors)

Distribution and localization
T-primary[8]
- Pyloric area   50%
- Lesser curvature   25%
- Cardia   10%
- Fundus and body   10%
- Greater curvature   3%–5%

N-lymph nodes[9]
- Locoregional
- Retropancreatic
- Portal
- Paraaortic
- Mesenteric
- Retroperitoneal

M-distant metastasis[2]
- Locally advanced cancer or distant metastases at presentation in 80%–90%
- Most common sites:
  - Liver   38%–100%
  - Lung   40%–60%
  - Bone   20%–35%
  - Peritoneum   10%

TNM Classification[10]

The TNM classification and staging guidelines for gastric cancer are given in Tables 4.1 and 4.2.

Guidelines[10,11]

European Society for Medical Oncology (ESMO) and National Comprehensive Cancer Network (NCCN) guidelines for gastric cancer are given in Table 4.3.

Evidence-Based Viewpoints

- Fludeoxyglucose (FDG) PET/CT can evaluate gastric cancer more accurately and is helpful for the

evaluation of tumor biologic characteristics, detection of lymph node and distant metastases, and assessment of tumor response to therapy and prediction of prognosis.[12]
- FDG PET/CT scan is recommended for the preoperative assessment of gastric cancer if there is no evidence of M1 on conventional imaging.[10]
- FDG PET/CT is highly valuable in the evaluation of gastric cancer recurrence after surgical resection.[13]
- The major advantage of FDG PET/CT is in the detection of distant metastases to the liver, lungs, and skeleton.[14]
- FDG PET/CT is recommended for staging or restaging of esophagogastric carcinoma, including in patients who have received neoadjuvant treatment, and for the evaluation of suspected recurrence of esophagogastric tumors when other imaging is negative or equivocal.[15]

Cost-Effectiveness

There are few investigations on the cost-effectiveness of using FDG PET/CT for gastric cancer. An economic modeling revealed that adding FDG PET/CT to the standard evaluation of locally advanced gastric cancer can determine occult metastatic disease in 10% of patients

TABLE 4.1
Gastric Cancer TNM Classification

TNM	T1	T2	T3	T4a	T4b
N0	IA	IB	IIA	IIB	IIIB
N1	IB	IIA	IIB	IIIA	IIIB
N2	IIA	IIB	IIIA	IIIB	IIIC
N3	IIB	IIIA	IIIB	IIIC	IIIC
M1	IV	IV	IV	IV	IV

TABLE 4.2
Gastric Cancer TNM Staging Guidelines

Primary Tumor (T)	Lymph Nodes (N)	Distant Metastasis (M)
T0: No evidence of primary tumor	N0: No regional lymph node metastasis	M0: No distant metastasis
T1: Tumor invades lamina propria, muscularis mucosae, or submucosa	N1: Metastasis in 1 to 2 regional lymph nodes	M1: Distant metastasis
T2: Tumor invades muscularis propria	N2: Metastasis in 3 to 6 regional lymph nodes	
T3: Tumor penetrates subserosal connective tissue without invasion of visceral peritoneum or adjacent structures	N3: Metastasis in 7 or more regional lymph nodes	
T4: Tumor invades serosa (visceral peritoneum) or adjacent structures		

TABLE 4.3
Gastric Cancer ESMO and NCCN Guidelines

Clinical Guidelines	T	N	M
ESMO	Not recommended	Recommended[a]	Recommended[a]
NCCN	Recommended[b]	Not recommended	Not recommended

ESMO, European Society for Medical Oncology; *NCCN*, National Comprehensive Cancer Network.
[a]May not be informative in mucinous-type adenocarcinoma.
[b]If no evidence of M1 disease.

and result in less futile surgeries, which ultimately will save $13,000 per patient.[16] However, more investigations are needed to clarify the cost-effectiveness of using FDG PET/CT for imaging this type of cancer.

Clinical Point of View

Initial staging is of crucial importance for the management of patients with gastric cancer, because the prognosis and the rate of surgical curability are determined by the presence or absence of lymph node metastases. In recent years, systemic approaches, including chemotherapy (and to a certain extent also radiotherapy in patients with suboptimal lymph node resection other than D2), have been tested to improve outcome in potentially resectable gastric cancer.

However, at least in Western studies, dose density and tolerance were better in patients who underwent preoperative chemotherapy, whereas in the postoperative setting, 40%–50% of patients were not able to complete the scheduled therapy.

With this in mind, three groups have to be distinguished for the determination of management:
1. Patients with localized gastric cancer without lymph node or distant metastases, who are candidates for immediate potentially curative surgery
2. Patients with local lymph node metastases only, who are candidates for (neo)adjuvant chemotherapy
3. Patients with distant metastases, who would not undergo surgical intervention and would only receive palliative chemotherapy

In addition, noninvasive measurement of response to neoadjuvant therapy becomes increasingly important to potentially switch ineffective (toxic) therapy or not delay surgery if it is indicated. In addition, early recognition of nonresponders to palliative chemotherapy would also be helpful in these relatively frail patients who are prone to potential side effects of therapy.

Pitfalls[17,18]

False positive
- Postsurgical inflammatory changes
- Physiologic gastric uptake
- Inflammatory/infectious disease: granulomatous disease, diverticulitis, gastritis, benign tumors, reactive lymph nodes
- Acute fractures for bone metastases

False negative
- Signet ring cell carcinoma (SRC)
- Mucinous adenocarcinoma

- Poorly differentiated cancers with diffuse infiltrative pattern
- Common in all cancers: early-stage malignancy, hyperglycemic state, small lesions (<8 mm)

Discussion

Gastric cancer is a common malignancy across the world, particularly in Far East Asian countries. Given the poor outcome, early detection and precise assessment of patients are of importance for patients' management and prognosis. However, various studies have shown a huge difference between Asian and Western patient populations in terms of biology, outcome, and response or tolerance to therapies, suggesting that findings from these different geographic regions have to be interpreted with caution and should not be uncritically extrapolated.

Early diagnosis is achieved by the widespread use of upper GI tract endoscopy. However, for further treatment, the patients need to be staged for primary tumor, lymph node involvement, and distant metastases. Conventional imaging methods such as CT and endoscopic ultrasound have been used so far; however, they cannot be used independently for this purpose because of technical limitations. On the other hand, FDG PET/CT was increasingly utilized successfully during the last decade for the evaluation of different malignancies by merging tumor anatomic and biologic data. Nonetheless, in contrast to most other malignancies, the sensitivity of this modality for the detection of primary gastric cancer is limited because of physiologic radiotracer uptake in the stomach and low FDG uptake, particularly in signet ring cell carcinoma and mucinous adenocarcinoma subtypes. However, the use of gastric distension FDG PET/CT is recommended, which is able to increase the sensitivity from 80% to 90%. The technique causes a significant decrease in gastric wall physiologic FDG avidity but has minimal effect on tumor pathologic FDG uptake, leading to an increased tumor to normal gastric background ratio and a better detection rate.[19–21]

Staging

Although some types of gastric cancer are not highly FDG avid and FDG PET/CT is not recommended by some authors[22] and major guidelines such as ESMO,[11] there is a widely accepted consensus of the usefulness of FDG PET/CT in staging of gastric cancer.[23–27]

Some authors even considered a promising role for FDG PET/CT in staging of primary gastric cancer. In a retrospective study comparing the roles of contrast-enhanced CT (CE-CT) and FDG PET/CT in detecting primary gastric cancer, respective sensitivity, specificity, negative predictive value (NPV), positive predictive value (PPV), and accuracy values of 92%, 57%, 57%, 92%, and 87% and 82%, 86%, 46%, 97%, and 82% were calculated. FDG PET/CT was also significantly more specific for detecting both lymph nodes (95% vs. 62%) and distant metastases (89% vs. 63%).[28]

However, the detection of low-FDG-avid primary tumors and corresponding lymph node metastatic disease is a flaw of this technique. For instance, only 30%–40% of metastatic lymph nodes from non-FDG-avid primary tumors accumulate FDG, which is another factor for false-negative images.[29] Therefore, the use of FDG PET/CT in some special types of gastric cancer (i.e., signet cell carcinoma and mucinous carcinoma) should be designated only for special cases with unclear findings on other imaging modalities.

In the assessment of solid organ metastases, FDG PET/CT showed an accuracy, sensitivity, and specificity of 97%, 95%, and 100%, respectively.[30] However, MRI and CE-CT may provide better sensitivity in the detection of small hepatic metastases and tiny peritoneal carcinomatosis, respectively.

FDG PET/CT is also a promising surveillance method after surgery for detecting gastric cancer recurrence with an approximate sensitivity of 85% and specificity of 88%.[13,31] In a meta-analysis of eight studies and 500 patients, the pooled sensitivity and specificity were 86% and 88% for this modality in the detection of recurrent gastric cancer.[32]

In a study of 113 patients with locally advanced gastric cancer, FDG PET/CT discovered occult distant metastases in 10% of patients, preventing unnecessary interventions.[16]

In contrast to intestinal-type or tubular adenocarcinoma, mucinous and signet ring cell carcinomas are not highly FDG avid. Some investigators revealed that the tumors arising from the proximal part of the stomach are much more frequently detected by FDG PET/CT than the tumors in the distal region, most likely because of a high incidence of intestinal-type malignancy in this territory.[33]

In addition, the role of FDG PET/CT in staging of primary gastric lymphoma is well discussed and approved in the medical literature. Lymphoma accounts for less than 5% of gastric malignancies, and the stomach is the most common organ for both extranodal and GI tract lymphoma.[34] The technique is also able to upstage 16% and downstage 14% of patients.[35]

Another tumor that arises in the stomach in two-thirds of cases is gastrointestinal stromal tumors (GISTs), which are less malignant than the same tumor in the rest of the GI tract. However, GISTs should be discussed and managed in a manner completely different from the above-mentioned approaches for gastroesophageal adenocarcinoma. Nevertheless, it is important to mention that FDG PET/CT is considered as the gold standard imaging modality for the assessment of this malignancy.[36] A systematic review and meta-analysis results revealed that the modality has a high value in predicting early response to tyrosine kinase inhibitors such as imatinib (Gleevec), with a pooled sensitivity of 90% and specificity of 62%.[37–40]

Therapy monitoring and prognostic value

FDG PET/CT is a useful modality to differentiate responders from nonresponders to neoadjuvant therapies to prevent side effects of unnecessary treatments and to optimize treatment approach by changing therapy to a second-line regimen. In a retrospective study of 130 patients, the patients' management altered in 15% of the cases based on FDG PET/CT findings.[17]

Also, FDG PET/CT provides prognostic information in gastric cancers. In a prospective study comprising 44 patients with locally advanced gastric cancer, the authors calculated a 2-year survival of 90% versus 25% for metabolic responders and nonresponders, respectively, 2 weeks after commencement of cisplatin-based chemotherapy ($P = .002$).[41] The early diminished FDG uptake of primary gastric cancer is a prognostic factor representing favorable response to therapy,[42] and better prognosis is presumed for patients with gastric cancer who experience a complete metabolic response to chemotherapy.[21]

Moreover, there is a significant correlation between a high standardized uptake value (SUV) of the primary gastric malignancy on FDG PET/CT and poor overall survival.[30] In a retrospective study of 151 patients with metastatic lymph nodes from gastric cancer, Song et al. shared the point that the preoperative SUV_{max} of the involved lymph nodes on FDG PET/CT is an independent prognostic factor for both overall and recurrence-free survival.[43] In addition, a high SUV of the primary gastric tumor was correlated with malignant nodal involvement and noncurative surgery.[44]

Radiotracers beyond FDG

[18]F-fluorothymidine (FLT) uptake, which represents cancer cell proliferation, has been used to investigate gastric cancer. ^{18}F-FLT showed better sensitivity than FDG PET/CT in the evaluation of primary gastric

malignancies, particularly those cancers with a low FDG uptake.[45] In a study with 104 patients with gastric cancer evaluated by ^{18}F-FLT PET/CT, a higher tumor to background ratio is reported in malignancy compared with normal gastric mucosa.[46]

Moreover, ^{18}F-FLT PET/CT was superior to CE-CT in the evaluation of the primary tumor and regional lymph node metastases and demonstrated promising results in the assessment of response to neoadjuvant therapy.[45,47] Also, it was able to change patients' management and prevent futile surgeries.[47]

The human epidermal growth factor receptor 2 (HER2) status predicts the response of gastric cancer to treatment with anti-HER2 antibodies. In a retrospective study of 64 patients who underwent FDG PET/CT, the authors recognized a markedly higher SUV_{max} in the HER2-negative group than in the HER2-positive group. They predicted HER2 expression with an accuracy of approximately 64%, with an SUV_{max} cutoff of 6.2, which helped in treatment planning in these patients.[48]

PET imaging using ^{89}Zr-trastuzumab has been examined to delineate HER2-positive gastric cancer and monitor the pharmacodynamic effects of treatment with tyrosine kinase inhibitors.[49]

ESOPHAGEAL CANCER
Background
General[50]
- Esophageal cancer is the eighth most common cancer worldwide.
- Esophageal cancer is the seventh leading cause of cancer-related death worldwide.
- There is a threefold higher prevalence in men compared with women, commonly over the age of 60 years.
- Metastatic disease is the first presentation in more than one-third of patients with squamous cell carcinoma (SCC).

Early clinical symptoms[51]
- Dysphagia, odynophagia, weight loss

Primary diagnostic procedure[51,52]
- Barium esophagram, esophagoscopy with ultrasound (for local and regional lymph node assessment), and biopsy

Standard treatment[53,54]
- Stage 0: Surgery
- Stage I: Chemoradiation therapy + surgery
- Stage II: Chemoradiation therapy + surgery, chemoradiation or surgery alone

- Stage III: Chemoradiation therapy + surgery or chemoradiation
- Stage IV: Palliative therapy with esophageal stent, radiation therapy laser surgery, chemotherapy, or clinical trials

Prognostic factors[55]
- Size of the tumor
- Tumor grade and stage
- Lymph node involvement
- Esophageal cancer positive family history
- Response to neoadjuvant therapy

Five-year survival[56,57]
- Stage 0   >90%
- Stage I   >70%
- Stage IIA   15%–30%
- Stage IIB   10%–30%
- Stage III   10%–25%
- Stage IV   <4%

Tumor Characteristics and Typical Behavior
Histopathology (United States)[58]
- Adenocarcinoma   >70%
- Squamous cell carcinoma <30%

Histopathology (worldwide)[58]
- Adenocarcinoma   20%–30%
- Squamous cell carcinoma 60%–70%

Distribution and localization
T-primary[59]
- Cervical   10%
- Middle and upper thoracic 40%
- Lower thoracic   50%

N-lymph nodes[60]
- Cervical
  - Supraclavicular and infraclavicular   6%
  - Peritracheal and periesophageal   69%
  - Abdominal   9%
- Upper thoracic
  - Superior mediastinal   29%
  - Middle mediastinal   27%
  - Lower mediastinal   29%
  - Abdominal   32%
- Middle thoracic
  - Superior mediastinal   11%
  - Middle mediastinal   21%
  - Lower mediastinal   18%
  - Abdominal   40%
- Lower thoracic
  - Superior mediastinal   10%

- Middle mediastinal   14%
- Lower mediastinal   27%
- Abdominal   70%

M-distant metastasis[60]
- Liver
- Lung
- Adrenal

TNM Classification[61]

The TNM classification and staging guidelines for esophageal cancer are given in Tables 4.4 and 4.5.

Guidelines[61,62]

ESMO and NCCN guidelines for esophageal cancer are given in Table 4.6.

Evidence-Based Viewpoints

- FDG PET/CT should routinely be used as an additional tool for staging esophageal cancer and is beneficial mostly because it prevents futile surgeries.[1]
- FDG PET/CT is recommended for staging and restaging of esophageal cancer and for evaluation after neoadjuvant therapy.[15,63]

- FDG PET/CT is recommended for providing more accurate M-staging of patients with esophageal cancer before curative therapy.[64,65]
- FDG PET/CT is a strong predictor of therapy response and an independent predictor of overall survival in patients with nonmetastatic esophageal cancer.[61,66]

Cost-Effectiveness

In a study of 156 patients, FDG PET/CT scan could detect distant metastases in about 11% of patients, which prevented futile surgeries and reduced healthcare expenses of each patient by more than $2000.[64] However, there is moderate evidence that the use of FDG PET/CT will likely improve important healthcare outcomes.[1]

Clinical Points of View

In the treatment of gastric cancer, one of the main sources of information at diagnosis is correct staging to differentiate the (rare) percentage of patients with curative potential (i.e., resectable cancer) from patients with more advanced disease, who should best be spared surgical intervention (stage IV disease) or undergo radio/chemotherapy in case of lymph node involvement before reassessing surgical possibilities.

Although most of the primary tumors are readily amenable to histologic reassessment after neoadjuvant therapy, involved lymph nodes still present a challenge in terms of response assessment.

In the palliative setting, evaluating response and potentially recognizing nonresponders early in the course of therapy would be of high interest, because the regimens used for the treatment of esophageal cancers are characterized by a relatively high toxicity. This is probably also because patients with esophageal cancer have a relatively high rate of relevant comorbidities (caused by the risk factors of smoking and alcohol intake) and thus are probably more susceptible to side effects than patients with other types of cancer.

TABLE 4.4
Esophageal Cancer TNM Classification

TNM	T1	T2	T3	T4a	T4b
N0	IA,IB	IB,IIA,IIB	IB,IIA,IIB	IIIA	IIIC
N1	IIB	IIB	IIIA	IIIC	IIIC
N2	IIIA	IIIA	IIIB	IIIC	IIIC
N3	IIIC	IIIC	IIIC	IIIC	IIIC
M1	IV	IV	IV	IV	IV

Classification of T1-3N0 based on the tumor grade and location.

TABLE 4.5
Esophageal Cancer TNM Staging Guidelines

Primary Tumor (T)	Lymph Nodes (N)	Distant Metastasis (M)
T1: Invasion of lamina propria, muscularis mucosae, or submucosa	N0: Absent	M0: Absent
T2: Invasion of muscularis propria	N1: 1 to 2 regional lymph nodes (LNs)	M1: Present
T3: Invasion of adventitia	N2: 3 to 6 regional LNs	
T4: Invasion of adjacent structures	N3: ≥7 regional LNs	
• T4a: Resectable (pleura, pericardium, or diaphragm)		
• T4b: Unresectable (aorta, vertebral body, or trachea)		

Pitfalls[67,68]

False positive

- Inflammatory lesions (Barrett esophagus, sarcoidosis, postradiation esophagitis and ulceration)
- Physiologic uptake of brown fat tissue
- Asymmetric uptake in the vocal cords
- Vessel atherosclerosis
- Heterogeneous FDG uptake by tumor, resembling lymph node involvement

False negative

- Small tumor size (<1 cm)
- Small intracapsular locoregional metastases
- Low-grade malignancy
- Diffuse, nonintestinal growth–type adenocarcinoma
- Mucin-producing adenocarcinoma
- Lymph nodes adjacent to the primary tumor (≤3 cm)

Discussion

Staging

According to major practice guidelines, and similar to many other malignancies, FDG PET/CT plays an important role in staging and restaging of esophageal cancer. SCC is strongly FDG avid; however, the rate of false-negative adenocarcinoma subtype is higher for several reasons, such as slow-growing type, mucin-producing tumors, and well-differentiated malignancy.

FDG PET/CT is more accurate than conventional imaging modalities in staging esophageal cancer. It has been shown to improve lymph node staging and detection of stage IV esophageal cancer.[65,69–71]

Another potent alternative that is still widely used for staging of esophageal cancer and assessment of regional lymph nodes is endoscopic ultrasonography, particularly if combined with fine-needle aspiration. Its sensitivity for the evaluation of the primary tumor and nodal involvement is 85%–95% and 70%–80%, respectively.[72] Therefore, in candidates for surgical resection, endoscopic ultrasound and FDG PET/CT are recommended to evaluate the T- and N-staging of the tumor.[62]

Furthermore, FDG PET/CT is superior to stand-alone CT scan as a standard diagnostic procedure for the evaluation of primary esophageal cancer and nodal involvement. In a prospective study of 47 patients, the authors found a greater sensitivity and accuracy for FDG PET compared with CT in the evaluation of lymph node involvement. The calculated sensitivity, specificity, and accuracy were reported as 52%, 94%, and 84% for FDG PET, compared with 15%, 97%, and 77% for CT scan, respectively.[72]

However, some reported data do not support the use of FDG PET/CT in staging of early-stage esophageal cancer (e.g., cTisN0 and cT1N0). It may yield a low sensitivity for nodal assessment and high false-positive results for distant metastases.[73]

In addition, FDG PET/CT was successfully used in restaging and for the assessment of recurrent esophageal cancer.[74] In a meta-analysis and systematic review, the calculated pooled sensitivity and specificity were 96% and 78% for recurrent cancer, respectively.[75] One study with a large patient population showed high accuracy of FDG PET/CT with a sensitivity, specificity, PPV, NPV, and accuracy of 96%, 81%, 92%, 89%, and 91% in the detection of suspected recurrence in patients with esophageal carcinoma.[76] It was also more specific than and was superior to CE-CT in the detection of nodal recurrence.

TABLE 4.6
Esophageal Cancer ESMO and NCCN Guidelines

Clinical Guidelines	T	N	M
ESMO	Recommended • Staging to assess resectability • Evaluation of response to therapy before surgery	Preferred to CT scan	Recommended (if no evidence of M1 on CT)
NCCN	Recommended • Staging to assess resectability • Treatment response in neoadjuvant chemotherapy and/or radiation[a] and definitive chemoradiation • Planning for radiation therapy • Principles of surveillance	Preferred to CT scan	Recommended (if no evidence of M1 on CT)

ESMO, European Society for Medical Oncology; *NCCN*, National Comprehensive Cancer Network.
[a]FDG PET/CT should not be used for the selection of patients for surgery following preoperative chemoradiation.

Therapy monitoring and prognostic value

The potential role of FDG PET/CT has already been shown in the evaluation of response to therapy in esophageal cancer, particularly in patients who undergo neoadjuvant chemoradiation therapy.[66,70,71] It is also more sensitive ($P = .005$) than stand-alone CT in the determination of disease progression, leading to prevention of futile surgery.[69,77]

Moreover, semiquantitative evaluation may help to differentiate between responders and nonresponders, which is of critical importance for continuing the ongoing treatment.[78] In a study of 40 patients with esophageal adenocarcinoma, a significant drop of >35% in the SUV of the primary tumor was seen in responders 2 weeks after therapy.[79]

FDG PET/CT also has prognostic values in esophageal cancer imaging. The postchemoradiation SUV_{max} is the main predictor for survival in patients with esophageal cancer.[80] A higher SUV of the primary tumor is associated with poorer disease-specific survival rates.[81]

Although FDG PET/CT may be useful for radiation planning in selected patients, its role as a standard imaging modality for the delineation of gross tumor volume is not verified yet.[6]

Radiotracers beyond FDG

The value of ^{18}F-FLT PET/CT was compared with that of FDG PET/CT in the assessment of esophageal cancer. Despite the superiority of FDG PET/CT for TNM stratification,[82] the interim ^{18}F-FLT PET/CT is more competent in the prediction of 2-year progression-free survival of patients with esophageal SCC.[83]

The use of ^{18}F-3-fluoro-alpha-methyl tyrosine (^{18}F-FAMT) has been investigated in patients with esophageal cancer.[84] The authors demonstrated that the tumor avidity to this radiotracer correlates significantly with tumor progression factors. They also found a higher specificity and PPV for ^{18}F-FAMT compared with FDG PET/CT in the evaluation of metastatic lymph nodes.

Teaching Cases

Case 1: Staging esophageal cancer

Findings. A 67-year-old male with lower thoracic esophageal adenocarcinoma. FDG PET/CT shows a tracer-avid primary tumor in the distal esophagus (A,B; arrow). There are several small FDG-avid pulmonary nodules, consistent with metastases (C, arrow). Of incidental note are a cutaneous lesion and multiple FDG-avid small cervical lymph nodes (D, arrow), likely inflammatory in nature (Fig. 4.1).

Teaching points

- The lung is a common site of distant metastases.
- Distant metastases can be evident without apparent locoregional lymph node involvement.
- Patients are considered nonresectable if they present with distant metastases.

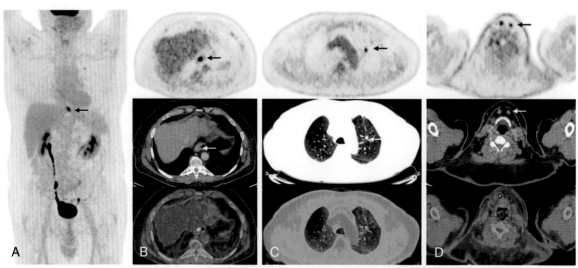

FIG. 4.1 FDG PET/CT showing a tracer-avid primary tumor in the distal esophagus (A,B; *arrow*). There are several small FDG-avid pulmonary nodules, consistent with metastases (C, *arrow*). Of incidental note are a cutaneous lesion and multiple FDG-avid small cervical lymph nodes (D, *arrow*), likely inflammatory in nature.

Pitfalls

- Submental lymphadenopathy is not a common pattern of esophageal cancer spread. However, FDG-positive level I cervical lymph nodes should be further clarified to rule out primary head and neck malignancy. A symmetric pattern is useful for the differentiation of inflammatory from malignant origin of the lymph nodes.

Case 2: Treatment monitoring

Findings. A 67-year-old male with esophageal adenocarcinoma (HER2/neu positive) and liver and lung metastases (A,C; arrows). Interim FDG PET/CT shows significant metabolic response to therapy (B,D; arrows) (Fig. 4.2).

Teaching points

- FDG PET/CT is superior to stand-alone CT in the evaluation of response to therapy.

- The posttreatment reduction of FDG uptake is the main predictor for survival in patients with esophageal cancer.
- The HER2/neu status predicts the response of esophageal cancer to treatment with anti-HER2 antibodies. It can be used as the target for a theranostic approach.
- FDG PET/CT can differentiate between necrotic tumor tissue and viable malignancy.
- The liver is the most common site for distant metastases of adenocarcinoma (the second most common for SCC) and the lung is the most common site for distant metastases from SCC (the second most common for adenocarcinoma).

Case 3: Recurrent gastric cancer

Findings. An 87-year-old male with gastric adenocarcinoma. FDG PET/CT shows tracer-avid local recurrence (C, arrow) and multiple liver metastases (A, arrow) (Fig. 4.3).

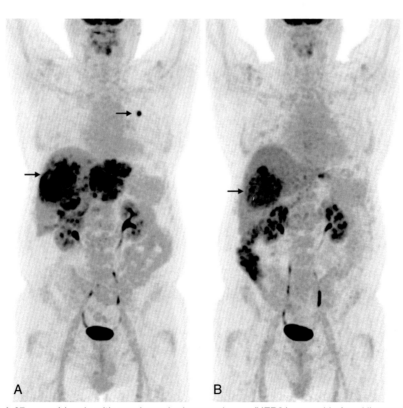

FIG. 4.2 A 67-year-old male with esophageal adenocarcinoma (HER2/neu positive) and liver and lung metastases (A,C; *arrows*). Interim FDG PET/CT shows a significant metabolic response to therapy (B,D; *arrows*).

Continued

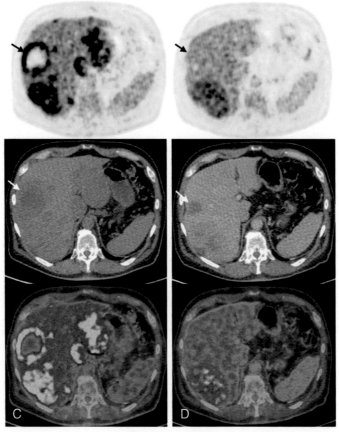

Fig. 4.2, cont'd

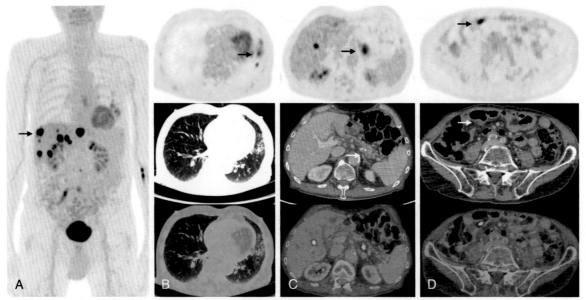

FIG. 4.3 FDG PET/CT showing tracer-avid local recurrence (C, *arrow*) and multiple liver metastases (A, *arrow*). B, C, and D, FDG PET/CT and fused axial images.

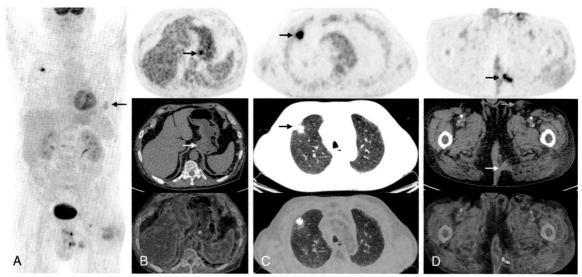

FIG. 4.4 FDG PET/CT showing a primary cancer with a low FDG uptake (B, *arrow*). There is a tracer-avid solitary right lung metastasis (C, *arrows*). A diffuse pattern of mildly FDG-avid left lung involvement is most likely inflammatory in nature. A focal FDG uptake in the right parotid gland is nonspecific. There is an FDG-avid rectal fistula formation (D, *black and white arrows*). The heterogeneous uptake in left gluteal muscles is nonspecific. There are mildly FDG-avid left and non-FDG-avid right inguinal lymph nodes (D, *blue arrows*), most likely reactive in nature. A, FDG PET MIP image.

- There are also FDG-avid small aortocaval lymph nodes and peritoneal carcinomatosis (D, arrow).
- Multiple mildly FDG-avid lesions of the left lung are inflammatory in nature (B, arrow).
- Of incidental note is a focal uptake in midesophagus, nonspecific and most likely inflammatory in nature.

Teaching points
- FDG PET/CT has additional value to stand-alone CT for the evaluation of recurrent disease.
- Gastric cancer has a higher incidence among men.

Pitfalls
- Inflammatory lung lesions should not be interpreted as metastatic disease.
- Midesophageal inflammatory uptake may cause a false-positive report.

Case 4: Staging signet ring cell cancer
Findings. A 64-year-old male with signet ring cell carcinoma of the gastroesophageal junction. FDG PET/CT shows a primary cancer with low FDG uptake

(B, arrow). There is a tracer-avid solitary right lung metastasis (C, arrows). A diffuse pattern of mildly FDG-avid left lung involvement is most likely inflammatory in nature. A focal FDG uptake in the right parotid gland is nonspecific. There is an FDG-avid rectal fistula formation (D, black and white arrows). The heterogeneous uptake in the left gluteal muscles is nonspecific. There are mildly FDG-avid left and non-FDG-avid right inguinal lymph nodes (D, blue arrows), most likely reactive in nature. An FDG uptake in the left fifth rib is most likely degenerative in nature (Fig. 4.4).

Teaching points
- Owing to different characteristics, metastatic lesions from a low-FDG-avid primary tumor may avidly take up FDG.
- FDG PET/CT is a useful modality for the evaluation of metastatic disease in very-low-FDG-avid primary cancers.

Pitfalls
- Nonmalignant FDG-avid lesions (left lung pneumonia, right parotid focal uptake, rectal fistula formation, left gluteal muscle uptake, reactive

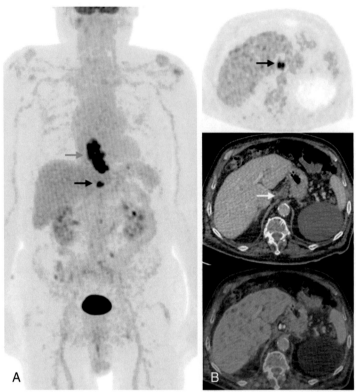

FIG. 4.5 FDG PET/CT showing a tracer-avid primary cancer (A, *blue arrow*) with an avid metastatic gastrohepatic lymph node (A,B; *black and white arrows*).

inguinal lymph nodes, and degenerative changes in the left rib) are the sources of a false-positive report.

Case 5: N-staging, esophageal cancer

Findings. A 64-year-old male with lower thoracic esophageal adenocarcinoma. FDG PET/CT shows a tracer-avid primary cancer (A, blue arrow) with avid metastatic gastrohepatic lymph node (A,B; black and white arrows) (Fig. 4.5).

Teaching points

- FDG PET/CT is valuable for nodal staging of esophageal cancer.
- It is able to define the field of radiotherapy in selected patients.
- The most common sites of nodal metastases in patients with lower thoracic esophageal cancer are abdominal lymph node stations (70%).
- About 75% of patients are diagnosed in the advanced stages with lymph node metastases.

Case 6: Staging, upper thoracic esophageal cancer

Findings. A 74-year-old male with upper thoracic esophageal SCC. FDG PET/CT shows a tracer-avid primary cancer (A, blue arrow) with a metabolically active upper mediastinal metastatic lymph node (A,B; black and white arrows). Of incidental note are faintly FDG-avid right rib fractures (Fig. 4.6).

Teaching points

- SCC is more FDG avid than adenocarcinoma.
- The upper thoracic esophageal cancers commonly metastasize to the superior (29%), middle (27%), and lower (29%) mediastinal as well as abdominal (32%) lymph nodes.
- The lung is the most common site of metastases from SCC.

Pitfalls

- There is physiologic uptake at the percutaneous endoscopic gastrostomy (PEG) tube insertion site.

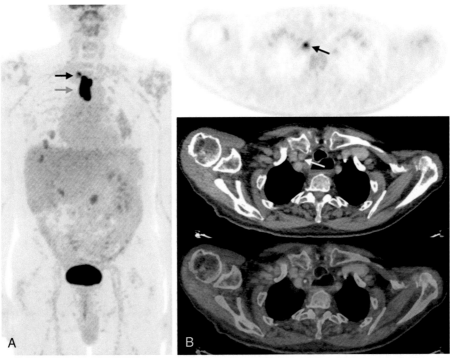

FIG. 4.6 FDG PET/CT showing a tracer-avid primary cancer (A, *blue arrow*) with a metabolically active upper mediastinal metastatic lymph node (A,B; *black and white arrows*).

Close attention should be paid to correct the location of the PEG tube at the time of image review.

Case 7: Staging gastric cancer

Findings. An 81-year-old male with signet ring cell cancer of the gastric antrum. FDG PET/CT shows a diffuse tracer uptake in the stomach, with accentuation in the antrum (C, arrow), which could be suggestive of primary tumor. There are multiple tracer-avid bone metastases with no corresponding morphologic lesions on CT of the vertebral bodies (B, black and white arrows). There is bilateral pneumonia with increased FDG uptake (A, black arrow). FDG-avid mediastinal lymph nodes are most likely inflammatory in nature. Of incidental note is a focal FDG uptake in the prostate gland (A, blue arrow), suspicious for malignancy (Fig. 4.7).

Teaching points
- Because of physiologic uptake in the gastric wall, the determination of malignant gastric tumors may be difficult in some cases.
- Special preparation of patients with the gastric distention technique significantly decreases the gastric

wall uptake and is able to increase the sensitivity from 80% to 90%.
- FDG PET/CT is superior to stand-alone CT in the detection of early osseous metastases.

Pitfalls
- Diffuse gastric uptake may obscure malignant lesions with low FDG uptake and cause a false-negative result.

Case 8: Treatment monitoring

Findings. A 69-year-old female with poorly differentiated SCC of the middle thoracic esophagus. FDG PET/CT shows a tracer-avid primary cancer (A, blue arrow) and several small FDG-avid locoregional, upper mediastinal, supraclavicular, and axillary lymph nodes with excellent response to chemoradiation therapy. A focal FDG uptake in the left thigh is confirmed to be a metastatic disease on pathology. Of incidental note is an FDG-avid soft tissue lesion within the ascending colon, which was a tubular adenoma on pathology (A,B; black arrows) (Fig. 4.8).

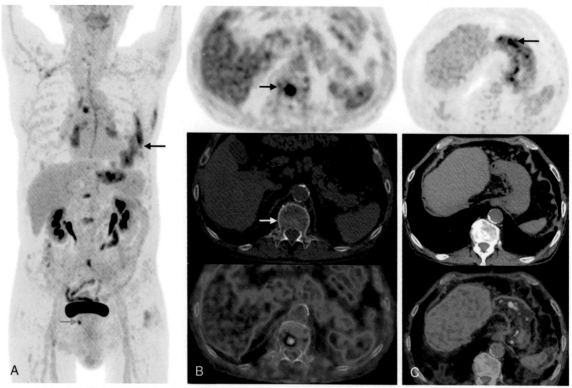

FIG. 4.7 FDG PET/CT showing a diffuse tracer uptake in the stomach, with accentuation in the antrum (C, *arrow*), which could be suggestive of primary tumor. There are multiple tracer-avid bone metastases with no corresponding morphologic lesions on CT of the vertebral bodies (B, *black and white arrows*). There is bilateral pneumonia with increased FDG uptake (A, *black arrow*). FDG-avid mediastinal lymph nodes are most likely inflammatory in nature. Of incidental note is a focal FDG uptake in the prostate gland (A, *blue arrow*), suspicious for malignancy.

Teaching points

- FDG PET/CT can upstage patients if avid supraclavicular lymph nodes are discovered.
- FDG PET/CT may play an important role in N-staging of patients with tracer-avid small lymph nodes.

Pitfalls

- Some benign lesions such as colon adenomas may be FDG avid and should not be interpreted as metastatic disease. Further evaluation of these lesions with colonoscopy is warranted.

Case 9: Staging—atypical distant metastasis
Findings. A 27-year-old female with upper thoracic esophageal cancer. FDG PET/CT shows a tracer-avid primary cancer (A,B; blue arrows) with metabolically active left adrenal metastasis (A,C; black arrows). There is an FDG-avid small right cervical lymph node (B, black arrow), which is overlapped by adjacent vessels in the transaxial view. Of

incidental note is a horseshoe kidney. Bilateral FDG-avid pneumonia is also noted (A, green arrow) (Fig. 4.9).

Teaching points

- FDG PET/CT is more accurate in staging of esophageal cancer for distant metastases and for the evaluation of equivocal findings than stand-alone CT.
- Patients with distant metastases are considered non-resectable. FDG PET/CT is a cost-effective modality because it prevents futile surgeries.
- The coronal view of CT could be more useful in the evaluation of small cervical lymph nodes neighboring the great vessels.

Pitfalls

- FDG-avid aspiration pneumonia is a common pitfall in upper thoracic esophageal cancer.
- Of incidental note is FDG uptake at the tip of the portal catheter, likely caused by a small radioactive clot.

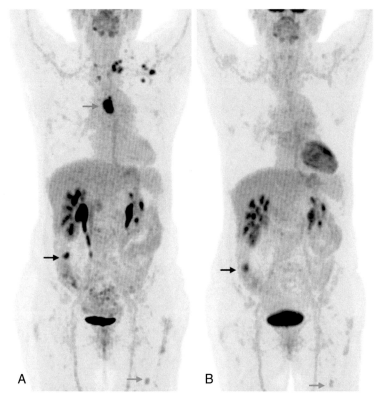

FIG. 4.8 FDG PET/CT showing a tracer-avid primary cancer (A, *blue arrow*) and several small FDG-avid locoregional, upper mediastinal, supraclavicular, and axillary lymph nodes with excellent response to chemoradiation therapy. A focal FDG uptake in the left thigh is confirmed to be a metastatic disease on pathology. Of incidental note is an FDG-avid soft tissue lesion within the ascending colon, which was a tubular adenoma on pathology (A,B; *black arrows*).

Case 10: Atypical lymph node metastases
Findings. A 70-year-old female with middle thoracic esophageal SCC. FDG PET/CT shows the tracer-avid primary tumor with numerous metabolically active cervical, thoracic, abdominal, and pelvic lymph node metastases (Fig. 4.10).

Teaching points
- The sensitivity of FDG PET/CT for the evaluation of primary esophageal cancer is >90%.
- Differential diagnosis consists of a second cancer, such as lymphoma, or general inflammatory or infectious process, such as granulomatous disease.

Case 11: Staging, FDG PET/CT versus CT
Findings. A 65-year-old male with lower thoracic esophageal SCC. FDG PET/CT shows a tracer-avid primary tumor (B, black and white arrows) with small metabolically active celiac lymph node metastasis (C, red arrow). There are also multiple small non-FDG-avid abdominal lymph nodes. Of incidental note are two FDG-avid polyps in the sigmoid colon, which were confirmed to be adenoma on pathology. The FDG-avid rectal lesion was confirmed to be adenocarcinoma on pathology (A, blue arrow) (Fig. 4.11).

Teaching points
- FDG PET/CT is superior to stand-alone CT in the detection of small metastatic lymph nodes, if tracer avid.
- However, if the lesions are too small (<8 mm), it may be negative on PET because of partial-volume effects.

Pitfalls
- Small non-FDG-avid lymph nodes can cause false-negative results on FDG PET/CT.
- Colorectal FDG-avid lesions could be benign, premalignant, or malignant, and further evaluation with colonoscopy and histopathology examination is warranted, particularly in high-risk patients.

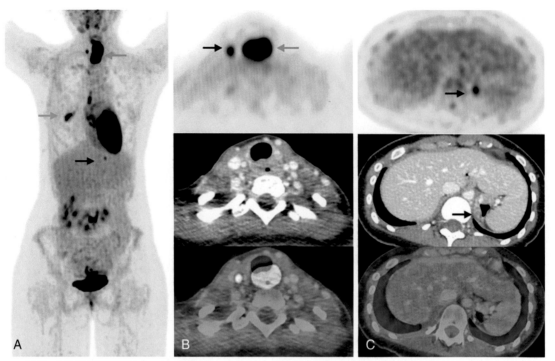

FIG. 4.9 FDG PET/CT showing a tracer-avid primary cancer (A,B; *blue arrows*) with metabolically active left adrenal metastasis (A,C; *black arrows*). There is an FDG-avid small right cervical lymph node (B, *black arrow*), which is overlapped by adjacent vessels in the transaxial view. Of incidental note is a horseshoe kidney. Bilateral FDG-avid pneumonia is also noted (A, *green arrow*).

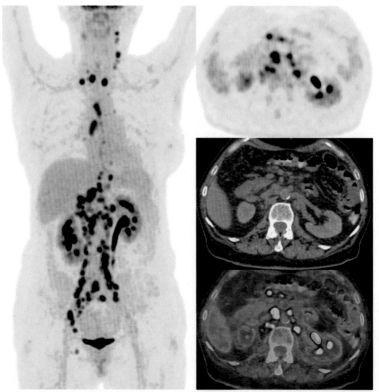

FIG. 4.10 FDG PET/CT showing a tracer-avid primary tumor with numerous metabolically active cervical, thoracic, abdominal, and pelvic lymph node metastases.

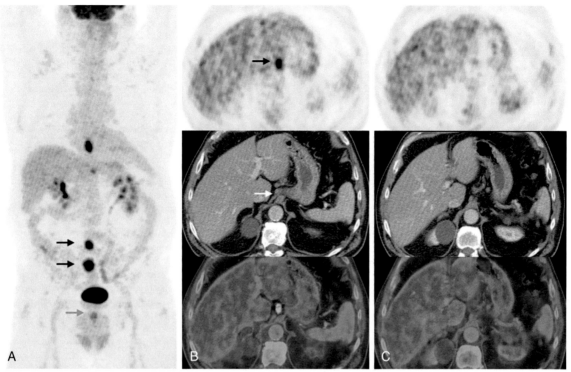

FIG. 4.11 FDG PET/CT showing a tracer-avid primary tumor (B, *black and white arrows*) with small metabolically active celiac lymph node metastasis (C, *red arrow*). There are also multiple small non-FDG-avid abdominal lymph nodes. Of incidental note are two FDG-avid polyps in the sigmoid colon, which were confirmed to be adenoma on pathology. The FDG-avid rectal lesion was confirmed to be adenocarcinoma on pathology (A, *blue arrow*).

REFERENCES

1. Fletcher JW, Djulbegovic B, Soares HP, et al. Recommendations on the use of 18F-FDG PET in oncology. *Journal of Nuclear Medicine: Official Publication, Society of Nuclear Medicine.* March 2008;49(3):480–508.
2. Dicken BJ, Bigam DL, Cass C, Mackey JR, Joy AA, Hamilton SM. Gastric adenocarcinoma: review and considerations for future directions. *Annals of Surgery.* January 2005;241(1):27–39.
3. Gastric cancer signs and symptoms. http://www.cancer.org/cancer/stomachcancer/detailedguide/stomach-cancer-signs-symptoms.
4. Gastic cancer diagnostic procedures. http://www.cancer.org/cancer/stomachcancer/detailedguide/stomach-cancer-diagnosis.
5. Low VH, Levine MS, Rubesin SE, Laufer I, Herlinger H. Diagnosis of gastric carcinoma: sensitivity of double-contrast barium studies. *American Journal of Roentgenology.* February 1994;162(2):329–334.
6. Muijs CT, Beukema JC, Pruim J, et al. A systematic review on the role of FDG-PET/CT in tumour delineation and radiotherapy planning in patients with esophageal cancer. *Radiotherapy and Oncology: Journal of the European Society for Therapeutic Radiology and Oncology.* November 2010;97(2):165–171.
7. Gastric cancer survival. http://www.cancer.org/cancer/stomachcancer/detailedguide/stomach-cancer-survival-rates.
8. Nandi A, Biswas P, Kar M, Sinha S. Clinicopathological profile of gastric cancer in a tertiary care hospital in Eastern India: a prospective 2 year study. *Clinical Cancer Investigation Journal.* 2014;3(1):14–20.
9. Di Leo A, Marrelli D, Roviello F, et al. Lymph node involvement in gastric cancer for different tumor sites and T stage: Italian Research Group for Gastric Cancer (IRGGC) experience. *Journal of Gastrointestinal Surgery: Official Journal of the Society for Surgery of the Alimentary Tract.* September 2007;11(9):1146–1153.
10. NCCN Clinical Practice Guidelines in Oncology. *Gastric Cancer.* 2016. Version 1. www.NCCN.org.
11. Waddell T, Verheij M, Allum W, et al. Gastric cancer: ESMO-ESSO-ESTRO Clinical Practice Guidelines for diagnosis, treatment and follow-up. *Annals of Oncology: Official Journal of the European Society for Medical Oncology.* October 2013;24(suppl 6):vi57–vi63.

12. Agrawal A, Rangarajan V. Appropriateness criteria of FDG PET/CT in oncology. *The Indian Journal of Radiology & Imaging.* April-June 2015;25(2):88–101.

13. Li P, Liu Q, Wang C, et al. Fluorine-18-fluorodeoxyglucose positron emission tomography to evaluate recurrent gastric cancer after surgical resection: a systematic review and meta-analysis. *Annals of Nuclear Medicine.* April 2016;30(3):179–187.

14. Kinkel K, Lu Y, Both M, Warren RS, Thoeni RF. Detection of hepatic metastases from cancers of the gastrointestinal tract by using noninvasive imaging methods (US, CT, MR imaging, PET): a meta-analysis. *Radiology.* September 2002;224(3):748–756.

15. The Royal College of Physicians and the Royal College of Radiologists. *Evidence-Based Indications for the Usage of PET-CT in the UK.* London: RCP, RCR; 2016.

16. Smyth E, Schoder H, Strong VE, et al. A prospective evaluation of the utility of 2-deoxy-2-[(18) F]fluoro-D-glucose positron emission tomography and computed tomography in staging locally advanced gastric cancer. *Cancer.* November 15, 2012;118(22):5481–5488.

17. Cayvarli H, Bekis R, Akman T, Altun D. The Role of 18F-FDG PET/CT in the evaluation of gastric cancer recurrence. *Molecular Imaging and Radionuclide Therapy.* October 5, 2014;23(3):76–83.

18. Long NM, Smith CS. Causes and imaging features of false positives and false negatives on F-PET/CT in oncologic imaging. *Insights into Imaging.* December 2011;2(6):679–698.

19. Kamimura K, Nagamachi S, Wakamatsu H, et al. Role of gastric distention with additional water in differentiating locally advanced gastric carcinomas from physiological uptake in the stomach on 18F-fluoro-2-deoxy-D-glucose PET. *Nuclear Medicine Communications.* June 2009;30(6):431–439.

20. Le Roux PY, Duong CP, Cabalag CS, Parameswaran BK, Callahan J, Hicks RJ. Incremental diagnostic utility of gastric distension FDG PET/CT. *European Journal of Nuclear Medicine and Molecular Imaging.* April 2016;43(4):644–653.

21. Yun M, Choi HS, Yoo E, Bong JK, Ryu YH, Lee JD. The role of gastric distention in differentiating recurrent tumor from physiologic uptake in the remnant stomach on 18F-FDG PET. *Journal of Nuclear Medicine: Official Publication, Society of Nuclear Medicine.* June 2005;46(6):953–957.

22. Hopkins S, Yang GY. FDG PET imaging in the staging and management of gastric cancer. *Journal of Gastrointestinal Oncology.* March 2011;2(1):39–44.

23. Kawanaka Y, Kitajima K, Fukushima K, et al. Added value of pretreatment (18)F-FDG PET/CT for staging of advanced gastric cancer: comparison with contrast-enhanced MDCT. *European Journal of Radiology.* May 2016;85(5):989–995.

24. Lim JS, Yun MJ, Kim MJ, et al. CT and PET in stomach cancer: preoperative staging and monitoring of response to therapy. *Radiographics: A Review Publication of the Radiological Society of North America, Inc.* January-February 2006;26(1):143–156.

25. Malibari N, Hickeson M, Lisbona R. PET/computed tomography in the diagnosis and staging of gastric cancers. *PET Clinics.* July 2015;10(3):311–326.

26. Okumura Y, Aikou S, Onoyama H, et al. Evaluation of 18F-FDG uptake for detecting lymph node metastasis of gastric cancer: a prospective pilot study for one-to-one comparison of radiation dose and pathological findings. *World Journal of Surgical Oncology.* 2015;13:327.

27. Serrano OK, Love C, Goldman I, et al. The value of FDG-PET in the staging of gastric adenocarcinoma: a single institution retrospective review. *Journal of Surgical Oncology.* May 2016;113(6):640–646.

28. Altini C, Niccoli Asabella A, Di Palo A, et al. 18F-FDG PET/CT role in staging of gastric carcinomas: comparison with conventional contrast enhancement computed tomography. *Medicine.* May 2015;94(20):e864.

29. Kim EY, Lee WJ, Choi D, et al. The value of PET/CT for preoperative staging of advanced gastric cancer: comparison with contrast-enhanced CT. *European Journal of Radiology.* August 2011;79(2):183–188.

30. Chung HW, Lee EJ, Cho YH, et al. High FDG uptake in PET/CT predicts worse prognosis in patients with metastatic gastric adenocarcinoma. *Journal of Cancer Research and Clinical Oncology.* December 2010;136(12):1929–1935.

31. Lee JW, Lee SM, Son MW, Lee MS. Diagnostic performance of FDG PET/CT for surveillance in asymptomatic gastric cancer patients after curative surgical resection. *European Journal of Nuclear Medicine and Molecular Imaging.* May 2016;43(5):881–888.

32. Zou H, Zhao Y. 18FDG PET-CT for detecting gastric cancer recurrence after surgical resection: a meta-analysis. *Surgical Oncology.* September 2013;22(3):162–166.

33. Stahl A, Ott K, Weber WA, et al. FDG PET imaging of locally advanced gastric carcinomas: correlation with endoscopic and histopathological findings. *European Journal of Nuclear Medicine and Molecular Imaging.* February 2003;30(2):288–295.

34. Koch P, del Valle F, Berdel WE, et al. Primary gastrointestinal non-Hodgkin's lymphoma: I. Anatomic and histologic distribution, clinical features, and survival data of 371 patients registered in the German Multicenter Study GIT NHL 01/92. *Journal of Clinical Oncology: Official Journal of the American Society of Clinical Oncology.* September 15, 2001;19(18):3861–3873.

35. Yi JH, Kim SJ, Choi JY, Ko YH, Kim BT, Kim WS. 18F-FDG uptake and its clinical relevance in primary gastric lymphoma. *Hematological Oncology.* June 2010;28(2):57–61.

36. Valls-Ferrusola E, Garcia-Garzon JR, Ponce-Lopez A, et al. Patterns of extension of gastrointestinal stromal tumors (GIST) treated with imatinib (Gleevec(R)) by 18F-FDG PET/CT. *Revista espanola de enfermedades digestivas: organo oficial de la Sociedad Espanola de Patologia Digestiva.* July 2012;104(7):360–366.

37. Banzo I, Quirce R, Martinez-Rodriguez I, et al. 18F-FDG PET/CT in response evaluation of gastrointestinal stromal tumours treated with imatinib. *Revista espanola de medicina nuclear.* May-June 2008;27(3):168–175.

38. Chacon M, Eleta M, Espindola AR, et al. Assessment of early response to imatinib 800 mg after 400 mg progression by (1)(8)F-fluorodeoxyglucose PET in patients with metastatic gastrointestinal stromal tumors. *Future Oncology.* 2015;11(6):953–964.

39. Hassanzadeh-Rad A, Yousefifard M, Katal S, et al. The value of (18) F-fluorodeoxyglucose positron emission tomography for prediction of treatment response in gastrointestinal stromal tumors: a systematic review and meta-analysis. *Journal of Gastroenterology and Hepatology.* May 2016;31(5):929–935.

40. Schima W, Kurtaran A. GIST: imaging diagnosis, staging, and response assessment. *Wiener medizinische Wochenschrift.* 2009;159(15–16):408–413.

41. Ott K, Fink U, Becker K, et al. Prediction of response to preoperative chemotherapy in gastric carcinoma by metabolic imaging: results of a prospective trial. *Journal of Clinical Oncology: Official Journal of the American Society of Clinical Oncology.* December 15, 2003;21(24):4604–4610.

42. Wang C, Guo W, Zhou M, et al. The predictive and prognostic value of early metabolic response assessed by positron emission tomography in advanced gastric cancer treated with chemotherapy. *Clinical Cancer Research: An Official Journal of the American Association for Cancer Research.* April 1, 2016;22(7):1603–1610.

43. Song BI, Kim HW, Won KS, Ryu SW, Sohn SS, Kang YN. Preoperative standardized uptake value of metastatic lymph nodes measured by 18F-FDG PET/CT improves the prediction of prognosis in gastric cancer. *Medicine.* July 2015;94(26):e1037.

44. Choi JY, Shim KN, Kim SE, Jung HK, Jung SA, Yoo K. The clinical value of 18F-fluorodeoxyglucose uptake on positron emission tomography/computed tomography for predicting regional lymph node metastasis and non-curative surgery in primary gastric carcinoma. *The Korean Journal of Gastroenterology, Taehan Sohwagi Hakhoe chi.* December 2014;64(6):340–347.

45. Herrmann K, Ott K, Buck AK, et al. Imaging gastric cancer with PET and the radiotracers 18F-FLT and 18F-FDG: a comparative analysis. *Journal of Nuclear Medicine: Official Publication, Society of Nuclear Medicine.* December 2007;48(12):1945–1950.

46. Malkowski B, Staniuk T, Srutek E, Gorycki T, Zegarski W, Studniarek M. (18)F-FLT PET/CT in patients with gastric carcinoma. *Gastroenterology Research and Practice.* 2013;2013:696423.

47. Staniuk T, Zegarski W, Malkowski B, Jankowski M, Klag M, Pietrzak T. Evaluation of FLT-PET/CT usefulness in diagnosis and qualification for surgical treatment of gastric cancer. *Contemporary Oncology.* 2013;17(2):165–170.

48. Chen R, Zhou X, Liu J, Huang G. Relationship between 18F-FDG PET-CT scans and HER2 expression in gastric cancer. *Journal of Nuclear Medicine: Official Publication, Society of Nuclear Medicine.* July 2016;57(7):1040–1044.

49. Janjigian YY, Viola-Villegas N, Holland JP, et al. Monitoring afatinib treatment in HER2-positive gastric cancer with 18F-FDG and 89Zr-trastuzumab PET. *Journal of*

Nuclear Medicine: Official Publication, Society of Nuclear Medicine. June 2013;54(6):936–943.

50. *Cancer Facts & Figures.* American Cancer Society; 2016. Available at: http://www.cancer.org/acs/groups/content/@editorial/documents/document/acspc-044552.pdf.

51. Feldman M, Friedman L, Brandt L. *Sleisenger & Fordtran's Gastrointestinal and Liver Disease.* 9th ed. Philadelphia: Saunders; 2010:745–767.

52. Ferri F. *Esophageal Tumors. Ferri's clinical advisor 2013.* Philadelphia: Mosby: Elsevier; 2012:389–391.

53. Cleveland Clinic Treatment for Esophageal Cancer. http://www.clevelandclinicmeded.com/medicalpubs/diseasemanagement/hematology-oncology/esophageal-cancer/.

54. Jeong Y, Kim JH, Kim SB, et al. Role of surgical resection in complete responders on FDG-PET after chemoradiotherapy for locally advanced esophageal squamous cell carcinoma. *Journal of Surgical Oncology.* April 2014;109(5):472–477.

55. Yuequan J, Shifeng C, Bing Z. Prognostic factors and family history for survival of esophageal squamous cell carcinoma patients after surgery. *The Annals of Thoracic Surgery.* September 2010;90(3):908–913.

56. Hwang J, Lyer R, Salo J. Cancer Management. *Esophageal Cancer.* 2015. http://www.cancernetwork.com/cancer-management/esophageal/page/0/3.

57. Survival rates for cancer of the esophagus by stage. http://www.cancer.org/cancer/esophaguscancer/detailedguide/esophagus-cancer-survival-rates.

58. Kirby TJ, Rice TW. The epidemiology of esophageal carcinoma. The changing face of a disease. *Chest Surgery Clinics of North America.* May 1994;4(2):217–225.

59. Alberts S, Goldberg R. Gastrointestinal tract cancers. In: Casciato D, ed. *Manual of Clinical Oncology.* 5th ed. Philadelphia, USA: LWW; 2004:185–232.

60. Thoracic esophagus. In: Robin P, Hansen JT, eds. *TNM Staging Atlas with Oncoanatomy.* 2nd ed. Philadelphia, USA: Wolters Kluwer/LWW; 2012:226–235.

61. NCCN clinical practice guidelines in oncology. *Esophageal and Esophagogastric Junction Cancer.* 2016. Version 1. www.NCCN.org.

62. Stahl M, Mariette C, Haustermans K, Cervantes A, Arnold D, Group EGW. Oesophageal cancer: ESMO clinical practice guidelines for diagnosis, treatment and follow-up. *Annals of Oncology: Official Journal of the European Society for Medical Oncology.* October 2013;24(suppl 6):vi51–vi56.

63. Westerterp M, van Westreenen HL, Reitsma JB, et al. Esophageal cancer: CT, endoscopic US, and FDG PET for assessment of response to neoadjuvant therapy–systematic review. *Radiology.* September 2005;236(3):841–851.

64. Anderegg MC, de Groof EJ, Gisbertz SS, et al. 18F-FDG PET-CT after neoadjuvant chemoradiotherapy in esophageal cancer patients to optimize surgical decision making. *PLoS One.* 2015;10(11):e0133690.

65. Wong R, Walker-Dilks C, Raifu A. Evidence-based guideline recommendations on the use of positron emission tomography imaging in oesophageal cancer. *Clinical Oncology.* March 2012;24(2):86–104.

66. Shridhar R, Imani-Shikhabadi R, Davis B, Streeter OA, Thomas Jr CR. Curative treatment of esophageal cancer; an evidenced based review. *Journal of Gastrointestinal Cancer*. December 2013;44(4):375–384.

67. Bruzzi JF, Munden RF, Truong MT, et al. PET/CT of esophageal cancer: its role in clinical management. *Radiographics: A Review Publication of the Radiological Society of North America, Inc.* November-December 2007;27(6):1635–1652.

68. Yang GY, Wagner TD, Jobe BA, Thomas CR. The role of positron emission tomography in esophageal cancer. *Gastrointestinal Cancer Research*. January 2008;2(1):3–9.

69. Lin J, Kligerman S, Goel R, Sajedi P, Suntharalingam M, Chuong MD. State-of-the-art molecular imaging in esophageal cancer management: implications for diagnosis, prognosis, and treatment. *Journal of Gastrointestinal Oncology*. February 2015;6(1):3–19.

70. Lordick F, Ott K, Krause BJ. New trends for staging and therapy for localized gastroesophageal cancer: the role of PET. *Annals of Oncology: Official Journal of the European Society for Medical Oncology*. October 2010;21(suppl 7):vii294–vii299.

71. Munden RF, Macapinlac HA, Erasmus JJ. Esophageal cancer: the role of integrated CT-PET in initial staging and response assessment after preoperative therapy. *Journal of Thoracic Imaging*. May 2006;21(2):137–145.

72. Kim K, Park SJ, Kim BT, Lee KS, Shim YM. Evaluation of lymph node metastases in squamous cell carcinoma of the esophagus with positron emission tomography. *The Annals of Thoracic Surgery*. January 2001;71(1):290–294.

73. Cuellar SL, Carter BW, Macapinlac HA, et al. Clinical staging of patients with early esophageal adenocarcinoma: does FDG-PET/CT have a role? *Journal of Thoracic Oncology: Official Publication of the International Association for the Study of Lung Cancer*. August 2014;9(8):1202–1206.

74. Guo H, Zhu H, Xi Y, et al. Diagnostic and prognostic value of 18F-FDG PET/CT for patients with suspected recurrence from squamous cell carcinoma of the esophagus. *Journal of Nuclear Medicine: Official Publication, Society of Nuclear Medicine*. August 2007;48(8):1251–1258.

75. Goense L, van Rossum PS, Reitsma JB, et al. Diagnostic Performance of (1)(8)F-FDG PET and PET/CT for the detection of recurrent esophageal cancer after treatment with curative intent: a systematic review and meta-analysis. *Journal of Nuclear Medicine: Official Publication, Society of Nuclear Medicine*. July 2015;56(7):995–1002.

76. Sharma P, Jain S, Karunanithi S, et al. Diagnostic accuracy of (1)(8)F-FDG PET/CT for detection of suspected recurrence in patients with oesophageal carcinoma. *European Journal of Nuclear Medicine and Molecular Imaging*. June 2014;41(6):1084–1092.

77. Findlay JM, Gillies RS, Franklin JM, et al. Restaging oesophageal cancer after neoadjuvant therapy with F-FDG PET-CT: identifying interval metastases and predicting incurable disease at surgery. *European Radiology*. October 2016;26(10):3519–3533.

78. Baksh K, Prithviraj G, Kim Y, et al. Correlation between standardized uptake value in preneoadjuvant and postneoadjuvant chemoradiotherapy and tumor regression grade in patients with locally advanced esophageal cancer. *American Journal of Clinical Oncology*. December 22, 2015.

79. Weber WA, Ott K, Becker K, et al. Prediction of response to preoperative chemotherapy in adenocarcinomas of the esophagogastric junction by metabolic imaging. *Journal of Clinical Oncology: Official Journal of the American Society of Clinical Oncology*. June 15, 2001;19(12):3058–3065.

80. Lomas H, Hoffe S, Weber J, Dilling T, Chuong M. Post chemoradiation PET SUV is highly predictive of overall survival in esophageal cancer. *Journal of Nuclear Medicine & Radiation Therapy*. 2012;3(125).

81. Omloo JM, Sloof GW, Boellaard R, et al. Importance of fluorodeoxyglucose-positron emission tomography (FDG-PET) and endoscopic ultrasonography parameters in predicting survival following surgery for esophageal cancer. *Endoscopy*. June 2008;40(6):464–471.

82. Ma C, Li D, Yin Y, Cao J. Comparison of characteristics of 18F-fluorodeoxyglucose and 18F-fluorothymidine PET during staging of esophageal squamous cell carcinoma. *Nuclear Medicine Communications*. December 2015;36(12):1181–1186.

83. Chen H, Li Y, Wu H, et al. 3'-deoxy-3'-[(1)(8)F]-fluorothymidine PET/CT in early determination of prognosis in patients with esophageal squamous cell cancer: comparison with [(1)(8)F]-FDG PET/CT. *Strahlentherapie und Onkologie : Organ der Deutschen Rontgengesellschaft*. February 2015; 191(2):141–152.

84. Sohda M, Sakai M, Honjyo H, et al. Use of pre-treatment 18F-FAMT PET to predict patient survival in squamous cell carcinoma of the esophagus treated by curative surgery. *Anticancer Research*. July 2014;34(7):3623–3628.

CHAPTER 5

Gastroenteropancreatic Neuroendocrine Neoplasms

MOHSEN BEHESHTI • ALIREZA REZAEE • MARKUS RADERER • WERNER LANGSTEGER

BACKGROUND
General

- Neuroendocrine neoplasms (NENs) could arise from anywhere in the body but they arise mainly (about 70%) from the gastroenteropancreatic (GEP) system.[1,2] Other locations include the lung as well as endocrine organs, such as adrenal medulla, pituitary, thyroid, and parathyroid.[3]
- They are equally distributed among males and females.[4]
- The majority of GEP-NENs arise from the small intestine, particularly the ileum, and secrete biogenic amines and peptides, predominantly serotonin peptides, which often create characteristic hormonal syndromes.[5-7] However, it may be different in diverse geographic locations worldwide.
- GEP-NENs express multiple somatostatin receptor (SSTR) subtypes, with SSTR-2 predominance.[8,9]
- Synchronous or metachronous cancers occur in approximately 29% of patients with small intestinal NENs.[3] The most common metachronous malignancies include those of the prostate (26%), breast (14%), colon (9%), lung (6%), and bladder (5%).[10]
- The major NENs of the pancreas (P-NENs) are insulinoma, gastrinoma, VIPoma (which secretes vasoactive intestinal peptide), somatostatinoma, glucagonoma, and nonfunctional tumors (e.g., pancreatic peptidoma).[11]
- About 64% of patients with P-NEN present with distant metastases at the time of diagnosis (most common with glucagonoma, VIPoma, and somatostatinoma; less common with gastrinoma and insulinoma).[2,5,12]
- About 22% of gastrointestinal (GI)-NENs present with distant metastasis, half of which have no known primaries.[13]
- NENs are usually small (<1 cm) and slow growing.[14]

- The Ki-67 proliferative index is a prognostic factor in NENs and a predictor of progression-free survival. Currently, it is used for grading of these tumors. The level is ≤2 for G1 or well-differentiated, 3–20 for G2 or moderately differentiated, and >20 for G3 or poorly differentiated neoplasms (cancers). Circulating tumor cells are another promising prognostic marker in these patients.[15-18]
- Main risk factors for GEP-NENs[13,19-21]:
  - Multiple endocrine neoplasia (MEN) syndrome (particularly MEN-1)
  - Race (more common in African-Americans)
  - Gender (more common in black males than in black females, but equal in white males and females)
  - Older age (average age of 55–65 years at diagnosis)
  - Family history of carcinoid tumor
  - Pernicious anemia (for gastric NENs)
  - Positive family history of any kind of cancer (for P-NENs)
  - Smoking
  - Prolonged history of diabetes mellitus (for P-NENs)

Clinical Symptoms

- The condition is asymptomatic or has vague, nonspecific symptoms in the early stages. In view of this, the median time from initial symptoms to diagnosis was 5–7 years in most series.[11]
- Functional P-NENs release hormones with the corresponding symptoms[11]:
  - Insulinoma: Fasting hypoglycemia
  - Gastrinoma: Diarrhea, Zollinger-Ellison syndrome
  - VIPoma: Watery diarrhea
  - Somatostatinoma: Steatorrhea, weight loss, glucose intolerance, gallbladder disease
  - Glucagonoma: Skin rash, diabetes, thrombophlebitis

- Nonfunctioning tumors secreting nonactive pancreatic peptides (PPomas): Epigastric pain, dyspepsia, jaundice, abdominal mass
- Thirty percent of GI-NENs secrete serotonin with resultant carcinoid syndrome; the condition clinically manifests with diarrhea, flushing, bronchoconstriction, and occasionally right-sided valvular heart disease. The symptoms, however, may be variable, and the full-fledged symptomatic triad is hardly ever encountered.[7]

Primary Diagnostic Procedures[11,22–24]

- Biochemical laboratory evaluation (particularly the chromogranin-A as the gold standard of chemical tests and serotonin, as well as urinary 5-hydroxyindoleacetic acid)
- Endoscopic ultrasonography (EUS)
- Anatomic conventional imaging modalities, such as triphasic computed tomography (CT), magnetic resonance imaging (MRI), magnetic resonance cholangiopancreatography, or endoscopic retrograde cholangiopancreatography
- Functional imaging by scintigraphy with a radio-labeled somatostatin analogue (e.g., octreotide), replaced by ^{68}Ga-DOTA-peptides or ^{18}F-dihydroxyphenylalanine (DOPA) positron emission tomography/computed tomography (PET/CT) if available
- Imaging (EUS)-guided biopsy

Standard Treatment[12,25–27]

- Surgery is the only curative treatment.
- Various palliative and symptomatic forms of therapy, including application of somatostatin analogues (SST-A), chemotherapy, radiation therapy, peptide receptor radionuclide therapy, ^{131}I-metaiodobenzylguanidine (MIBG) radiolabeled therapy, or targeted therapies, may apply, based on grading and site of origin of the tumor.

Prognostic Factors

- Grading is the most relevant prognostic factor in NEN irrespective of origin; G3 neuroendocrine carcinomas (NECs) are highly aggressive neoplasms, whereas neuroendocrine tumors (NETs) G1 and G2 run a more indolent course.
- GI-NETs[28]
  - Age (worse if ≥50 years)
  - Stage of the disease (worse in metastatic malignancy)
  - Gender (worse in males)
  - Tumor depth (worse if deeper)

- Tumor size (worse if larger)
- Tumor primary site (worse long-term survival with ileojejunal cancers)
- P-NETs[29–34]
  - Stage and grade of malignancy (doubled likelihood of death with distant metastatic disease or high-grade tumor)
  - Age (worse if >55 years)
  - Serum level of chromogranin-A and neuron-specific enolase (worse if not normalized during therapy)
  - Tumor type (worse if nonfunctional)

Five-Year Survival

GI-NETs[13,35]

• Overall:	70%–80%
• Localized:	93%
• Lymph node metastasis:	74%
• Distant organ metastasis:	20%–30%

P-NETs[a,36]

• Stage I:	61%
• Stage II:	52%
• Stage III:	41%
• Stage IV:	16%

[a]For patients treated with surgery.

TUMOR CHARACTERISTICS AND TYPICAL BEHAVIOR
Histopathology of P-NETs[11,37]

- Insulinoma: 50%
- Gastrinoma: 30%
- Nonfunctioning (PPomas): >15%
- VIPoma, glucagonoma, somatostatinoma: 5%–10%
- Tumors secreting growth hormone-releasing hormone (GHRH), adrenocorticotropic hormone, corticotropin-releasing factor, parathyroid hormone-related peptide: <5%

Distribution and Localization
T-primary NETs[4,38,39]

Distribution and Localization[a]

GEP-NENs:	61%
• Small intestine:	31%
• Rectum:	26%
• Colon:	18%
• Pancreas:	12%
• Stomach:	6%
• Appendix:	6%
• Others:	4%

Non-GEP-NENs:	39%
• Respiratory system:	69%
• Unclassified:	24%
• Female genitourinary:	5%
• Breast:	1%
• Urinary system:	1%
• Prostate:	<1%

[a]May be different in diverse geographic locations worldwide.

N-P-NETs lymph nodes[40]

- Regional lymph nodes
  - Splenic hilum
  - Suprapancreatic
  - Left gastropancreatic fold
  - Hepatic artery
  - Inferior pancreatic
  - Paraaortic
  - Anterior pancreatic-duodenal
  - Posterior pancreatic-duodenal
  - Celiac
- Distant lymph nodes
  - Mediastinal
  - Iliac

M-P-NETs distant metastasis[40]

• Liver:	45%–80%
• Lungs:	40%–60%
• Bone:	20%–35%

TNM CLASSIFICATION FOR P-NENS[41,42]

The classification is provided in Table 5.1.

Primary tumor (T)

T1: Tumor limited to the pancreas, <2 cm in the greatest diameter

T2: Tumor limited to the pancreas, >2 cm in the greatest diameter

T3: Tumor extends beyond the pancreas but does not involve the celiac axis or superior mesenteric artery

T4: Tumor involves the celiac axis or superior mesenteric artery (unresectable tumor)

Regional lymph nodes (N)

N0: No regional lymph node metastasis

N1: Regional lymph node metastasis

Distant metastasis (M)

M0: No distant metastasis

M1: Distant metastasis

TNM CLASSIFICATION FOR GI-NENS[42]

The classification is provided in Table 5.2.

Primary tumor (T)

T1: Tumor invades lamina propria or submucosa and size ≤2 cm

- **T1a:** Tumor size <1 cm in the greatest diameter
- **T1b:** Tumor size 1–2 cm in the greatest diameter

T2: Tumor invades muscularis propria or size >2 cm with invasion of lamina propria or submucosa

T3: Tumor invades through the muscularis propria into the subserosa, or into nonperitonealized pericolic or perirectal tissues

T4: Tumor invades peritoneum or other organs

Regional lymph nodes (N)

N0: No regional lymph node metastasis

N1: Regional lymph node metastasis

Distant metastasis (M)

M0: No distant metastasis

M1: Distant metastasis

GUIDELINES

European Society for Medical Oncology, National Comprehensive Cancer Network, and European Neuroendocrine Tumor Society guidelines for initial diagnosis and staging are given in Table 5.3.

EVIDENCE-BASED VIEWPOINTS

- In patients with suspicious thoracic and GEP-NETs, ^{68}Ga-SSTR PET/CT shows high sensitivity, specificity, and accuracy and should be considered as first-line diagnostic imaging modality.[45]

TABLE 5.1
TNM Classification for P-NENs

TNM	T1	T2	T3	T4
N0	IA	IB	IIA	III
N1	IIB	IIB	IIB	III
M1	IV	IV	IV	IV

TABLE 5.2
TNM Classification for GI-NENs[a]

TNM	T1	T2	T3	T4
N0	I	IIA	IIB	IIIA
N1	IIIB	IIIB	IIIB	IIIB
M1	IV	IV	IV	IV

[a]For appendiceal carcinoid staging, refer to NCCN Guideline.[42]

TABLE 5.3
Guidelines

Clinical Guideline	Initial Diagnosis (Primary Tumor), N-staging, and M-staging

ESMO[43]	• Recommended (if expression of somatostatin receptor [SSTR] 2 has been proved)
	  • 68Ga-DOTA-TOC/-NOC/-TATE PET/CT or MR for staging
	  • Follow-up after 18–24 months
	• Complementary 11C-5-HTP, 18F-DOPA, or 18F-FDG PET/CT

NCCN[42]	• Staging NENs: SSTR imaging (scintigraphy or PET/CT) if clinically indicated • PRRT planning: 68Ga-DOTA-peptides for SSTR status if clinically indicated • NENs with unknown primary: is optional if conventional imaging method is negative • Poorly differentiated NENs of unknown primary: FDG PET/CT is recommended
ENETS[44]	• FDG PET/CT may be considered in patients in whom radical surgery is being pursued or if clarification of equivocal findings on conventional imaging may change the therapeutic approach. FDG PET/CT may be useful in resectable cases for whole-body assessment

CT, computed tomography; *DOPA*, dihydroxyphenylalanine; *ENETS*, European Neuroendocrine Tumor Society; *ESMO*, European Society for Medical Oncology; *FDG*, fludeoxyglucose; *HTP*, hydroxytryptophan; *MR*, magnetic resonance; *NCCN*, National Comprehensive Cancer Network; *NEN*, neuroendocrine neoplasm; *NOC*, NaI3-octreotide; *PET*, positron emission tomography; *PRRT*, peptide receptor radionuclide therapy; *TATE*, Tyr3-octreotate; *TOC*, Phe1-Tyr3-octreotide.

- 68Ga-SSTR PET/CT is promising for assessing SSTRs before peptide receptor radiolabeled therapy (PRRT) and therapy evaluation after PRRT.[46]
- 68Ga-labeled SSTR PET/CT is recommended for staging and assessment of suspected recurrence in NENs. Also, 18F-DOPA PET/CT is recommended in selected cases of NENs.[47]
- 18F-DOPA PET/CT is an accurate method in diagnosing patients with proven or suspected NENs.[38]
- FDG PET/CT is recommended for staging and restaging of selected patients with poorly differentiated NENs, such as NECs G3.[47]
- FDG PET/CT may be useful to characterize tumor aggressiveness with higher FDG uptake (higher standard uptake value [SUV]), which indicates worse prognosis.[48]

COST-EFFECTIVENESS

Overall costs for the evaluation of GEP-NENs with 68Ga-DOTA Phe1-Tyr3-octreotide (TOC) PET/CT is markedly lower than with 111In-DTPA-octreotide scan (548€ versus 827€, respectively). Moreover, imaging with 68Ga-DOTATOC PET/CT obviates the need for additional examinations such as MRI in most of the cases, which dramatically reduces the consequential costs.[49] However, further researches are warranted regarding the latter statement when liver resection is planned.

CLINICAL POINT OF VIEW

Management and prognosis of NENs are primarily based on histologic grading, with G3 tumors/NECs being highly aggressive diseases mostly treated according to small cell lung cancer treatment regimen, that is, cisplatin-based chemotherapy.

In highly differentiated NENs (i.e., NET G1 and G2), the approach is more sophisticated and based on various factors:

1. **Extent of disease/stage**: As surgery is the only curative therapy, all patients with a diagnosis of NET should be assessed for resectability. Since even patients with approved metastatic lesions (e.g., to the liver) have a better outcome following an attempt of radical surgery, precise staging with localization of the primary tumor is mandatory. However, even in patients with disseminated disease not amenable to radical surgery, resection of the primary tumor has also been shown to be beneficial if it is located in the small intestine (to avoid local complications due to fibrosis), as well as in selected cases with the tumor in the pancreas.

2. **Location of the primary tumor**: The origin of the primary tumor has an impact on both surgical and palliative management of patients with metastatic NETs. Both the appropriate type of somatostatin analogue (SST-A) agents and origin of the primary tumor should be considered to achieve a favorable treatment response. Although chemotherapy based on streptozotocin or temozolomide is virtually ineffective in patients with intestinal NETs, it is a valid option in patients with P-NETs. The application of the mTOR (mammalian target of rapamycin) inhibitor everolimus has now been approved for progressive pancreatic, intestinal, and pulmonary NETs as well as cancer of unknown pri-

mary, whereas the tyrosine-kinase inhibitor sunitinib is only effective on patients with progressive P-NETs.

3. **Functionality**: As mentioned before, the functional tumors have better prognosis than nonfunctional tumors, and patients with functional tumors are candidates for therapy with SST-A irrespective of the SSTR status of tumor cells. Contrary to common misconceptions, functionality is defined only by the presence of respective symptoms rather than biochemical or histologic parameters.

4. **Somatostatin receptor status**: Recent data have shown that SST-A shows antineoplastic effects in patients with nonoperable nonfunctioning NETs with SSTR. For example, ocreotide and lanreotide are effective on small bowel NETs, whereas patients with pancreatic NETs and cancers of unknown primary benefit from the latter. These therapies proved to significantly prolong progression-free survival. Although SST-As have pleiotropic functions and their activity might not be confined to patients with positive SSTR imaging, the current state of approval for octreotide and lanreotide requires confirmed in vivo SSTR presence. In addition, a certain number of receptors is required on tumor cells for PRRT to be successful.

PITFALLS

False Positive (⁶⁸Ga-DOTA-Peptide PET/CT)

- Uptake in exocrine pancreas[50]
- Physiologic uptake in the pancreas uncinate process[51]
- Physiologic uptake in adrenal glands[52]
- Inflammation (prostatitis, postradiation change)[53,54]
- Reactive lymph nodes[55]
- Active bone remodeling (osteoarthritis, recent fracture, vertebral hemangioma with rim bone remodeling, fibrous dysplasia)[53]
- Epiphyseal growth plates[54]
- Splenosis[53]

False Negative (⁶⁸Ga-DOTA-Peptide PET/CT)[54]

- Atypical SSTR subtype expression
- Poorly differentiated tumors
- Masked lesions by physiologic pancreatic activity
- Small-sized lesions (<5 mm)

False Positive (FDG PET/CT)[56]

- Chronic active pancreatitis
- Serous cystadenoma

False Negative (FDG PET/CT)[57]

- Well-differentiated, slow-growing tumors

DISCUSSION

High expression of predominantly SSTR-2 and SSTR-5 on more than 70% of GI-NENs makes them excellent targets for imaging with radiolabeled somatostatin analogues like ¹¹¹In-octreotide, with overall sensitivity of 80%–90% in detecting primary and metastatic NEN lesions if they are large enough and adequately express receptors. It is double sensitive for this purpose when compared with ¹²³I-MIBG scintigraphy. However, the sensitivity of this technique for detection of unknown primary tumors is unpromising and less than 25%.[10,58]

FDG PET/CT

Given low proliferation and high differentiation, NETs are usually faintly FDG avid. Nonetheless, FDG PET/CT is substantially valuable for highly aggressive, poorly differentiated GEP-NENs[34,59-62] and has both diagnostic and prognostic value and the ability to help in therapy planning in this setting.[8,10,63,64] Hence, these patients with high Ki-67 index and cellular proliferation show high FDG uptake and will most likely better respond to chemotherapy than to somatostatin analogues.[52]

FDG PET/CT plays an essential role in the assessment of primary poorly differentiated NECs and their distant metastases with a sensitivity of 90% and 91%, respectively. This study, which was performed on 31 patients, showed that the management has been changed in 26% of the cases based on FDG PET/CT information.[65]

On the other hand, ductal adenocarcinoma as the most common pancreatic cancer (90% versus 5% for P-NENs) is localized to the gland, locally advanced, or advanced with metastases in 9%, 29%, and 52% of patients, with a 5-year relative survival of 29%, 11%, and 3%, respectively. The tumor stage is unknown in 10% of cases, with a 5-year relative survival of 5%.[11,37,66] Usually, this kind of cancer demonstrates an intense FDG uptake and FDG PET/CT has been successfully used for staging and determination of resectability of the primary tumor and corresponding nodal, liver, and other distant metastases. It also helps in differentiating benign from malignant pancreatic masses, evaluation of malignancy recurrence, therapy response monitoring, planning for imaging-guided biopsy, clarification of equivocal CT findings or indeterminate pathology examination in suspected pancreatic cancers, and differentiation of postsurgical fibrosis from malignancy recurrence.[56,57,67-70] In a retrospective study by Lemke and colleagues, they found FDG PET/CT superior to both FDG PET and stand-alone CT in the detection of pancreatic cancers with sensitivity and specificity of approximately 89% and 64% vs 84% and 61% vs 77% and 64%, respectively.[71]

The limitations of FDG PET/CT motivated the scientists for production of other radiotracers to image this kind of tumors. ^{68}Ga-DOTA-peptides, ^{18}F-DOPA, and ^{11}C-5-HTP are the commonly used positron emitters for the assessment of NENs.[13]

^{68}Ga-DOTA-Peptide Conjugates PET/CT

^{68}Ga-DOTA-peptide PET/CT has multitude advantages over conventional ^{111}In-octreotide scan, such as easy production by generator versus cyclotron, faster acquisition time of 2 h versus 4 plus 24 h, better spatial resolution of 3–6 mm versus 10–15 mm, 10-fold higher affinity for SSTRs, broad-spectrum affinity of ^{68}Ga-DOTANOC to SSTR2/3/5 versus SSTR-2 only, and potential semiquantitative evaluation of lesions by SUV, which can be used for response monitoring and prognostication.[27,52,61,72,73] Its other advantages include lack of major toxicity as well as lower radiation dose for patients.[74,75] Accordingly, ^{68}Ga-DOTA-peptide PET/CT has been shown to be highly useful for imaging of GEP-NETs and probably will surpass somatostatin receptor scintigraphy (SRS) in the future for the assessment of these neoplasms.[52,76] The three peptides used in ^{68}Ga-labeled PET/CT are DOTA-Tyr^3-octreotate (TATE), DOTA-Phe^1-Tyr^3-octreotide (TOC), and DOTA-NaI^3-octreotide (NOC) with minimal differences in the imaging setting.[52,77] They all have affinity for SSTR-2; however, DOTATATE has additional affinity for SSTR-3 and DOTANOC shows good affinity for all SSTR-2, 3, and 5.[78]

A meta-analysis of 16 studies and 567 patients that evaluated the diagnostic performance of modality in thoracic and GEP-NENs revealed a patient-based sensitivity and specificity of 93% and 91%, respectively.[45] These values reach 97% and 100% for the evaluation of distant metastases. This prospective study also demonstrated that the management strategy was altered in 19% and supported in 29% of patients.[79]

^{68}Ga-DOTA-peptide conjugates PET/CT is also superior to conventional anatomic imaging (CT/MRI) and ^{111}In-pentetreotide single-photon emission CT/CT for the detection of GEP-NETs,[51,75,80] with a sensitivity of 95%, 45% and 31%, respectively.[80] It is also superior in N- and M-staging, with a sensitivity of 64%, 39%, and 22%, respectively.[80] Naswa and colleagues evaluated 109 patients with GEP-NETs and compared the role of ^{68}Ga-DOTANOC PET/CT with that of conventional imaging

(contrast-enhanced [CE]-CT, MRI, and ultrasound) in primary tumor and its metastases. For the assessment of primary tumor, they calculated a sensitivity, specificity, PPV, NPV, and accuracy of approximately 78%, 93%, 95%, 71%, and 84% for PET/CT versus 64%, 93%, 94%, 60%, and 74%, respectively. For metastatic disease, those values were 98%, 100%, 100%, 94%, and 98% for PET/CT versus 82%, 100%, 100%, 70%, and 87% for conventional imaging, respectively.[79] Moreover, ^{68}Ga-DOTATATE PET/CT is a promising imaging method for the evaluation of GEP-NETs with sensitivity, specificity, PPV, NPV, and accuracy of 94%, 89%, 85%, 96%, and 91%, respectively.[81]

As ^{68}Ga-DOTANOC PET/CT is a potent technique, the SUV$_{max}$ on this technique is a prognostic factor in these patients.[82] Also, a decreased ^{68}Ga-DOTATATE uptake in tumors after the first cycle of peptide receptor radionuclide therapy (PRRT) delta SUV (tumor/spleen) predicts time to progression and correlated with an improvement in clinical symptoms.[83]

Even with physiologic uptake of PET radiotracer in the uncinated process of the pancreas, the detection rate of P-NENs is higher (67%), compared with multiphase CE-CT (56%).[51] Although the physiologic tracer distribution within the pancreas gland can be either diffuse or focal, any focal uptake would be suspicious for malignancy.[77] Obtaining a delayed scan may improve diagnostic confidence in these circumstances[84]; nonetheless, it might be limited due to the short half-life of [68]Ga (68 min).

In addition, several studies confirmed the ability of ^{68}Ga-DOTA-peptide conjugates PET/CT in altering managements in approximately 33%–36% of patients with GEP NETs.[74,77,80]

Dual-Imaging FDG and ^{68}Ga-DOTA PET/CT

Considering the different potentials of FDG and ^{68}Ga-DOTA PET/CT in the detection of well- versus poorly differentiated NENs, some authorities suggested the dual, comparative PET/CT imaging approach with both radiotracers to better assess this kind of malignancy and more accurately detect the locations of well- and poorly differentiated disease. Indeed, the role of two tracers is complementary.[34,53] Kayani and colleagues calculated a sensitivity of 82% and 66% for ^{68}Ga-DOTATATE and FDG PET/CT for the detection of NETs. Interestingly, this rose to 92% with the dual-imaging protocol.[85]

Utilization of this dual-imaging protocol could be pivotal in guiding biopsy to get fewer false-negative results.[53] It also results in optimal patient management with theranostic application of peptide receptor radionuclide treatments as well as posttherapy restaging.[53,60]

^{18}F-DOPA and ^{11}C-5-HTP PET/CT

The NEN cells are capable of taking up decarboxylate amine precursors (e.g., L-DOPA and hydroxytrypto-phan or [5-HTP]) to produce catecholamine and sero-tonin.[38] Thus these molecules can be used in metabolic imaging of those cancers.

^{18}F-DOPA PET/CT is an encouraging modality to evaluate small lesions of primary NENs and corre-sponding lymph node metastases.[13,72,86–88] A patient-based sensitivity of 95% was reported in the literature for this method for staging of NENs. In comparison, the region-based sensitivity was calculated as 95%, 71%, 62%, and 61% for ^{18}F-DOPA PET/CT, SRS + CT, SRS, and CT, respectively.[89,90] The PET/CT contributed to management in 57% of patients.[90]

To enhance accuracy, pretreatment with carbidopa may help subside high background radiotracer uptake by a sixfold decrease in renal excretion but three-fold increase in tumor radiotracer uptake.[72,91] How-ever, since the medication increases washout in both healthy and cancerous pancreatic tissue, preparation with pretreatment carbidopa is not favored in patients with P-NENs.[92]

In addition, ^{11}C-5-HTP PET/CT is successfully uti-lized for the tumor staging as well as surveillance and therapy monitoring.[13] Some authorities calculated a sensitivity of 100% for this modality and concluded that it should be applied as a universal method for detecting NENs.[93] In another investigation, the same group calculated sensitivity, specificity, and PPV of about 84%, 100%, and 100% in staging of patients with NEN and it was the only imaging modality to guide the surgeons in discovering the primary lesion in 29% of cases.[94]

In addition, in specific P-NENs, per-lesion analysis revealed that the sensitivity of modalities for the detec-tion of pancreatic NENs reaches 96%, 80%, 46%, 77%, and 68% for ^{11}C-5-HTP PET/CT, ^{18}F-DOPA PET/CT, SRS, SRS/CT, and stand-alone CT, respectively, which introduces the ^{11}C-5-HTP PET/CT as an optimal imag-ing technique.[87]

Although ^{11}C-5-HTP is superior to ^{18}F-DOPA PET/CT in the assessment of differentiated P-NETs, its use is restricted due to its complex production and less availability.[60]

Octreoscan, ^{68}Ga-DOTA-peptide, ^{18}F-DOPA, and ^{11}C-5-HTP PET/CT are reported to be more sensitive than standard stand-alone multiple detector computed tomography or MRI and may change management in one-third to half of patients if additional lesions are discovered.[10] The detection rate by CT and MRI ranges from 76%–100% and 67%–100%, respectively.[58]

^{64}Cu-DOTATATE PET/CT

This is another modality that uses radiolabeled soma-tostatin analogues for visualization of NENs. ^{64}Cu-DOTATATE is a ligand that is attached to a radioisotope with intermediate half-life (12.7 h) and avidly binds to SSTRs.[95]

It is significantly superior to Octreoscan for this pur-pose, with sensitivity and accuracy of 97% and 97% versus 87% and 88%, respectively.[96] In comparison with Octreoscan, it provides excellent imaging quality with better sensitivity but less radiation exposure for patients.[95]

The Role of PET/CT in Other Neuroendocrine Neoplasms
Medullary thyroid cancer

Medullary thyroid cancer (MTC) is a rare NET that accounts for 5% of all thyroid cancers and expresses SSTR s (predominantly SSTR-2) and produces calci-tonin. It is primarily diagnosed clinically followed by ultrasound and fine-needle aspiration biopsy. Surgery is the primary curative approach; however, there is an up to 50% risk of biochemical recurrence.[97,98] There-fore, accurate detection and localization of recurrent disease or metastases are of crucial importance, as sur-gery remains the mainstay of therapy even in relapsed cancers.

^{68}Ga-DOTATATE PET/CT is an extremely useful method in the early detection of disease recurrence in this type of cancer. However, the detection rate is cor-related with serum calcitonin levels, with best imaging results at levels >500 pg/mL. Another benefit of this imaging method is referral of positive but inoperable patients to PRRT.[97,99,100] Overall, since the ^{68}Ga-DOTA-peptide conjugates PET/CT represents SRS of NEN cells, it is an essential imaging to be performed before start-ing therapy with somatostatin analogues.[101] Naswa and colleagues calculated a sensitivity of 81% and PPV of 100% for ^{68}Ga-DOTANOC PET/CT in evaluating recur-rent MTC.[102]

^{18}F-DOPA PET/CT can be used for imaging tumors with even low expression of SSTR such as medullary thyroid carcinoma.[101] It is capable of detecting meta-static disease from well-differentiated tumors, early in the course of MTC. However, it may provide limited sensitivity for the detection of postsurgical residual disease.[103] Both ^{18}F-DOPA- and FDG PET/CT modali-ties may be useful in clarification of equivocal find-ings on CIM.[104] However, it is shown that ^{18}F-DOPA is superior to FDG PET/CT in staging and surveillance of MTC cases, with a patient-based sensitivity of 81% vs 58% and accuracy of 94% vs 62%, respectively.[105]

^{18}F-DOPA PET/CT is also able to alter management in 27% of patients.[105] Nonetheless, its difficult and expensive production may limit ^{18}F-DOPA PET/CT clinical application.[101] FDG PET/CT is supposed to play a complementary role for ^{18}F-DOPA PET/CT in patients with recurrent aggressive MTC.[106]

A meta-analysis of 24 studies and 538 patients revealed that FDG PET/CT is more sensitive in patients with recurrent MTC with high serum calcitonin (>1000 pg/mL) and short calcitonin doubling times (<2 years)[107] but of limited use in levels <500 pg/mL.[108] Treglia and colleagues calculated a pooled detection rate of 75% with calcitonin level >1000 ng/mL but only 40% when the level was <150 ng/mL.[107] The modality can alter the management of patients with recurrent MTC and this is quite important because normally, this imaging is performed after negative conventional methods.[99,107] It is less sensitive than ^{18}F-DOPA PET/CT for MTC metastases with sensitivity of 58% versus 81%.[99] In addition, FDG PET/CT is superior to conventional imaging such as CT, MRI, and ^{131}I-MIBG for localizing involved lymph nodes, particularly in cervical, mediastinal, and supraclavicular stations.[109]

Pheochromocytoma/paraganglioma

Pheochromocytoma and paraganglioma are rare catecholamine-producing tumors derived of the sympathetic nervous system and located in the adrenal medulla in the majority of cases; they most commonly metastasize to lymph nodes, bones, lungs, and liver.[110]

Expression of SSTR (particularly type 2) by these malignancies makes them good targets for imaging with ^{68}Ga-DOTA-peptides PET/CT.[111] ^{68}Ga-DOTANOC PET/CT is highly accurate and even superior to ^{131}I-MIBG scintigraphy for the evaluation of pheochromocytoma with lesion-based sensitivity, specificity, PPV, NPV, and accuracy of approximately 94%, 86%, 94%, 86%, and 91% for PET/CT versus 61%, 79%, 86%, 48%, and 67% for scintigraphy, respectively. It is 100% accurate in MEN2-associated and malignant tumor.[112] Janssen and colleagues found ^{68}Ga-DOTATATE PET/CT to be superior to other imaging modalities[113,114] in the localization of sporadic metastatic PCCs and PGLs with lesion-based detection rate of approximately 98%, 82%, 78%, 75%, and 49% for ^{68}Ga-DOTATATE PET/CT, CT/MRI, ^{18}F-FDA (fluorodopamine), ^{18}F-DOPA, and ^{18}F-FDG PET/CT, respectively.[113] It is also superior to other functional PET imaging as well as anatomic modalities (CT/MRI) in the detection of hereditary PCC/PGL metastatic disease.[115]

Also, ^{18}F-DOPA PET/CT has a higher sensitivity than (82% vs 68%) but comparable (100%) specificity with ^{131}I-MIBG scintigraphy for localization of PCC.

It is superior for the assessment of PGL as well.[116,117] This result was achieved in the initial evaluation of this method for the assessment of PCC as well.[118]

^{18}F-FDA PET/CT is another modality that is superior to [123/131]I-MIBG scintigraphy in metastatic PCC[119] and PGL.[120]

FDG PET/CT facilitates the assessment of metabolic tumor volume and total lesion glycolysis. One study showed that these two parameters serve as predictors of biochemical response in metastatic PCCs and PGLs.[18]

Nevertheless, it seems that PCC and PGL routinely do not demonstrate intense ^{18}F-FLT uptake, which could provide new information on biologic behavior of PGL and guide the management in these patients against antiproliferative therapies. Further clinical trials are warranted to clarify the value of ^{18}F-FLT PET/CT in the assessment of PCCs and PGLs.[121]

Metastatic neuroendocrine neoplasms with unknown primary

NENs account for approximately 2%–4% of carcinoma of unknown primary (CUP).[122] Given the low rate of glucose metabolism by NETs, it is believed that FDG PET/CT is not an optimal method for the assessment of CUP-NENs, particularly in well-differentiated types. However, there is little literature presenting its value in poorly differentiated NECs with a high proliferation rate, which complies with about 30% of NEC-CUP.[122] In contrast, ^{68}Ga-DOTANOC PET/CT is a promising and very accurate modality in identifying the primary site as well as corresponding metastatic lesions.[122–124] It is highly superior to Octreoscan for this purpose,[125,126] with a detection rate of 59% versus 39%.[125] An investigation showed that this technique could localize the primary site in 60% of patients with indeterminate conventional imaging modalities.[122] It can also alter management in patients with ^{68}Ga-DOTA-peptide-avid metastasis but unknown primary cancer[125,127] in up to 28% of cases.[127]

In addition, ^{18}F-DOPA PET/CT is also capable of accurately localizing the primary tumor in patients with CUP-NET and is superior to SRS for this purpose,[2,128] mainly for well-differentiated, serotonin-secreting tumors.[128]

Therapeutic Value of Radiolabeled Somatostatin Analogues in Gastroenteropancreatic Neuroendocrine Cancers

Peptide receptor or somatostatin analogues radionuclide therapy (PRRT) has been used as an efficient and well-accepted treatment for nonresectable (due to tumor size or vascular invasion) or metastatic well-differentiated

GEP-NENs in the recent two decades.[54,129,130] In patients with initially unresectable pancreatic NENs, neoadjuvant therapy with ^{177}Lu-octreotate could increase the chance for successful later surgery.[130] Expectedly, the patients with positive ^{18}F-DOPA PET/CT, ^{68}Ga-DOTA-peptide conjugates PET/CT, or SRS are good candidates for this therapy method.[54] Nonetheless, there is only one randomized trial and PRRT has not been approved yet, although it is highly valuable in individual patients failing approved standard therapies.[131]

The most commonly used radiopeptides for this purpose are ^{177}Lu-octreotate and ^{90}Y-octreotide. In patients with GEP-NENs, this therapy causes tumor remission in 46% of patients, including minor response.[132] This modality led to disease control rates of 68%–94%, with quite similar progression-free and overall survival rates, compared with chemotherapy, somatostatin analogues, and newer targeted therapies. Generally, PRRT is well tolerated, with moderate toxicity in most patients.[129] One of the side effects is renal toxicity, most likely after therapy with ^{90}Y-labeled somatostatin analogues, which is more prevalent in older patients with diabetes and hypertension.[133] It also has relatively rare hematologic side effects.[134,135] The side effects may subside with the administration of appropriate dosage and coadministration of amino acids as well as use of renal protective agents.[136,137]

In a retrospective study on 74 patients with metastatic GEP-NEN, the investigators revealed that the patients with well-differentiated grade 1 and 2 neoplasms who underwent therapy with ^{177}Lu-octreotate showed favorable response and notable long-term outcome, even with a Ki-67 index of >10%.[138]

Nevertheless, further randomized controlled trials are warranted to standardize the therapy, facilitate comparison with other available treatment strategies, and establish its position in the treatment algorithm of NENs.[129,136] As mentioned before, the randomized trial (NETTER-1) on treatment of midgut NETs with ^{177}Lu-DOTATATE (^{177}Lu-DOTA[0]-Tyr[3]-octreotate or Lutathera) provides evidence for a clinically meaningful and statistically significant improvement of progression-free and overall survival, compared with Sandostatin LAR (octreotide) therapy.[131] It has the potential to become the treatment of choice for metastatic or inoperable GEP-NENs.[137]

TEACHING CASES
Case 1: ^{18}F-DOPA PET/CT: Staging GI-NEN
Findings
A 68-year-old female, referred with biopsy-proven diagnosis of terminal ileum NEN G2, proliferation index 2%–5%. ^{18}F-DOPA PET/CT shows the tracer-avid primary tumor in terminal ileum (Fig. 5.1A and B; yellow arrows) as well as several metastatic regional lymph nodes (Fig. 5.1A, arrowheads). There are multiple ^{18}F-DOPA-avid liver metastases with no corresponding morphologic lesions on CT (Fig. 5.1A and C; white arrows).

Teaching points
- ^{18}F-DOPA PET/CT is a promising modality for the evaluation of GEP-NEN, especially hormone-producing types.
- It is highly sensitive (95%) for detecting primary tumor as well as N- and M-staging.
- ^{18}F-DOPA PET/CT changed the patient's management in 57% of G1 or G2 NENs.

Pitfalls
- Physiologic intensive ^{18}F-DOPA uptake may be seen in the gallbladder and uncinate process of the pancreas.
- The patient is imaged with arms down by the sides, with resultant beam hardening artifact on CT.

Case 2: ^{18}F-DOPA PET/CT: Staging Paraganglioma
Findings
A 58-year-old female with primary right jugular paraganglioma that showed intensive ^{18}F-DOPA uptake (Fig. 5.2A and B; green arrows). ^{18}F-DOPA PET/CT depicted two additional sites of tracer-avid primary tumors (Fig. 5.2A and C; white arrows) suggestive of jugulotympanic paragangliomas, which were not detectable on CIM (CT and MRI). A metastatic mediastinal lymph node is also seen in mediastinum (Fig. 5.2A, yellow arrow).

Teaching points
- ^{18}F-DOPA PET/CT is superior to conventional imaging modalities for the evaluation of small paragangliomas.
- ^{18}F-DOPA PET/CT is an encouraging modality with a high sensitivity of 95% to evaluate small lesions of primary NENs and corresponding lymph node metastases, particularly if the tumor produces hormones.
- Jugulotympanic paraganglioma (glomus jugulare/tympanicum tumor) is the most common tumor of the middle ear. It often occurs in women of age 40–69 years. Its common locations include the jugular bulb (85%), tympanic branch of glossopharyngeal nerve (Jacobson nerve) (12%), and posterior auricular branch of vagus nerve (Arnold nerve) (3%). It is rarely malignant with cervical lymph nodes, lung, and liver metastases.

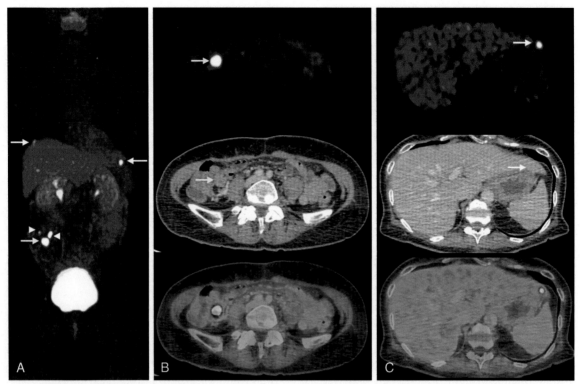

FIG. 5.1 ^{18}F-dihydroxyphenylalanine (DOPA) positron emission tomography/computed tomography (CT) showing the tracer-avid primary tumor in terminal ileum (A and B; *yellow arrows*) as well as several metastatic regional lymph nodes (A, *arrowheads*). There are multiple ^{18}F-DOPA-avid liver metastases with no corresponding morphologic lesions on CT (A and C; *white arrows*).

Case 3: ^{18}F-DOPA PET/CT: Lung NEN (Carcinoid)

Findings

A 30-year-old male with hormone-producing (GHRH) pulmonary NEN G1 with history of type I diabetes mellitus and uncontrolled plasma glucose levels. ^{18}F-DOPA PET/CT shows tracer-avid primary tumor in the right lung (Fig. 5.3A and B; arrows).

Teaching points

- ^{18}F-DOPA PET/CT is useful for the assessment of well- and moderately differentiated hormone-producing NENs.
- Typical lung carcinoids comprise 90% of lung carcinoids and are the most slow-growing pulmonary NETs compared with small cell lung cancer, large cell NEC, and atypical carcinoid tumors. This explains their very low FDG uptake. They are the most common NENs after the GEP type and rarely metastasize beyond the lung.

Case 4: ^{68}Ga-DOTANOC PET/CT: GI-NEN

Findings

A 73-year-old female with terminal ileum NEN G1. ^{68}Ga-DOTANOC PET/CT shows tracer-avid primary tumor (Fig. 5.4A and B; arrows). Tracer uptakes in the dorsal part of the pancreas (Fig. 5.4C, arrows) as well as symmetric uptake in the adrenal glands (Fig. 5.4A, arrowheads) are physiologic.

Teaching points

- ^{68}Ga-DOTANOC PET/CT is a promising modality to exclude metastatic disease in patients with G1 NEN.
- It provides high diagnostic performance for the evaluation of G1 GEP-NEN.

Pitfalls

- Mild diffuse ^{68}Ga-DOTANOC uptake in the prostate gland and intensive spleen uptake are physiologic.

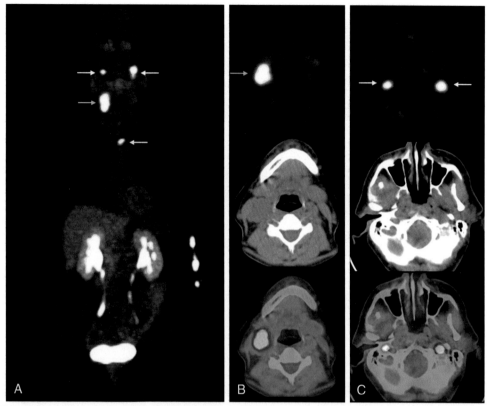

FIG. 5.2 A 58-year-old female with primary right jugular paraganglioma, which showed intensive ^{18}F-dihydroxyphenylalanine (DOPA) uptake (A and B; *green arrows*). ^{18}F-DOPA positron emission tomography/computed tomography (CT) depicted two additional sites of tracer-avid primary tumors (A and C; *white arrows*) suggestive of jugulotympanic paragangliomas, which were not detectable on CIM (CT and magnetic resonance imaging). A metastatic mediastinal lymph node is also seen in mediastinum (A, *yellow arrow*).

Case 5: FDG Versus ^{68}Ga-DOTANOC PET/CT: Staging Gastric NEN

Findings

A 61-year-old male with gastric NEN G2. FDG PET/CT shows a mildly tracer-avid primary tumor and few liver metastases (Fig. 5.5A and C; arrows). ^{68}Ga-DOTANOC PET/CT shows an intensely tracer-avid primary tumor with more liver lesions compared with FDG PET/CT (Fig. 5.5B and D; arrows).

Teaching points

- ^{68}Ga-DOTA-peptide is superior to FDG PET/CT for the evaluation of well- and moderately differentiated NENs.
- For the assessment of well-differentiated tumors with a proliferation index (PI) of ≤2, both ^{68}Ga-DOTA-peptide and ^{18}F-DOPA PET/CT are utilized.

However, the latter is favored for hormone-producing neoplasms.

- For the evaluation of moderately differentiated tumors with PI of 3–20, FDG with either ^{68}Ga-DOTA-peptide or ^{18}F-DOPA PET/CT should be used.
- For poorly differentiated tumors with PI>20, FDG PET/CT is the best molecular diagnostic method.
- ^{68}Ga-DOTA-peptide PET/CT also has theranostic values for intensely tracer-avid neoplasms.

Case 6: ^{68}Ga-DOTANOC PET/CT: Restaging—Gastric NEN

Findings

A 62-year-old male with gastric NEN G1, status post partial gastrectomy. ^{68}Ga-DOTANOC PET/CT shows intensely tracer-avid small gastrohepatic lymph node, which was too small to be suspicious on CT (Fig. 5.6A and B; arrows).

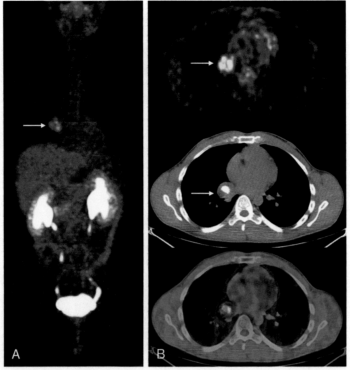

FIG. 5.3 ^{18}F-dihydroxyphenylalanine positron emission tomography/computed tomography showing tracer-avid primary tumor in the right lung (A and B; *arrows*).

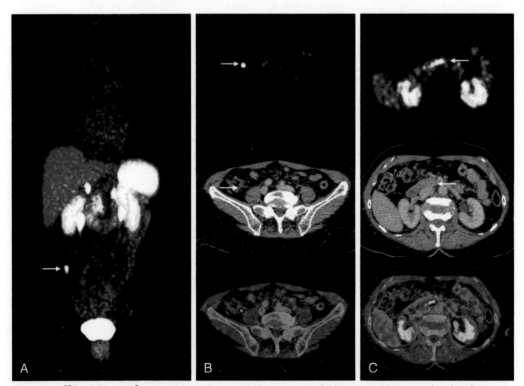

FIG. 5.4 ^{68}Ga-DOTA-NaI^3-octreotide positron emission tomography/computed tomography showing tracer-avid primary tumor (A and B; *arrows*). Tracer uptakes in the dorsal part of pancreas (C, *arrows*) as well as symmetric uptake in adrenal glands (A, *arrowheads*) are physiologic.

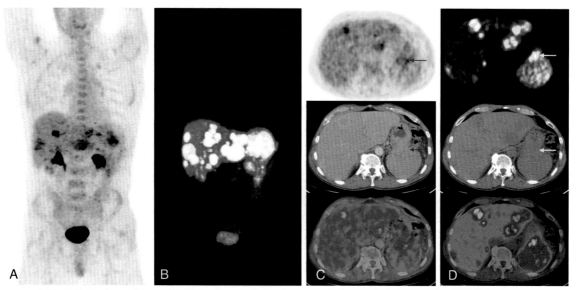

FIG. 5.5 Fludeoxyglucose (FDG) positron emission tomography/computed tomography (PET/CT) showing mildly tracer-avid primary tumor and few liver metastases (A and C; *arrows*). ^{68}Ga-DOTA-NaI^3-octreotide PET/CT shows intensely tracer-avid primary tumor with more liver lesions compared with FDG PET/CT (D, *arrows*).

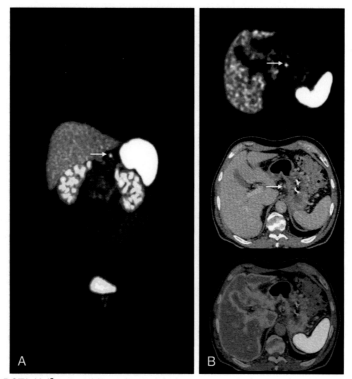

FIG. 5.6 ^{68}Ga-DOTA-NaI^3-octreotide positron emission tomography/computed tomography (CT) showing intensely tracer-avid small gastrohepatic lymph node, which was too small to be suspicious on CT (A and B; *arrows*).

Teaching points
- ⁶⁸Ga-DOTA-peptide PET/CT is superior to stand-alone CT in the evaluation of NENs.
- It provides excellent performance with a sensitivity and specificity of 93% and 91%, respectively, for the assessment of regional involvement as well as distant metastases.

Case 7: ⁶⁸Ga-DOTANOC PET/CT: Lung NEN Recurrence

Findings

A 27-year-old male with lung NEN G1, status post surgical resection. ⁶⁸Ga-DOTANOC PET/CT shows tracer-avid recurrent mediastinal nodal involvement with too small lymph nodes to be suspicious on CT (Fig. 5.7A and B; white arrows). These were confirmed to be metastatic disease on histopathology. There is a very faint focal uptake in the right supraclavicular region, which was proved to be a metastasis with increased uptake on follow-up ⁶⁸Ga-DOTANOC PET/CT (Fig. 5.7A, yellow arrow).

Teaching points
- ⁶⁸Ga-DOTANOC PET/CT is superior to stand-alone CT and MRI for early detection of recurrent NENs.
- ⁶⁸Ga-DOTANOC PET/CT is highly sensitive for small NEN lesions, long before they meet the pathologic criteria on conventional imaging modalities.

Pitfalls
- ⁶⁸Ga-DOTA-peptide uptake in pituitary gland is physiologic (Fig. 5.7A, arrowhead).

Case 8: FDG Versus ⁶⁸Ga-DOTA-Peptide PET/CT: Recurrent NEN

Findings

A 76-year-old female with moderately differentiated pancreatic NEN (PI = 10%–20%), status post resection. FDG PET/CT is unremarkable. Faint tracer uptake in the gastroesophageal junction is physiologic (Fig. 5.8A, arrow). ⁶⁸Ga-DOTANOC PET/CT shows a significantly better performance, showing multiple tracer-avid liver metastases (Fig. 5.8B, arrows) as well as small

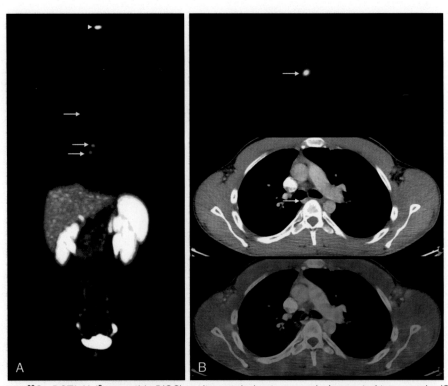

FIG. 5.7 ⁶⁸Ga-DOTA-Nal³-octreotide (NOC) positron emission tomography/computed tomography (CT) showing tracer-avid recurrent mediastinal nodal involvement with too small lymph nodes to be suspicious on CT (A and B; *white arrows*). There is a very faint focal uptake in the right supraclavicular region, which was proved to be a metastasis with increased uptake on follow-up ⁶⁸Ga-DOTANOC PET/CT (A, *yellow arrow*).

tracer-avid recurrent primary tumor (Fig. 5.8D, arrows). It is able to detect a positive tiny upper abdominal mesenteric lymph node, which is too small to be suspicious on CT (Fig. 5.8F, arrows). Intense ^{68}Ga uptake in bilateral adrenal glands is physiologic (Fig. 5.8).

Teaching points
- ^{68}Ga-DOTA-peptide is superior to FDG PET/CT as well as stand-alone CT in the evaluation of recurrent well-differentiated NENs.
- It is able to accurately guide treatment approach in NEN recurrence.

Pitfalls
- Mild ^{68}Ga-DOTA-peptide uptake in thyroid gland is physiologic.
- Physiologic intense uptake of ^{68}Ga-DOTA-peptide in adrenal glands is a limitation for this modality to evaluate metastases to this organ.
- Mild uptake of FDG in the gastroesophageal junction can be physiologic or inflammatory in nature.

Case 9: FDG Versus ^{68}Ga-DOTANOC PET/CT: Recurrent NEN
Findings

A 54-year-old male with recurrent mediastinal NEN G1-2. FDG PET/CT shows physiologic distribution of radiotracer with no metabolic evidence of malignancy (Fig. 5.9A and C). ^{68}Ga-DOTANOC PET/CT performed at 2 days interval shows tracer-avid local recurrent neoplasm (Fig. 5.9B and D; arrows) as well as numerous distant cervical, abdominal, and liver metastases.

Teaching points
- FDG PET/CT may be helpful to determine if any poorly differentiated tumor is localized in the body before the patient undergoes peptide receptor radionuclide therapy (PRRT) based on highly positive ^{68}Ga-DOTANOC PET/CT. A positive FDG PET/CT can alter the planned management in this setting.

Case 10: FDG Versus ^{68}Ga-DOTANOC PET/CT: Rectal NEN
Findings

An 80-year-old male with moderately differentiated (G2) rectal NEN. The primary tumor is more intense on ^{68}Ga-DOTANOC (Fig. 5.10B and D; arrows) than on FDG PET/CT (which was performed 1 day later). However, liver, bone, and lung metastases are more avid on FDG compared with ^{68}Ga-DOTANOC PET/CT (Fig. 5.10A and B). FDG uptake in prostate cancer is most likely inflammatory in nature (Fig. 5.10A, arrow).

Teaching points
- Although the primary tumor is better depicted in ^{68}Ga-DOTANOC, the corresponding metastases are vice versa. It indicates that the primary tumor may have diverse characteristics from its own metastases.

Pitfalls
- ^{68}Ga-DOTA-peptide in the uncinate process of the pancreas and spleen is physiologic and should not be interpreted as malignancy.

Case 11: FDG PET/CT: Staging Lung NEC
Findings

An 81-year-old male with poorly differentiated pulmonary NEC, G3, PI: 60%–70%. FDG PET/CT shows tracer-avid primary tumor in the upper lobe of the right lung (Fig. 5.11A and B; arrows). There is a faintly FDG-avid left hilar lymph node, which was proved to be metastasis based on follow-up images (Fig. 5.11C, arrows). Focal FDG uptake in the right lower abdomen was clarified to be a benign polyp in colon (Fig. 5.11D, arrows).

Teaching points
- FDG PET/CT is a promising method for the assessment of poorly differentiated NECs.
- It provides high diagnostic performance in G3 NENs with high proliferation index (i.e., >20%).
- A solitary FDG-avid hilar lymph node should be followed closely to exclude malignancy.

Pitfalls
- Benign lesions such as GI polyps could be FDG avid.

Case 12: ^{18}F-DOPA Versus ^{68}Ga-DOTANOC PET/CT: Recurrent Medullary Thyroid Cancer
Findings

A 28-year-old male with MTC, with calcitonin of 9617 pg/mL (normal <10 pg/mL) and carcinoembryonic antigen of 30 ng/mL (normal <3.4 ng/mL). The images show recurrent disease with disseminated metastases, more prominent on ^{18}F-DOPA (Fig. 5.12A) compared with ^{68}Ga-DOTANOC PET/CT (Fig. 5.12B) with 1 day interval. ^{18}F-DOPA uptake in brain basal ganglia is physiologic (Fig. 5.12A, arrow). ^{68}Ga-DOTA-peptide uptake in pituitary gland is physiologic (Fig. 5.12B, arrow).

Teaching point
- ^{18}F-DOPA is superior to ^{68}Ga-DOTA-peptide as well as FDG PET/CT for the assessment of MTC.

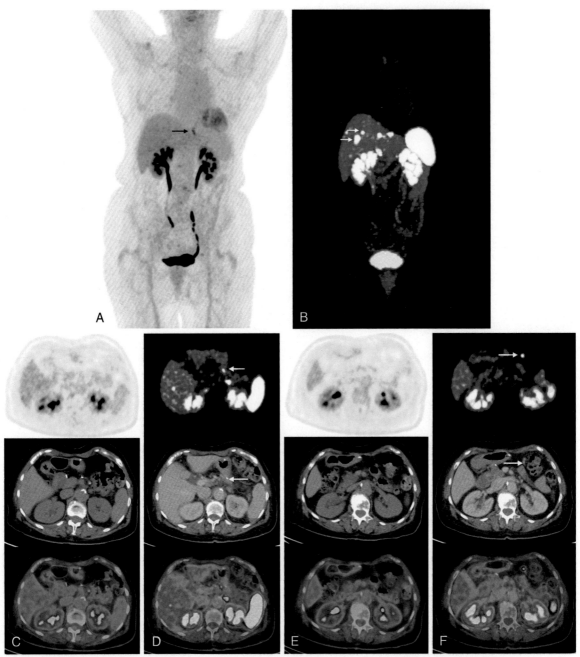

FIG. 5.8 Fludeoxyglucose positron emission tomography/computed tomography (PET/CT) is unremarkable. Faint tracer uptake in gastroesophageal junction is physiologic (A, *arrow*). ^{68}Ga-DOTA-NaI^3-octreotide PET/CT shows significantly better performance, showing multiple tracer-avid liver metastases (B, *arrows*) as well as small tracer-avid recurrent primary tumor (D, *arrows*). It is able to detect a positive tiny upper abdominal mesenteric lymph node, which is too small to be suspicious on CT (F, *arrows*). C and E, FDG PET, CT, and fused axial images.

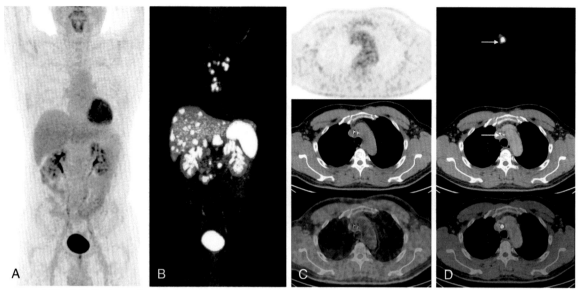

FIG. 5.9 Fludeoxyglucose positron emission tomography/computed tomography (PET/CT) showing physiologic distribution of radiotracer with no metabolic evidence of malignancy (A and C). ^{68}Ga-DOTA-Nal[3]-octreotide PET/CT performed at 2 days interval shows tracer-avid local recurrent neoplasm (D; *arrows*) as well as numerous distant cervical, abdominal, and liver metastases.

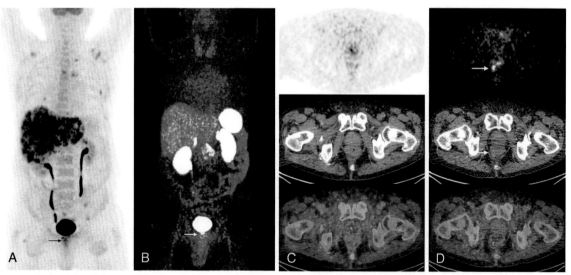

FIG. 5.10 Primary tumor is more intense on ^{68}Ga-DOTA-Nal[3]-octreotide (NOC) (B and D; *arrows*) compared with fludeoxyglucose (FDG) positron emission tomography/computed tomography (PET/CT) (which was performed 1 day later). However, liver, bone, and lung metastases are more avid on FDG compared with ^{68}Ga-DOTANOC PET/CT (A and B). FDG uptake in prostate cancer is most likely inflammatory in nature (A, *arrow*). C, FDG PET, CT, and fused axial images.

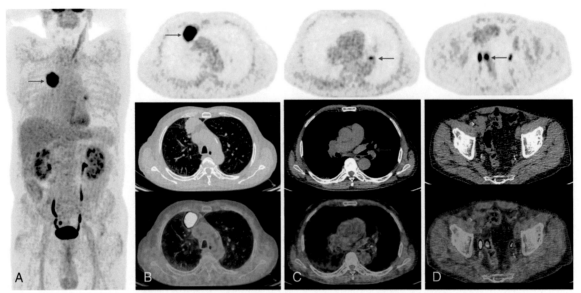

FIG. 5.11 Fludeoxyglucose (FDG) positron emission tomography/computed tomography showing tracer-avid primary tumor in the upper lobe of the right lung (A and B; *arrows*). There is a faintly FDG-avid left hilar lymph node, which was proved to be metastasis based on follow-up images (C, *arrows*). Focal FDG uptake in the right lower abdomen was clarified to be a benign polyp in colon (D, *arrows*).

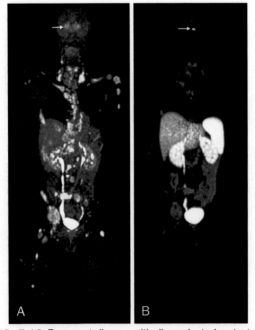

FIG. 5.12 Recurrent disease with disseminated metastases more prominent on ¹⁸F-dihydroxyphenylalanine (DOPA) (A) compared with ⁶⁸Ga-DOTA-Nal³-octreotide positron emission tomography/computed tomography (B) with 1 day interval. ¹⁸F-DOPA uptake in brain basal ganglia is physiologic (A, *arrow*). ⁶⁸Ga-DOTA-peptide uptake in pituitary gland is physiologic (B, *arrow*).

Case 13: FDG and ¹⁸F-DOPA PET/CT: Mass-Forming Pancreatitis

Findings

A 65-year-old male with pancreatic mass, measuring $50 \times 40 \times 30\,mm$, discovered on CIM. The known pancreatic head mass shows no tracer uptake either on FDG PET/CT (Fig. 5.13A and C; arrows) or on ¹⁸F-DOPA PET/CT (Fig. 5.13B and D; arrows) with 10 days interval. Pathology reported as negative for cancer; however, it was positive for chronic pancreatitis (Fig. 5.13).

Teaching points

- Mass-forming pancreatitis often develops in patients with a history of chronic pancreatitis. The main pathologic feature is a mass with progressive interstitial fibrosis and chronic inflammatory changes that both may explain its very low FDG uptake.
- The aforementioned modalities cannot replace pathology in differentiation of mass-forming pancreatitis from pancreatic tumors.

Pitfalls

- Knowledge of the physiologic distribution of various PET tracers is pivotal for correct interpretation.
- In contrast to FDG, ¹⁸F-DOPA PET is not positive for degenerative joint disease and minimal physiologic uptake in the GI tract. No uptake is seen in the pharyngeal region as well. Its uptake in liver and kidneys

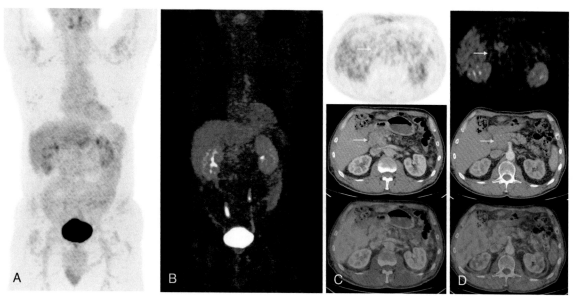

FIG. 5.13 The known pancreatic head mass shows no tracer uptake either on fludeoxyglucose positron emission tomography/computed tomography (PET/CT) (C; *arrows*) or on ^{18}F-dihydroxyphenylalanine PET/CT (D, *arrows*) with 10 days interval. Pathology was reported as negative for cancer; however, it was positive for chronic pancreatitis.

is more homogeneous and intense compared with FDG. Importantly, gallbladder can be highly ^{18}F-DOPA avid.

REFERENCES

1. Caplin ME, Buscombe JR, Hilson AJ, Jones AL, Watkinson AF, Burroughs AK. Carcinoid tumour. *Lancet.* September 5, 1998;352(9130):799–805.
2. Schillaci O. 18F-DOPA and other radiopharmaceuticals for imaging unknown primary neuroendocrine tumors. *Journal of Nuclear Medicine: Official Publication, Society of Nuclear Medicine.* March 2014;55(3):357–359.
3. Modlin IM, Lye KD, Kidd M. A 5-decade analysis of 13,715 carcinoid tumors. *Cancer.* February 15, 2003;97(4):934–959.
4. Dibble EH, Karantanis D, Mercier G, Peller PJ, Kachnic LA, Subramaniam RM. PET/CT of cancer patients: part 1, pancreatic neoplasms. *American Journal of Roentgenology.* November 2012;199(5):952–967.
5. Yao JC, Hassan M, Phan A, et al. One hundred years after "carcinoid": epidemiology of and prognostic factors for neuroendocrine tumors in 35,825 cases in the United States. *Journal of Clinical Oncology: Official Journal of the American Society of Clinical Oncology.* June 20, 2008;26(18):3063–3072.
6. Kimura W, Kuroda A, Morioka Y. Clinical pathology of endocrine tumors of the pancreas. Analysis of autopsy cases. *Digestive Diseases and Sciences.* July 1991;36(7):933–942.
7. Pinchot SN, Holen K, Sippel RS, Chen H. Carcinoid tumors. *The Oncologist.* December 2008;13(12):1255–1269.
8. Binderup T, Knigge U, Loft A, et al. Functional imaging of neuroendocrine tumors: a head-to-head comparison of somatostatin receptor scintigraphy, 123I-MIBG scintigraphy, and 18F-FDG PET. *Journal of Nuclear Medicine: Official Publication, Society of Nuclear Medicine.* May 2010;51(5):704–712.
9. de Herder WW, Hofland LJ, van der Lely AJ, Lamberts SW. Somatostatin receptors in gastroentero-pancreatic neuroendocrine tumours. *Endocrine-Related Cancer.* December 2003;10(4):451–458.
10. Ganeshan D, Bhosale P, Yang T, Kundra V. Imaging features of carcinoid tumors of the gastrointestinal tract. *American Journal of Roentgenology.* October 2013;201(4):773–786.
11. Pattou F, Proye C. Endocrine tumors of the pancreas. In: Holzheimer R, Mannick J, eds. *Surgical Treatment. Evidence-Based and Problem-Oriented.* Munich: Zuckschwerdt; 2001.
12. Kulke MH, Anthony LB, Bushnell DL, et al. NANETS treatment guidelines: well-differentiated neuroendocrine tumors of the stomach and pancreas. *Pancreas.* August 2010;39(6):735–752.
13. Zuetenhorst JM, Taal BG. Metastatic carcinoid tumors: a clinical review. *The Oncologist.* February 2005;10(2):123–131.
14. Mamikunian G, Vinik AI, O'Dorisio TM, et al. *Neuroendocrine Tumors: A Comprehensive Guide to Diagnosis and Management.* 4th ed. Inglewood, CA: Inter Science Institute; 2009.

15. Dhall D, Mertens R, Bresee C, et al. Ki-67 proliferative index predicts progression-free survival of patients with well-differentiated ileal neuroendocrine tumors. *Human Pathology.* April 2012;43(4):489–495.
16. Foltyn W, Zajecki W, Marek B, et al. The value of the Ki-67 proliferation marker as a prognostic factor in gastro-enteropancreatic neuroendocrine tumours. *Endokrynologia Polska.* 2012;63(5):362–366.
17. Khan MS, Kirkwood A, Tsigani T, et al. Circulating tumor cells as prognostic markers in neuroendocrine tumors. *Journal of Clinical Oncology: Official Journal of the American Society of Clinical Oncology.* January 20, 2013;31(3):365–372.
18. Patel D, Mehta A, Nilubol N, Dieckmann W, Pacak K, Kebebew E. Total 18F-FDG PET/CT metabolic tumor volume is associated with postoperative biochemical response in patients with metastatic pheochromocytomas and paragangliomas. *Annals of Surgical Oncology.* 2016;263(3):582–587.
19. Carcinoid Tumor-Risk Factors. http://www.cancer.net/cancer-types/carcinoid-tumor/risk-factors.
20. Risk Factors for Neuroendocrine Tumours. http://www.cancer.ca/en/cancer-information/cancer-type/neuroendocrine/risks/?region=on.
21. Hassan MM, Phan A, Li D, Dagohoy CG, Leary C, Yao JC. Risk factors associated with neuroendocrine tumors: a U.S.-based case-control study. *International Journal of Cancer.* August 15, 2008;123(4):867–873.
22. Tests for Pancreatic Cancer. http://www.cancer.org/cancer/pancreaticcancer/detailedguide/pancreatic-cancer-diagnosis.
23. van Eijck CH, Lamberts SW, Lemaire LC, et al. The use of somatostatin receptor scintigraphy in the differential diagnosis of pancreatic duct cancers and islet cell tumors. *Annals of Surgery.* August 1996;224(2):119–124.
24. A Review of Carcinoid Cancer. Diagnosis. http://www.carcinoid.org/for-patients/general-information/a-review-of-carcinoid-cancer/.
25. Reid MD, Bagci P, Ohike N, et al. Calculation of the Ki67 index in pancreatic neuroendocrine tumors: a comparative analysis of four counting methodologies. *Modern Pathology: An Official Journal of the United States and Canadian Academy of Pathology, Inc.* May 2015;28(5):686–694.
26. Pancreatic Neuroendocrine Tumors, Treatment. https://www.cancer.org/cancer/pancreatic-cancer/treating/medicine-pnets.html.
27. Oberg K, Sundin A. Imaging of neuroendocrine tumors. *Frontiers of Hormone Research.* 2016;45:142–151.
28. Shebani KO, Souba WW, Finkelstein DM, et al. Prognosis and survival in patients with gastrointestinal tract carcinoid tumors. *Annals of Surgery.* June 1999;229(6):815–821. discussion 822–813.
29. Bilimoria KY, Bentrem DJ, Merkow RP, et al. Application of the pancreatic adenocarcinoma staging system to pancreatic neuroendocrine tumors. *Journal of the American College of Surgeons.* October 2007;205(4):558–563.
30. Boyar Cetinkaya R, Vatn M, Aabakken L, Bergestuen DS, Thiis-Evensen E. Survival and prognostic factors in well-differentiated pancreatic neuroendocrine tumors. *Scandinavian Journal of Gastroenterology.* June 2014;49(6):734–741.
31. Halfdanarson TR, Rubin J, Farnell MB, Grant CS, Petersen GM. Pancreatic endocrine neoplasms: epidemiology and prognosis of pancreatic endocrine tumors. *Endocrine-Related Cancer.* June 2008;15(2):409–427.
32. Yao JC, Eisner MP, Leary C, et al. Population-based study of islet cell carcinoma. *Annals of Surgical Oncology.* December 2007;14(12):3492–3500.
33. Yao JC, Lombard-Bohas C, Baudin E, et al. Daily oral everolimus activity in patients with metastatic pancreatic neuroendocrine tumors after failure of cytotoxic chemotherapy: a phase II trial. *Journal of Clinical Oncology: Official Journal of the American Society of Clinical Oncology.* January 1, 2010;28(1):69–76.
34. Abdulrezzak U, Kurt YK, Kula M, Tutus A. Combined imaging with 68Ga-DOTA-TATE and 18F-FDG PET/CT on the basis of volumetric parameters in neuroendocrine tumors. *Nuclear Medicine Communications.* August 2016;37(8):874–881.
35. Survival Statistics for Carcinoid Tumours. http://www.cancerresearchuk.org/about-cancer/type/carcinoid/treatment/statistics-and-outlook-for-carcinoid#rIURqoW1jJxdTZeM.99.
36. Survival Rates for Neuroendocrine Pancreatic Tumors (Treated with Surgery). http://www.cancer.org/cancer/pancreaticcancer/detailedguide/pancreatic-cancer-survival-rates.
37. Hackeng WM, Hruban RH, Offerhaus GJ, Brosens LA. Surgical and molecular pathology of pancreatic neoplasms. *Diagnostic Pathology.* 2016;11(1):47.
38. Rufini V, Treglia G, Montravers F, Giordano A. Diagnostic accuracy of [18F]DOPA PET and PET/CT in patients with neuroendocrine tumors: a meta-analysis. *Clinical and Translational Imaging.* 2013;1(2):111–122.
39. Frilling A, Akerstrom G, Falconi M, et al. Neuroendocrine tumor disease: an evolving landscape. *Endocrine-Related Cancer.* October 2012;19(5):R163–R185.
40. Pancreas and ampulla of vater. In: Robin P, Hansen JT, eds. *TNM Staging Atlas with Oncoanatomy.* 2nd ed. Philadelphia, USA: Wolters Kluwer/LWW; 2012:310–323.
41. Exocrine and endocrine pancreas. In: Edge S, Byrd D, Compton C, Fritz A, Greene F, Trotti A, eds. *AJCC Cancer Staging Manual.* 7th ed. Berlin: Springer; 2010:241–249.
42. NCCN clinical practice guidelines in oncology. *Neuroendocrine Tumors.* 2016. Version 2. www.NCCN.org.
43. Oberg K, Knigge U, Kwekkeboom D, Perren A, Group EGW. Neuroendocrine gastro-entero-pancreatic tumors: ESMO Clinical Practice Guidelines for diagnosis, treatment and follow-up. *Annals of Oncology: Official Journal of the European Society for Medical Oncology/ESMO.* October 2012;23(suppl 7):vii124–130.
44. Garcia-Carbonero R, Sorbye H, Baudin E, et al. ENETS Consensus Guidelines for High-Grade Gastroenteropancreatic Neuroendocrine Tumors and Neuroendocrine Carcinomas. *Neuroendocrinology.* 2016;103(2):186–194.

45. Treglia G, Castaldi P, Rindi G, Giordano A, Rufini V. Diagnostic performance of Gallium-68 somatostatin receptor PET and PET/CT in patients with thoracic and gastroenteropancreatic neuroendocrine tumours: a meta-analysis. *Endocrine.* August 2012;42(1):80–87.

46. Kratochwil C, Stefanova M, Mavriopoulou E, et al. SUV of [68Ga]DOTATOC-PET/CT predicts response probability of PRRT in neuroendocrine tumors. *Molecular Imaging and Biology: The Official Publication of the Academy of Molecular Imaging.* June 2015;17(3):313–318.

47. The Royal College of Physicians and the Royal College of Radiologists. *Evidence-Based Indications for the Usage of PET-CT in the UK.* London: RCP, RCR; 2016. 2016.

48. Kapoor R, Bhattacharyya T, Gupta R, Mittal B, Kalra N. A systematic review of management of neuroendocrine tumors: an experience from a tertiary care center from India. *Clinical Cancer Investigation Journal.* 2014;3:363–372.

49. Schreiter NF, Brenner W, Nogami M, et al. Cost comparison of 111In-DTPA-octreotide scintigraphy and 68Ga-DOTATOC PET/CT for staging enteropancreatic neuroendocrine tumours. *European Journal of Nuclear Medicine and Molecular Imaging.* January 2012;39(1):72–82.

50. Castellucci P, Pou Ucha J, Fuccio C, et al. Incidence of increased 68Ga-DOTANOC uptake in the pancreatic head in a large series of extrapancreatic NET patients studied with sequential PET/CT. *Journal of Nuclear Medicine: Official Publication, Society of Nuclear Medicine.* June 2011;52(6):886–890.

51. Froeling V, Rottgen R, Collettini F, et al. Detection of pancreatic neuroendocrine tumors (PNET) using semi-quantitative [68Ga]DOTATOC PET in combination with multiphase contrast-enhanced CT. *The Quarterly Journal of Nuclear Medicine and Molecular Imaging: Official Publication of the Italian Association of Nuclear Medicine.* September 2014;58(3):310–318.

52. Sharma P, Singh H, Bal C, Kumar R. PET/CT imaging of neuroendocrine tumors with (68)Gallium-labeled somatostatin analogues: an overview and single institutional experience from India. *Indian Journal of Nuclear Medicine: The Official Journal of the Society of Nuclear Medicine, India.* January 2014;29(1):2–12.

53. Hofman MS, Lau WF, Hicks RJ. Somatostatin receptor imaging with 68Ga DOTATATE PET/CT: clinical utility, normal patterns, pearls, and pitfalls in interpretation. *Radiographics: A Review Publication of the Radiological Society of North America, Inc.* March–April 2015;35(2):500–516.

54. Hofman MS, Hicks RJ. Changing paradigms with molecular imaging of neuroendocrine tumors. *Discovery Medicine.* July 2012;14(74):71–81.

55. Shastry M, Kayani I, Wild D, et al. Distribution pattern of 68Ga-DOTATATE in disease-free patients. *Nuclear Medicine Communications.* December 2010;31(12):1025–1032.

56. Wassef H. Pancreatic cancer. In: Conti P, Cham D, eds. *PET-CT. A Case Based Approach.* Singapore: Springer Science+Business Media, Inc; 2005:258–263.

57. Sahani DV, Bonaffini PA, Catalano OA, Guimaraes AR, Blake MA. State-of-the-art PET/CT of the pancreas: current role and emerging indications. *Radiographics: A Review Publication of the Radiological Society of North America, Inc.* July–August 2012;32(4):1133–1158. discussion 1158–1160.

58. Gastrointestinal Carcinoid Tumors Treatment. Diagnostics: Biochemical Markers, Imaging, and Approach. http://www.cancer.gov/types/gi-carcinoid-tumors/hp/gi-carcinoid-treatment-pdq#link/_49_toc.

59. Diez M, Teule A, Salazar R. Gastroenteropancreatic neuroendocrine tumors: diagnosis and treatment. *Annals of Gastroenterology: Quarterly Publication of the Hellenic Society of Gastroenterology.* 2013;26(1):29–36.

60. Rufini V, Baum RP, Castaldi P, et al. Role of PET/CT in the functional imaging of endocrine pancreatic tumors. *Abdominal Imaging.* December 2012;37(6):1004–1020.

61. Sundin A, Eriksson B, Bergstrom M, Langstrom B, Oberg K, Orlefors H. PET in the diagnosis of neuroendocrine tumors. *Annals of the New York Academy of Sciences.* April 2004;1014:246–257.

62. Toumpanakis C, Kim MK, Rinke A, et al. Combination of cross-sectional and molecular imaging studies in the localization of gastroenteropancreatic neuroendocrine tumors. *Neuroendocrinology.* 2014;99(2):63–74.

63. Thapa P, Ranade R, Ostwal V, Shrikhande SV, Goel M, Basu S. Performance of 177Lu-DOTATATE-based peptide receptor radionuclide therapy in metastatic gastroenteropancreatic neuroendocrine tumor: a multiparametric response evaluation correlating with primary tumor site, tumor proliferation index, and dual tracer imaging characteristics. *Nuclear Medicine Communications.* May 27, 2016.

64. Nilica B, Waitz D, Stevanovic V, et al. Direct comparison of (68)Ga-DOTA-TOC and (18)F-FDG PET/CT in the follow-up of patients with neuroendocrine tumour treated with the first full peptide receptor radionuclide therapy cycle. *European Journal of Nuclear Medicine and Molecular Imaging.* August 2016;43(9):1585–1592.

65. Luo G, Liu Z, Guo M, et al. (18)F-FDG PET/CT can be used to detect non-functioning pancreatic neuroendocrine tumors. *International Journal of Oncology.* October 2014;45(4):1531–1536.

66. Howlader N, Noone A, Krapcho M, et al. *SEER Cancer Statistics Review, 1975-2013;* 2016. http://seer.cancer.gov/csr/1975_2013/.

67. Kalra MK, Maher MM, Boland GW, Saini S, Fischman AJ. Correlation of positron emission tomography and CT in evaluating pancreatic tumors: technical and clinical implications. *American Journal of Roentgenology.* August 2003;181(2):387–393.

68. Moadel RM, Blaufox MD, Freeman LM. The role of positron emission tomography in gastrointestinal imaging. *Gastroenterology Clinics of North America.* September 2002;31(3):841–861.

69. Tamm EP, Silverman PM, Charnsangavej C, Evans DB. Diagnosis, staging, and surveillance of pancreatic cancer. *American Journal of Roentgenology.* May 2003;180(5):1311–1323.

70. Valinas R, Barrier A, Montravers F, Houry S, Talbot JN, Huguier M. 18 F-fluorodeoxyglucose positron emission tomography for characterization and initial staging of pancreatic tumors. *Gastroenterologie Clinique et Biologique.* October 2002;26(10):888–892.

71. Lemke AJ, Niehues SM, Hosten N, et al. Retrospective digital image fusion of multidetector CT and 18F-FDG PET: clinical value in pancreatic lesions–a prospective study with 104 patients. *Journal of Nuclear Medicine: Official Publication, Society of Nuclear Medicine.* August 2004;45(8):1279–1286.

72. Santhanam P, Chandramahanti S, Kroiss A, et al. Nuclear imaging of neuroendocrine tumors with unknown primary: why, when and how? *European Journal of Nuclear Medicine and Molecular Imaging.* June 2015;42(7):1144–1155.

73. Kumar R, Sharma P, Garg P, et al. Role of (68)Ga-DOTA-TOC PET-CT in the diagnosis and staging of pancreatic neuroendocrine tumours. *European Radiology.* November 2011;21(11):2408–2416.

74. Deppen SA, Liu E, Blume JD, et al. Safety and efficacy of 68Ga-DOTATATE PET/CT for diagnosis, staging, and treatment management of neuroendocrine tumors. *Journal of Nuclear Medicine: Official Publication, Society of Nuclear Medicine.* May 2016;57(5):708–714.

75. Mojtahedi A, Thamake S, Tworowska I, Ranganathan D, Delpassand ES. The value of (68)Ga-DOTATATE PET/CT in diagnosis and management of neuroendocrine tumors compared to current FDA approved imaging modalities: a review of literature. *American Journal of Nuclear Medicine and Molecular Imaging.* 2014;4(5):426–434.

76. Srirajaskanthan R, Kayani I, Quigley AM, Soh J, Caplin ME, Bomanji J. The role of 68Ga-DOTATATE PET in patients with neuroendocrine tumors and negative or equivocal findings on 111In-DTPA-octreotide scintigraphy. *Journal of Nuclear Medicine: Official Publication, Society of Nuclear Medicine.* June 2010;51(6):875–882.

77. Virgolini I, Gabriel M, Kroiss A, et al. Current knowledge on the sensitivity of the (68)Ga-somatostatin receptor positron emission tomography and the SUV_{max} reference range for management of pancreatic neuroendocrine tumours. *European Journal of Nuclear Medicine and Molecular Imaging.* October 2016;43(11):2072–2083.

78. Wild D, Macke HR, Waser B, et al. 68Ga-DOTANOC: a first compound for PET imaging with high affinity for somatostatin receptor subtypes 2 and 5. *European Journal of Nuclear Medicine and Molecular Imaging.* June 2005;32(6):724.

79. Naswa N, Sharma P, Kumar A, et al. Gallium-68-DOTA-NOC PET/CT of patients with gastroenteropancreatic neuroendocrine tumors: a prospective single-center study. *American Journal of Roentgenology.* November 2011;197(5):1221–1228.

80. Sadowski SM, Neychev V, Millo C, et al. Prospective study of 68Ga-DOTATATE positron emission tomography/computed tomography for detecting gastro-enteropancreatic neuroendocrine tumors and unknown primary sites. *Journal of Clinical Oncology: Official Journal of the American Society of Clinical Oncology.* February 20, 2016;34(6):588–596.

81. Haug AR, Cindea-Drimus R, Auernhammer CJ, et al. Neuroendocrine tumor recurrence: diagnosis with 68 Ga-DOTATATE PET/CT. *Radiology.* February 2014;270(2):517–525.

82. Campana D, Ambrosini V, Pezzilli R, et al. Standardized uptake values of (68)Ga-DOTANOC PET: a promising prognostic tool in neuroendocrine tumors. *Journal of Nuclear Medicine: Official Publication, Society of Nuclear Medicine.* March 2010;51(3):353–359.

83. Haug AR, Auernhammer CJ, Wangler B, et al. 68Ga-DOTATATE PET/CT for the early prediction of response to somatostatin receptor-mediated radionuclide therapy in patients with well-differentiated neuroendocrine tumors. *Journal of Nuclear Medicine: Official Publication, Society of Nuclear Medicine.* September 2010;51(9):1349–1356.

84. Nakamoto Y, Ishimori T, Sano K, et al. Clinical efficacy of dual-phase scanning using 68Ga-DOTATOC-PET/CT in the detection of neuroendocrine tumours. *Clinical Radiology.* October 2016;71(10):1069.e1–1069.e5.

85. Kayani I, Bomanji JB, Groves A, et al. Functional imaging of neuroendocrine tumors with combined PET/CT using 68Ga-DOTATATE (DOTA-DPhe1,Tyr3-octreotate) and 18F-FDG. *Cancer.* June 2008;112(11):2447–2455.

86. Hoegerle S, Altehoefer C, Ghanem N, et al. Whole-body 18F dopa PET for detection of gastrointestinal carcinoid tumors. *Radiology.* August 2001;220(2):373–380.

87. Koopmans KP, Neels OC, Kema IP, et al. Improved staging of patients with carcinoid and islet cell tumors with 18F-dihydroxy-phenyl-alanine and 11C-5-hydroxy-tryptophan positron emission tomography. *Journal of Clinical Oncology: Official Journal of the American Society of Clinical Oncology.* March 20, 2008;26(9):1489–1495.

88. Nanni C, Fanti S, Rubello D. 18F-DOPA PET and PET/CT. *Journal of Nuclear Medicine: Official Publication, Society of Nuclear Medicine.* October 2007;48(10):1577–1579.

89. Koopmans KP, de Vries EG, Kema IP, et al. Staging of carcinoid tumours with 18F-DOPA PET: a prospective, diagnostic accuracy study. *The Lancet. Oncology.* September 2006;7(9):728–734.

90. Yakemchuk VN, Jager PL, Chirakal R, Reid R, Major P, Gulenchyn KY. PET/CT using (1)(8)F-FDOPA provides improved staging of carcinoid tumor patients in a Canadian setting. *Nuclear Medicine Communications.* March 2012;33(3):322–330.

91. Eriksson B, Orlefors H, Oberg K, Sundin A, Bergstrom M, Langstrom B. Developments in PET for the detection of endocrine tumours. *Best Practice & Research. Clinical Endocrinology & Metabolism.* June 2005;19(2):311–324.

92. Imperiale A, Bahougne T, Goichot B, Bachellier P, Taieb D, Namer IJ. Dynamic 18F-FDOPA PET findings after carbidopa premedication in 2 adult patients with insulinoma-related hyperinsulinemic hypoglycemia. *Clinical Nuclear Medicine*. August 2015;40(8):682–684.

93. Orlefors H, Sundin A, Garske U, et al. Whole-body (11) C-5-hydroxytryptophan positron emission tomography as a universal imaging technique for neuroendocrine tumors: comparison with somatostatin receptor scintigraphy and computed tomography. *The Journal of Clinical Endocrinology and Metabolism*. June 2005;90(6):3392–3400.

94. Orlefors H, Sundin A, Eriksson B, et al. PET-guided surgery – high correlation between positron emission tomography with 11C-5-hydroxytryptophane (5-HTP) and surgical findings in abdominal neuroendocrine tumours. *Cancers*. 2012;4(1):100–112.

95. Pfeifer A, Knigge U, Mortensen J, et al. Clinical PET of neuroendocrine tumors using 64Cu-DOTATATE: first-in-humans study. *Journal of Nuclear Medicine: Official Publication, Society of Nuclear Medicine*. August 2012;53(8):1207–1215.

96. Pfeifer A, Knigge U, Binderup T, et al. 64Cu-DOTATATE PET for neuroendocrine tumors: a prospective head-to-head comparison with 111In-DTPA-octreotide in 112 patients. *Journal of Nuclear Medicine: Official Publication, Society of Nuclear Medicine*. June 2015;56(6):847–854.

97. Tran K, Khan S, Taghizadehasl M, et al. Gallium-68 Dotatate PET/CT is superior to other imaging modalities in the detection of medullary carcinoma of the thyroid in the presence of high serum calcitonin. *Hellenic Journal of Nuclear Medicine*. January–April 2015;18(1):19–24.

98. Medullary Thyroid Cancer. Diagnosis. http://columbiasurgery.org/conditions-and-treatments/medullary-thyroid-cancer.

99. Ganeshan D, Paulson E, Duran C, Cabanillas ME, Busaidy NL, Charnsangavej C. Current update on medullary thyroid carcinoma. *American Journal of Roentgenology*. December 2013;201(6):W867–W876.

100. Conry BG, Papathanasiou ND, Prakash V, et al. Comparison of (68)Ga-DOTATATE and (18)F-fluorodeoxyglucose PET/CT in the detection of recurrent medullary thyroid carcinoma. *European Journal of Nuclear Medicine and Molecular Imaging*. January 2010;37(1):49–57.

101. Ambrosini V, Morigi JJ, Nanni C, Castellucci P, Fanti S. Current status of PET imaging of neuroendocrine tumours ([18F]FDOPA, [68Ga]tracers, [11C]/[18F]-HTP). *The Quarterly Journal of Nuclear Medicine and Molecular Imaging: Official Publication of the Italian Association of Nuclear Medicine*. March 2015;59(1):58–69.

102. Naswa N, Sharma P, Suman Kc S, et al. Prospective evaluation of 68Ga-DOTA-NOC PET-CT in patients with recurrent medullary thyroid carcinoma: comparison with 18F-FDG PET-CT. *Nuclear Medicine Communications*. July 2012;33(7):766–774.

103. Archier A, Heimburger C, Guerin C, et al. (18)F-DOPA PET/CT in the diagnosis and localization of persistent medullary thyroid carcinoma. *European Journal of Nuclear Medicine and Molecular Imaging*. June 2016;43(6):1027–1033.

104. Delorme S, Raue F. Medullary Thyroid Carcinoma: Imaging. *Recent Results in Cancer Research. Fortschritte der Krebsforschung. Progres dans les recherches sur le cancer*. 2015;204:91–116.

105. Beheshti M, Pocher S, Vali R, et al. The value of 18F-DOPA PET-CT in patients with medullary thyroid carcinoma: comparison with 18F-FDG PET-CT. *European Radiology*. June 2009;19(6):1425–1434.

106. Treglia G, Castaldi P, Villani MF, et al. Comparison of 18F-DOPA, 18F-FDG and 68Ga-somatostatin analogue PET/CT in patients with recurrent medullary thyroid carcinoma. *European Journal of Nuclear Medicine and Molecular Imaging*. April 2012;39(4):569–580.

107. Treglia G, Villani MF, Giordano A, Rufini V. Detection rate of recurrent medullary thyroid carcinoma using fluorine-18 fluorodeoxyglucose positron emission tomography: a meta-analysis. *Endocrine*. December 2012;42(3):535–545.

108. Ong SC, Schoder H, Patel SG, et al. Diagnostic accuracy of 18F-FDG PET in restaging patients with medullary thyroid carcinoma and elevated calcitonin levels. *Journal of Nuclear Medicine: Official Publication, Society of Nuclear Medicine*. April 2007;48(4):501–507.

109. Szakall Jr S, Esik O, Bajzik G, et al. 18F-FDG PET detection of lymph node metastases in medullary thyroid carcinoma. *Journal of Nuclear Medicine: Official Publication, Society of Nuclear Medicine*. January 2002;43(1):66–71.

110. Arora S, Agarwal KK, Karunanithi S, Tripathi M, Kumar R. Recurrent malignant pheochromocytoma with unusual omental metastasis: (68)Ga-DOTANOC PET/CT and (131)I-MIBG SPECT/CT scintigraphy findings. *Indian Journal of Nuclear Medicine: The Official Journal of the Society of Nuclear Medicine, India*. October 2014;29(4):286–288.

111. Mundschenk J, Unger N, Schulz S, et al. Somatostatin receptor subtypes in human pheochromocytoma: subcellular expression pattern and functional relevance for octreotide scintigraphy. *The Journal of Clinical Endocrinology and Metabolism*. November 2003;88(11):5150–5157.

112. Sharma P, Dhull VS, Arora S, et al. Diagnostic accuracy of (68)Ga-DOTANOC PET/CT imaging in pheochromocytoma. *European Journal of Nuclear Medicine and Molecular Imaging*. March 2014;41(3):494–504.

113. Janssen I, Chen CC, Millo CM, et al. PET/CT comparing (68)Ga-DOTATATE and other radiopharmaceuticals and in comparison with CT/MRI for the localization of sporadic metastatic pheochromocytoma and paraganglioma. *European Journal of Nuclear Medicine and Molecular Imaging*. September 2016;43(10):1784–1791.

114. Tan TH, Hussein Z, Saad FF, Shuaib IL. Diagnostic Performance of (68)Ga-DOTATATE PET/CT, (18)F-FDG PET/CT and (131)I-MIBG scintigraphy in mapping metastatic pheochromocytoma and paraganglioma. *Nuclear Medicine and Molecular Imaging.* June 2015;49(2):143–151.

115. Janssen I, Blanchet EM, Adams K, et al. Superiority of [68Ga]-DOTATATE PET/CT to other functional imaging modalities in the localization of SDHB-associated metastatic pheochromocytoma and paraganglioma. *Clinical Cancer Research: An Official Journal of the American Association for Cancer Research.* September 1, 2015;21(17):3888–3895.

116. Bandopadhyaya GP, Kumar A, Kumari J. Role of (18) F-DOPA PET/CT and (131)I-MIBG planar scintigraphy in evaluating patients with pheochromocytoma. *Hellenic Journal of Nuclear Medicine.* September–December 2015;18(suppl 1):141.

117. Taieb D, Sebag F, Barlier A, et al. 18F-FDG avidity of pheochromocytomas and paragangliomas: a new molecular imaging signature? *Journal of Nuclear Medicine: Official Publication, Society of Nuclear Medicine.* May 2009;50(5):711–717.

118. Hoegerle S, Nitzsche E, Altehoefer C, et al. Pheochromocytomas: detection with 18F DOPA whole body PET–initial results. *Radiology.* February 2002;222(2):507–512.

119. Timmers HJ, Eisenhofer G, Carrasquillo JA, et al. Use of 6-[18F]-fluorodopamine positron emission tomography (PET) as first-line investigation for the diagnosis and localization of non-metastatic and metastatic pheochromocytoma (PHEO). *Clinical Endocrinology.* July 2009;71(1):11–17.

120. Timmers HJ, Chen CC, Carrasquillo JA, et al. Comparison of 18F-fluoro-L-DOPA, 18F-fluoro-deoxyglucose, and 18F-fluorodopamine PET and 123I-MIBG scintigraphy in the localization of pheochromocytoma and paraganglioma. *The Journal of Clinical Endocrinology and Metabolism.* December 2009;94(12):4757–4767.

121. Blanchet EM, Taieb D, Millo C, et al. 18F-FLT PET/CT in the evaluation of pheochromocytomas and paragangliomas: a pilot study. *Journal of Nuclear Medicine: Official Publication, Society of Nuclear Medicine.* December 2015;56(12):1849–1854.

122. Naswa N, Sharma P, Kumar A, et al. (6)(8)Ga-DOTANOC PET/CT in patients with carcinoma of unknown primary of neuroendocrine origin. *Clinical Nuclear Medicine.* March 2012;37(3):245–251.

123. Pavlidis N, Khaled H, Gaafar R. A mini review on cancer of unknown primary site: a clinical puzzle for the oncologists. *Journal of Advanced Research.* May 2015;6(3):375–382.

124. Pruthi A, Pankaj P, Verma R, Jain A, Belho ES, Mahajan H. Ga-68 DOTANOC PET/CT imaging in detection of primary site in patients with metastatic neuroendocrine tumours of unknown origin and its impact on clinical decision making: experience from a tertiary care centre in India. *Journal of Gastrointestinal Oncology.* June 2016;7(3):449–461.

125. Prasad V, Ambrosini V, Hommann M, Hoersch D, Fanti S, Baum RP. Detection of unknown primary neuroendocrine tumours (CUP-NET) using (68)Ga-DOTA-NOC receptor PET/CT. *European Journal of Nuclear Medicine and Molecular Imaging.* January 2010;37(1):67–77.

126. Schreiter NF, Bartels AM, Froeling V, et al. Searching for primaries in patients with neuroendocrine tumors (NET) of unknown primary and clinically suspected NET: evaluation of Ga-68 DOTATOC PET/CT and In-111 DTPA octreotide SPECT/CT. *Radiology and Oncology.* December 2014;48(4):339–347.

127. Menda Y, O'Dorisio T, Graham M, et al. Role of Gallium-68 DOTATOC PET-CT in neuroendocrine tumors with unknown primary site. *Journal of Nuclear Medicine: Official Publication, Society of Nuclear Medicine.* 2015;56(suppl 3):143.

128. Imperiale A, Rust E, Gabriel S, et al. 18F-fluorodihydroxyphenylalanine PET/CT in patients with neuroendocrine tumors of unknown origin: relation to tumor origin and differentiation. *Journal of Nuclear Medicine: Official Publication, Society of Nuclear Medicine.* March 2014;55(3):367–372.

129. Bodei L, Kwekkeboom DJ, Kidd M, Modlin IM, Krenning EP. Radiolabeled somatostatin analogue therapy of gastroenteropancreatic cancer. *Seminars in Nuclear Medicine.* May 2016;46(3):225–238.

130. van Vliet EI, van Eijck CH, de Krijger RR, et al. Neoadjuvant treatment of nonfunctioning pancreatic neuroendocrine tumors with [^{177}Lu-DOTA^0,Tyr^3]octreotate. *Journal of Nuclear Medicine: Official Publication, Society of Nuclear Medicine.* November 2015;56(11):1647–1653.

131. Strosberg J, Wolin E, Chasen B, Kulke M. NETTER-1 phase III: progression-free survival, radiographic response, and preliminary overall survival results in patients with midgut neuroendocrine tumors treated with 177-Lu-Dotatate. *Journal of Clinical Oncology: Official Journal of the American Society of Clinical Oncology.* 2016;34(suppl 4S):194.

132. van Essen M, Krenning EP, Kam BL, de Herder WW, Feelders RA, Kwekkeboom DJ. Salvage therapy with (177)Lu-octreotate in patients with bronchial and gastroenteropancreatic neuroendocrine tumors. *Journal of Nuclear Medicine: Official Publication, Society of Nuclear Medicine.* March 2010;51(3):383–390.

133. Bergsma H, Konijnenberg MW, van der Zwan WA, et al. Nephrotoxicity after PRRT with (177)Lu-DOTA-octreotate. *European Journal of Nuclear Medicine and Molecular Imaging.* September 2016;43(10):1802–1811.

134. Gupta SK, Singla S, Bal C. Renal and hematological toxicity in patients of neuroendocrine tumors after peptide receptor radionuclide therapy with ^{177}Lu-DOTATATE. *Cancer Biotherapy & Radiopharmaceuticals.* November 2012;27(9):593–599.

135. Bodei L, Cremonesi M, Kidd M, et al. Peptide receptor radionuclide therapy for advanced neuroendocrine tumors. *Thoracic Surgery Clinics.* August 2014;24(3):333–349.

136. Bodei L, Kidd M, Prasad V, Modlin IM. Peptide receptor radionuclide therapy of neuroendocrine tumors. *Frontiers of Hormone Research*. 2015;44:198–215.

137. Kwekkeboom DJ, Kam BL, van Essen M, et al. Somatostatin-receptor-based imaging and therapy of gastroenteropancreatic neuroendocrine tumors. *Endocrine-Related Cancer*. March 2010;17(1):R53–R73.

138. Ezziddin S, Attassi M, Yong-Hing CJ, et al. Predictors of long-term outcome in patients with well-differentiated gastroenteropancreatic neuroendocrine tumors after peptide receptor radionuclide therapy with ^{177}Lu-octreotate. *Journal of Nuclear Medicine: Official Publication, Society of Nuclear Medicine*. February 2014;55(2):183–190.

CHAPTER 6

Colorectal Cancer

MOHSEN BEHESHTI • ALIREZA REZAEE • KEN HERRMANN •
MARKUS RADERER • WERNER LANGSTEGER

BACKGROUND[1–8]

- Colorectal cancer (CRC) is overall the third most common type of malignancy worldwide (8% of all cancers).
- CRC is the third most common cancer-related leading cause of death in the United States.
- There is a higher prevalence in men and in patients >60 years.
- Early clinical symptoms include:
  - Hematochezia/melena, abdominal pain, anemia, bowel habit alteration.
- Colonoscopy is the most accurate and preferred primary diagnostic procedure. CT colonography is an alternative.
- Metastatic disease is seen at first presentation in 20% of patients.
- Surgery is the standard treatment, with or without chemoradiation and/or targeted therapy:
  - Stage 0: Local surgical excision, occasional colectomy for very large tumors
  - Stage I: Partial colectomy and regional lymph node dissection
  - Stage II: Partial colectomy ± adjuvant chemotherapy or radiation therapy
  - Stage III: Partial colectomy + regional lymph node dissection + chemotherapy ± radiation therapy
  - Stage IV: Colectomy + neoadjuvant/adjuvant chemotherapy and/or targeted therapy + radiation therapy (in advanced cases)

Five-Year Survival[9]

- Stage I   (T1 or T2, N0, M0)   94%
- Stage II   (T3-4, N0, M0)   82%
- Stage III   (any T, N1-3, M0)   67%
- Stage IV   (any T, any N, M1)   11%

Prognostic Factors[10]

- Preoperative carcinoembryonic antigen (CEA)
- Tumor deposits
- Circumferential resection margin
- Perineural invasion
- Tumor regression grade after neoadjuvant therapy
- K-ras, BRAF, and DCC mutations
- Tumor stage
- Lymphovascular invasion

TUMOR CHARACTERISTICS AND TYPICAL BEHAVIOR

Histopathology[11]

- Adenocarcinoma >90%
- Neuroendocrine, squamous cell, adenosquamous, spindle cell, undifferentiated <10%

Cancer Distribution[12]

- Anorectal   29%
- Appendix, cecum, and ascending colon   23%
- Descending and sigmoid colon   23%
- Transverse colon   10%

COMMON PATTERN OF SPREAD

Lymph Nodes

- Ascending and transverse colon: pericolic, right colic, middle colic
- Descending colon: pericolic, left colic, inferior mesenteric, middle colic, sigmoidal
- Rectosigmoid: pericolic, inferior mesenteric, left colic, superior and middle rectal (hemorrhoidal), perirectal, sigmoid mesenteric, sigmoidal
- Rectum: perirectal; sigmoid mesenteric; inferior mesenteric; lateral and presacral; sacral promontory; internal iliac; superior, middle, and inferior rectal (hemorrhoidal)

Distant Metastasis[13]

- 20% at presentation
- Most common sites:
  - Liver   50%
  - Peritoneum   25%
  - Lung   10%–20%

TNM CLASSIFICATION

The TNM classification and cancer staging guidelines are given in Tables 6.1 and 6.2.

CLINICAL GUIDELINES[14–16]

The European Society for Medical Oncology (ESMO) and National Comprehensive Cancer Network (NCCN) clinical guidelines are given in Table 6.3.

EVIDENCE-BASED VIEWPOINTS[14,15,17]

- FDG PET/CT is appropriate for staging of stage IV disease and/or to rule out or detect synchronous metastases.
- FDG PET/CT is used in restaging of patients with CRC, especially in the case of rising tumor markers or clinical suspicion of recurrence but equivocal findings on conventional imaging modalities.

COST-EFFECTIVENESS[18–20]

- FDG PET/CT is cost-effective in the preoperative staging of recurrent colon and rectal cancers, as well as in the staging of metastatic disease, but not primary colon or rectal cancer.

CLINICAL POINT OF VIEW

Primary Staging

The primary decisive information in newly diagnosed CRC is the extent of disease to differentiate between:

a. Stages I-III (i.e., absence of metastatic disease beyond regional lymph nodes) and
b. Stage IV (i.e., metastatic disease)

Patients with stage I-III disease are candidates for primary resection with curative potential, whereas patients with stage IV disease can or should be spared resection of the primary in the absence of stenosis, because surgical treatment may provide no clinical benefit in this setting.

However, patients with operable metastatic lesions in the liver or lung may still undergo potentially curative surgery after neoadjuvant systemic therapy. Thus, in patients with stage IV CRC, not only the information about the presence of organ metastases but also the extent of metastases (i.e., diffuse versus potentially resectable) is of crucial clinical importance to guide patient management.

Follow-Up After Surgery

a. Patients with elevated tumor marker (i.e., CEA): defining the presence of recurrent disease in terms of (1) localization and (2) extent of disease to assess the possibility of potential reoperation, i.e., localized or operable recurrence versus diffusely metastatic disease.
b. Rectal cancer: differentiation between posttherapeutic scar tissue and viable tumors

---

TABLE 6.1
Colorectal Cancer TNM Classification

TNM	T1	T2	T3	T4a	T4b
N0	I	I	IIA	IIB	IIC
N1	IIIA	IIIA	IIIB	IIIB	IIIC
N2a	IIIA	IIIB	IIIB	IIIC	IIIC
N2b	IIIB	IIIB	IIIC	IIIC	IIIC
M1a	IVA	IVA	IVA	IVA	IVA
M1b	IVB	IVB	IVB	IVB	IVB

TABLE 6.2
Colorectal Cancer TNM Staging Guidelines

Primary Tumor (T)	Regional Lymph Nodes (N)	Distant Metastasis (M)
T0: No evidence of primary tumor **Tis:** Carcinoma in situ: intraepithelial or invasion of lamina propria **T1:** Tumor invades submucosa **T2:** Tumor invades muscularis propria **T3:** Tumor invades through the muscularis propria into pericolorectal tissues **T4a:** Tumor penetrates to the surface of the visceral peritoneum **T4b:** Tumor directly invades or is adherent to other organs or structures	**N0:** No regional lymph node metastasis **N1:** Metastasis in 1 to 3 regional lymph nodes **N1a:** Metastasis in 1 regional lymph node **N1b:** Metastasis in 2 to 3 regional lymph nodes **N1c:** Tumor deposit(s) in the subserosa, mesentery, or nonperitonealized pericolic or perirectal tissues without regional nodal metastasis **N2:** Metastasis in 4 or more regional lymph nodes **N2a:** Metastasis in 4 to 6 regional lymph nodes **N2b:** Metastasis in 7 or more regional lymph nodes	**M0:** No distant metastasis **M1:** Distant metastasis **M1a:** Metastasis confined to one organ or site (for example, liver, lung, ovary, nonregional node) **M1b:** Metastases in more than one organ/site or the peritoneum

Metastatic Disease

a. Before initiation of therapy: differentiation between potentially operable and palliative situations (see earlier discussion).

b. Response assessment:

Currently, systemic therapies including novel antibodies (e.g., anti–vascular endothelial growth factor or anti–epidermal growth factor receptor) and chemotherapies, such as irinotecan, oxaliplatin, and fluoropyrimidines, show promise regarding response rates and survival. However, such therapeutic approaches are associated with increased toxicities and costs. Thus, methods to identify responders from nonresponders would be highly valuable to select optimal therapy regimens for patients who may benefit from that and prevent unnecessary toxicities and costs.

PITFALLS[21]

False Positive

- Physiologic FDG uptake within the colon may be intense, specifically in the cecum, ascending colon, and rectal region.
- Physiologic FDG uptake in postoperatively posteriorly displaced pelvic organs may mimic rectal cancer recurrence. The false-positive interpretation rate is reduced by the anatomic coregistration of the CT component in modern PET/CT scanners.
- Hyperplastic and adenomatous polyps may have high FDG uptake.
- Fistula and sinus tracts, as well as abscesses, can have intense FDG uptake; correlation with the CT scan is helpful.
- Crohn disease, ulcerative colitis, typhlitis, and diverticulitis may represent false-positive FDG findings.

False Negative

- Mucinous adenocarcinoma
- Within 4 weeks of chemotherapy

TABLE 6.3
ESMO and NCCN Colorectal Cancer Clinical Guidelines

Clinical Guidelines	Initial Diagnosis (Primary Tumor)	M-Staging
ESMO	No	Yes
NCCN	No	Yes[a]

ESMO, European Society for Medical Oncology; *NCCN*, National Comprehensive Cancer Network.
[a]In case of inconclusive findings on CT or MRI, change the management.

- Small tumor and/or lymph node metastasis (<8 mm)
- Metformin consumption (It may cause a diffuse colonic FDG uptake and obscure the underlying malignancy.)
- Common false-negative results for all cancers: early-stage malignancy, hyperglycemic state, small lesions (<8 mm)

DISCUSSION

According to clinical guidelines, CT and MRI are suggested as standard imaging modalities for the assessment of patients with CRC. The staging accuracy of CT is about 50%–70% for colon cancer, which is almost similar to that of MRI, and even improves with higher tumor (T) stages. Corresponding accuracies for the detection of lymph node (N) improvement are similar for both modalities, with approximately 85% accuracy. However, MRI is slightly superior to CT in detecting liver metastases.[14]

Primary Staging/Restaging

FDG PET/CT has become an essential diagnostic procedure in evaluating most of the cancers before or after the treatment. However, there are no sufficient data to support the use of FDG PET/CT in the preoperative staging of primary, recurrent, and metastatic CRC. This is mainly because FDG PET/CT seems to have no significant impact on decision making for therapy.[20,22]

This aspect is also emphasized in the most recent major clinical guidelines, such as NCCN, American Society of Clinical Oncology, and ESMO. For example, the NCCN guideline mentioned that FDG PET/CT does not replace a contrast-enhanced diagnostic CT scan in the primary evaluation of nonmetastatic CRC. However, the use of FDG PET/CT could be considered in the case of inconclusive CT and/or MRI findings to rule out or confirm metastasis. If the CEA level is elevated after therapy, contrast-enhanced CT is the diagnostic procedure of choice. However, FDG PET/CT is recommended if CT fails to detect the location of disease recurrence or metastasis.[14–17,23]

In contrast to the current clinical practice, a meta-analysis including 2283 patients with primary CRC reported a very good performance of FDG PET/CT for primary tumor detection and T- and M-staging.[24] This is also approved by some other investigators.[25] However, its performance was only mediocre for N-staging, with a pooled sensitivity of only 43%. However, ^{18}F-FDG PET/CT is a valuable imaging modality for the evaluation of hepatic and extrahepatic metastases in patients with CRC.[26] This is also mentioned in major clinical guidelines, such as ESMO.[16] In a follow-up meta-analysis including 39 articles and 3391 patients with CRC, FDG PET/CT demonstrated a significantly higher sensitivity than CT scan for the detection of liver metastases from CRC (94% vs. 84%).[27] Kuehl and colleagues calculated a sensitivity and accuracy of 95% and 97% for FDG PET/CT in the detection of intrahepatic and extrahepatic metastases, whereas the values for CT scan were 97% and 94%, respectively. However, because of the limited spatial resolution of FDG PET/CT, MRI is still superior in the evaluation of liver lesions smaller than 1 cm.[28]

Moreover, FDG PET/CT has an impact on the treatment approach by upstaging 50% and downstaging 21% of patients with lower rectal malignancies.[29] Petersen and colleagues discovered a modification of the treatment plan based on the FDG PET/CT findings in 30% of the included 67 patients with CRC.[30]

Recurrent Disease

FDG PET/CT is recommended by the Royal College of Radiologists for patients with increasing tumor markers and/or clinical suspicion of recurrence but equivocal findings on other imaging modalities.[17]

Some published research studies demonstrated the usefulness of FDG PET/CT for restaging of patients with CRC. A prospective study with 75 patients reported a high accuracy and sensitivity for restaging of local and metastatic recurrent CRC.[25] Serial CEA measurements are used after surgery to detect cancer recurrence. However, this tumor marker has a relatively low sensitivity (about 80%) and specificity (about 70%).[31] Metser and colleagues retrospectively analyzed 50 patients with colorectal cancer and elevated posttherapy serum CEA levels and discovered that FDG PET/CT is superior to CT alone in detection of recurrent disease and diagnostic CT has a limited sensitivity for this purpose. The corresponding specificity was 94% for both modalities, whereas FDG PET/CT was more sensitive than contrast-enhanced multidetector CT (97% vs. 70%), respectively.[32]

Therapy Monitoring

FDG PET/CT had an impact in the accurate planning of external beam radiation therapy. It helps to protect normal tissue, especially in rectal cancer, in which radiation therapy is an essential part of the treatment.[33] Furthermore, FDG PET/CT allows for the evaluation of response to therapy. One study evaluated 42 patients with locally advanced rectal cancer by FDG PET/CT before and 12 days after the initiation of radiochemotherapy. The authors reported that the modality is an early predictor of tumor response to treatment. The important information provided by FDG PET/CT for monitoring response to therapy and changing patients' management has also been reported by numerous other researchers.[34]

Prognostic Value

The prognostic role of FDG PET/CT in patients with CRC is also well investigated. FDG PET/CT seems to be the superior prognosticator compared with conventional imaging. Avallone and colleagues demonstrated a significantly better 5-year relapse-free survival in responders compared with nonresponders to chemotherapy in 42 patients with locally advanced rectal cancer.[34] Ogawa and colleagues performed ^{18}F-FDG PET/CT in 325 patients with CRC before surgery and concluded that the patients with high total lesion glycolysis (TLG) and tumor metabolic volume have a poorer prognosis. They also determined TLG as one of the independent predictors of poor prognosis in such patients.[35]

Xia and colleagues analyzed 15 studies with 867 patients in a meta-analysis and claimed that FDG PET/CT is useful for predicting overall survival in patients with CRC with liver metastases.[36] A prospective study evaluated the metabolic activity of metastatic lesions from CRC in 152 patients and concluded that the lesions' standardized uptake value (SUV) is a prognosticator for overall survival independent of the consecutive therapy ($P = .002$). The median survival was significantly longer in patients with an SUV < 4.26 (32 months) compared with those with an SUV > 4.26 (19 months).[37]

Radiopharmaceuticals Beyond ^{18}F-FDG

Although FDG PET/CT is an established imaging method in patients with cancer, to mitigate its shortcomings in the differentiation between malignant and inflammatory lesions, development of more specific PET radiotracers is warranted. Proliferation biomarkers such as fluorothymidine (FLT) and hypoxia tracers such as ^{60}Cu-diacetyl-bis (N[4]-methylthiosemicarbazone) (^{60}Cu-ATSM) have been studied so far in CRC. Multiple studies showed that ^{18}F-FLT PET/CT is comparable with ^{18}F-FDG PET/CT in the evaluation of primary CRC and corresponding lymph node metastases.[38,39]

In a pilot study of 17 patients with rectal cancer who underwent ^{60}Cu-ATSM PET/CT, the authors concluded that this tracer may predict patients' survival and malignancy response to neoadjuvant chemotherapy. Other positron emitters are under investigation.[40]

CONCLUSION

FDG PET/CT seems to have no significant role in the primary staging of CRC, except in stage IV disease with distant metastases at presentation. FDG PET/CT is useful for restaging or evaluation of recurrence, as well as in patients who are presenting with distant metastatic disease. FDG PET/CT is also capable of predicting the patients' survival and prognosis, evaluating tumor response to therapy, and affecting patients' management.

TEACHING CASES

Case 1: Staging Colon Cancer, Distant Metastasis

Findings

A 76-year-old male with colon cancer. FDG PET/CT demonstrates a primary tumor in the ascending colon (B, arrow). FDG-avid bilateral adrenal (C, arrowhead), peritoneal (C, arrow), left pulmonary (D, arrow), and right hilar (E, arrow) metastases are noted (Fig. 6.1).

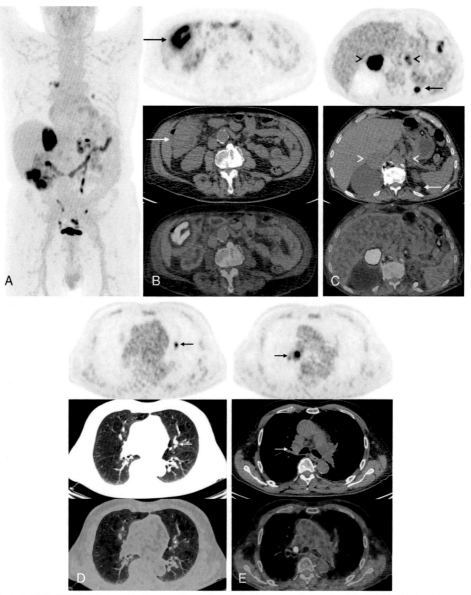

FIG. 6.1 FDG PET/CT demonstrating a primary tumor in the ascending colon (B, *arrow*). FDG-avid bilateral adrenal (C, *arrowhead*), peritoneal (C, *arrow*), left pulmonary (D, *arrow*), and right hilar (E, *arrow*) metastases are noted. A, FDG PET MIP image.

Teaching points
- Metastatic disease could be the first presentation in 20% of patients with advanced CRC.
- FDG PET/CT is superior to stand-alone CT in differentiating adrenal adenoma from metastasis and diagnosing the lymph node metastases especially in atypical locations and with borderline anatomic size.
- FDG PET/CT is superior to stand-alone CT in differentiating a splenule from metastatic lesions.
- Although the liver is the most common site of metastases, it is not involved in this patient.
- CRC is more prevalent among men and after the age of 60 years.

Case 2: Rectal Cancer, Radiotherapy Planning
Findings
A 75-year-old female with rectal cancer. FDG PET/CT demonstrates tracer-avid rectal wall thickening (B, arrowhead), compatible with the patient's known primary malignancy. There are multiple small FDG-avid metastatic pelvic lymph nodes (B,C; arrow). No distant metastasis is noted (Fig. 6.2).

Teaching points
- FDG PET/CT detects small lymph nodes that are not suspicious for metastases based on CT criteria, which have clinical relevance in the application of neoadjuvant treatment.
- Furthermore, it may help in better planning of external beam radiation.

Case 3: Sigmoid Colon Cancer, Atypical Metastases
Findings
A 76-year-old male with sigmoid cancer. FDG PET/CT shows a small FDG-avid eccentric sigmoid wall thickening (B, arrow), which was confirmed as colon adenocarcinoma in pathology. An extensive FDG-avid lesion is evident on the left scapula, which is proved as metastasis by biopsy (C, arrow) (Fig. 6.3).

Teaching points
- Eccentric primary tumor proliferation in the gastrointestinal tract may be missed by endoscopic evaluation, and FDG PET/CT imaging seems to provide more diagnostic accuracy in such cases.
- FDG PET/CT provides whole-body assessment in a single imaging and is able to better detect distant metastasis even without locoregional or liver involvement.

- Although 5-year survival is about 94% in stage I CRC, it reduces to about 11% in stage IV.

Pitfalls
- Traumatic changes or primary bone malignancies are in the differential diagnosis of osseous metastatic disease.
- A focal increased FDG uptake within the right pelvic region (B, arrowhead) is caused by the accumulation of radioactive urine within the ureter and should not be interpreted as metastatic disease.

Case 4: Staging Rectal Cancer, Pulmonary Metastasis
Findings
A 50-year-old male with rectal cancer. FDG PET/CT shows FDG-avid rectal wall thickening (B, arrowhead), representing the patient's known primary tumors. There are several tiny non-FDG-avid pelvic lymph nodes (B, arrows). An FDG-avid right pulmonary metastatic nodule is also evident (C, arrow) (Fig. 6.4).

Teaching points
- FDG PET/CT shows rectal cancer with distant metastases without liver involvement.
- CRC metastasizes to the lungs in 10%–20% of cases.

Pitfall
- No FDG uptake in the pelvic lymph nodes may be the result of an intense FDG uptake within the primary tumor and the resultant attenuation and small size of the nodes.

Case 5: Rectal Cancer, Treatment Evaluation
Findings
A 59-year-old male with rectal cancer. FDG PET/CT shows an FDG-avid primary tumor (A, arrow) with an excellent metabolic response to neoadjuvant chemoradiation therapy (B, arrow). An increased focal FDG uptake is noted in the anal region on follow-up images (C, arrow), suggestive of an inflammatory process caused by fistula formation after radiotherapy (Fig. 6.5).

Teaching points
- FDG PET/CT is a promising modality for radiotherapy planning and for the assessment of response to therapy. It is also able to exclude distant metastases if a curative surgical approach is contemplated.
- FDG PET/CT demonstrates a significant reduction of radiotracer in the primary tumor after therapy; however, no noticeable morphologic changes are noted

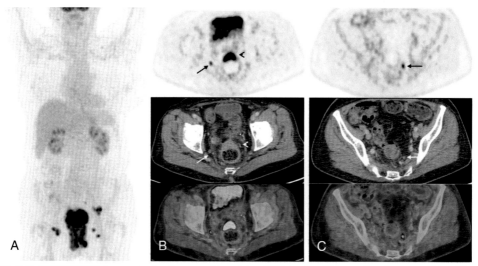

FIG. 6.2 FDG PET/CT demonstrating tracer-avid rectal wall thickening (B, *arrowhead*), compatible with the patient's known primary malignancy. There are multiple small FDG-avid metastatic pelvic lymph nodes (B,C; *arrow*). A, FDG PET MIP image.

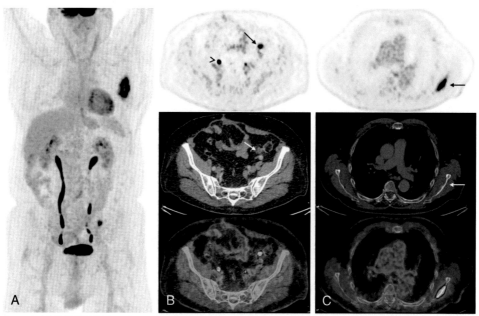

FIG. 6.3 FDG PET/CT showing a small FDG-avid eccentric sigmoid wall thickening (B, *arrow*), which was confirmed as colon adenocarcinoma in pathology. An extensive FDG-avid lesion is evident on the left scapula, which is proved as metastasis by biopsy (C, *arrow*).

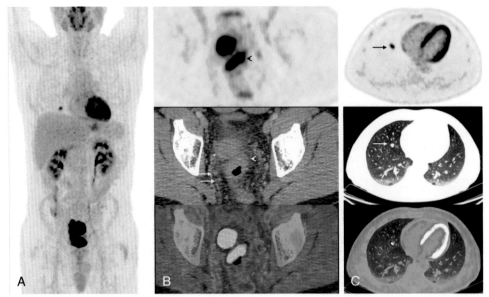

FIG. 6.4 FDG PET/CT showing FDG-avid rectal wall thickening (B, *arrowhead*), representing the patient's known primary tumors. There are several tiny non-FDG-avid pelvic lymph nodes (B, *arrows*). An FDG-avid right pulmonary metastatic nodule is also evident (C, *arrow*). A, FDG PET MIP image.

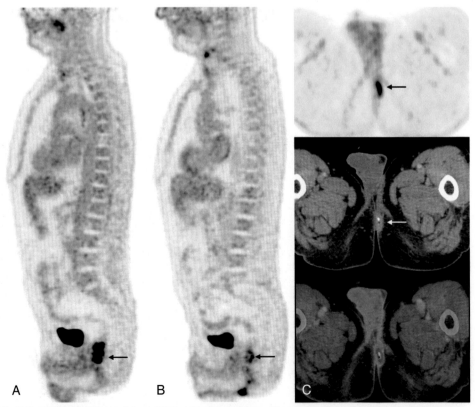

FIG. 6.5 FDG PET/CT showing an FDG-avid primary tumor (A, *arrow*) with an excellent metabolic response to neoadjuvant chemoradiation therapy (B, *arrow*). An increased focal FDG uptake is noted in the anal region on follow-up images (C, *arrow*), suggestive of inflammatory process caused by fistula formation after radiotherapy.

on CT. This shows the superiority of FDG PET/CT over stand-alone CT for the evaluation of response to treatment.

- Regression of the tumor and metabolic response after neoadjuvant therapy are favorable prognostic factors in CRC.

Pitfall
- Postradiation inflammatory process may cause an increased FDG uptake and false-positive findings and should be distinguished from local recurrence.

Case 6: Restaging Rectal Cancer, Treatment Evaluation—Flip-Flop Response
Findings
A 64-year-old female with rectal cancer. FDG PET/CT shows a tracer-avid primary rectal malignancy (C, arrow) with excellent metabolic response to radiation therapy (D, arrow). A very small FDG-avid presacral metastatic lymph node is noted on PET without suspicious finding on CT (E, arrow), which responded to radiotherapy (F). The follow-up scan demonstrates extensive FDG-avid bone marrow metastases (B) with no prominent corresponding morphologic changes on CT (G, arrow, primary staging; H, arrow, restaging). This emphasizes again the value of functional imaging in the early detection of distant metastasis (Fig. 6.6).

Teaching points
- FDG PET/CT is more accurate than stand-alone CT for the evaluation of response to therapy.
- FDG PET/CT is a potent modality for detecting bone marrow metastases.
- FDG PET/CT is superior to stand-alone CT scan in the evaluation of regional lymph node metastasis from rectal cancer.
- Approximately one-third of colorectal tumors arise from the anorectal region.

Case 7: Staging of Sigmoid Colon Cancer, Tubular Adenoma
Findings
A 72-year-old male with sigmoid cancer. FDG PET/CT shows a tracer-avid sigmoid wall thickening (B, arrow), compatible with the patient's known primary malignancy. There are two foci of increased FDG uptake within the cecum and descending colon (C, arrow), which were proved to be a premalignant tubular adenoma after colonoscopy and biopsy (Fig. 6.7).

Teaching points
- FDG-avid benign lesions could cause a false-positive result on PET/CT and are in the differential diagnosis of malignancies.
- The patients with an intense focal FDG uptake within the colon must be further evaluated with colonoscopy to exclude premalignant and malignant lesions, particularly if they are at high risk for malignancy.
- Colonoscopy is the most accurate and preferred diagnostic procedure for CRC.

Pitfalls
- Misregistration of PET and CT is a common pattern on the lower thoracic and upper abdominal regions (C, arrowhead).
- Tubular adenomatous lesions in the colon are usually FDG avid, which should be differentiated from malignancy.
- Focal versus diffuse pattern of FDG uptake may help to differentiate between premalignant or malignant lesions and physiologic uptake, respectively.

Case 8: Rectal Cancer Recurrence
Findings
A 48-year-old female with history of rectal cancer and postsurgical increased tumor markers. FDG PET/CT shows an increased tracer uptake of the anastomosis site (B, arrow). There is also a pathologic FDG-avid right supraclavicular lymph node (C, arrow), which is proved as metastasis on histopathologic examination (Fig. 6.8).

Teaching points
- An increased FDG uptake at the anastomosis site may represent an inflammatory process versus recurrent malignancy.
- FDG PET/CT is a valuable modality in the evaluation of patients with elevated tumor markers after CRC treatment to detect local recurrence versus distant metastases.

Pitfall
- Tissue biopsy of the anastomosis site was consistent with an inflammatory process, with no pathologic evidence of recurrent rectal cancer.

Case 9: Sigmoid Cancer—Biochemical Recurrence
Findings
A 54-year-old female with history of sigmoid cancer. FDG PET/CT shows a tracer-avid presacral soft tissue

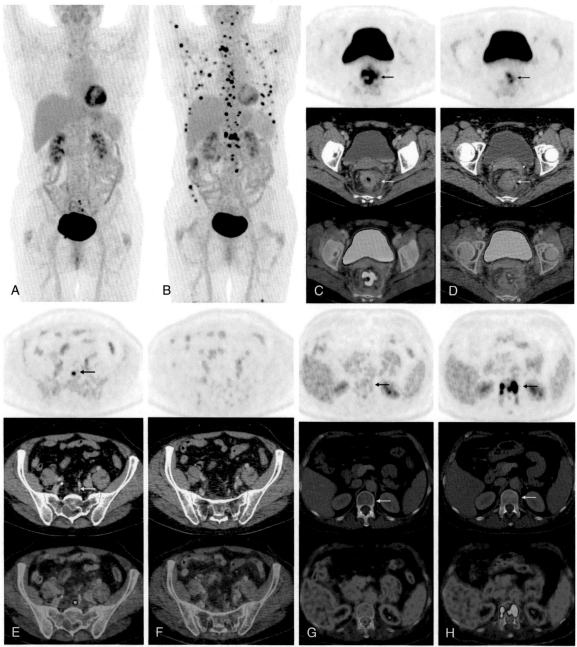

FIG. 6.6 FDG PET/CT showing tracer-avid primary rectal malignancy (C, *arrow*) with excellent metabolic response to radiation therapy (D, *arrow*). A very small FDG-avid presacral metastatic lymph node is noted on PET without suspicious finding on CT (E, *arrow*). It responded to radiotherapy (F). The follow-up scan demonstrates extensive FDG-avid bone marrow metastases (B), with no prominent corresponding morphologic changes on CT (G, *arrow*, primary staging; H, *arrow*, restaging).

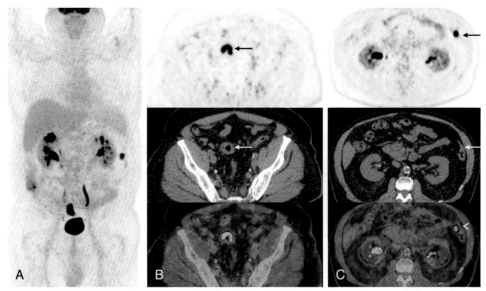

FIG. 6.7 FDG PET/CT showing a tracer-avid sigmoid wall thickening (B, *arrow*), compatible with the patient's known primary malignancy. There are two foci of increased FDG uptake within the cecum and descending colon (C, *arrow*), which were proved to be a premalignant tubular adenoma after colonoscopy and biopsy. A, FDG PET MIP image.

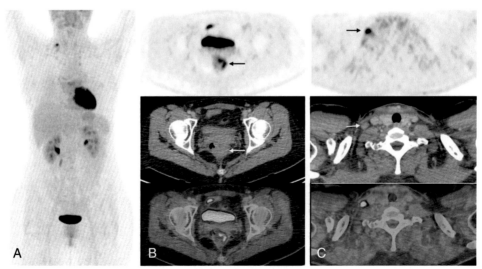

FIG. 6.8 FDG PET/CT showing an increased tracer uptake of the anastomosis site (B, *arrow*). There is also a pathologic FDG-avid right supraclavicular lymph node (C, *arrow*), which is proved as metastasis on histopathologic examination.

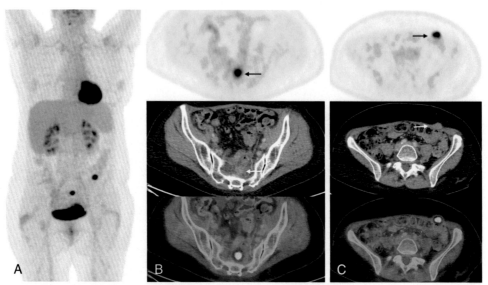

FIG. 6.9 FDG PET/CT showing a tracer-avid presacral soft tissue lesion (B, *arrow*), which was pathologically confirmed as recurrent sigmoid colon cancer. There is also an FDG-avid metastasis to the left abdominal wall (C, *arrow*). A, FDG PET MIP image.

lesion (B, arrow), which was pathologically confirmed as recurrent sigmoid colon cancer. There is also an FDG-avid metastasis to the left abdominal wall (C, arrow) (Fig. 6.9).

Teaching point
- Stand-alone CT scan has limited value for the differentiation of malignancy recurrence from posttreatment scar tissue particularly in the presacral region.

Pitfall
- Metastatic lesions to the abdominal wall and postsurgical inflammatory process from colostomy takedown may present similarly on FDG PET/CT and should be interpreted correctly.

Case 10: Colon Cancer With Surgical Mesh Repair
Findings
A 69-year-old female with history of colon cancer, status postresection and mesh repair. FDG PET/CT shows a diffuse tracer uptake corresponding to the site of mesh repair (B, arrow) (Fig. 6.10).

Pitfall
- Mesh can cause an inflammatory process, with a resultant increased FDG uptake on PET/CT, which may persist for years.

Case 11: Follow-Up, Equivocal Morphologic Findings on CT
Findings
A 35-year-old male with history of colon cancer. There are hypodense equivocal liver lesions on CT (B, arrow) without any pathologic FDG uptake (Fig. 6.11).

Teaching point
- FDG PET/CT is a promising modality to evaluate equivocal findings on conventional imaging in patients with cancer.

Pitfall
- The focal FDG uptake within the right pelvis is an accumulation of radioactive urine in the ureter (A, arrow).

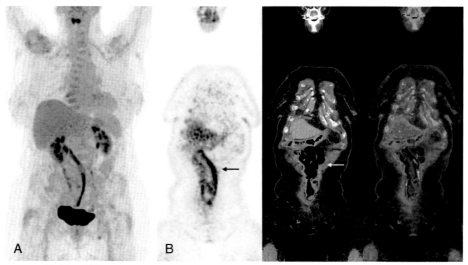

FIG. 6.10 FDG PET/CT showing diffuse tracer uptake corresponding to the site of mesh repair (B, *arrow*).

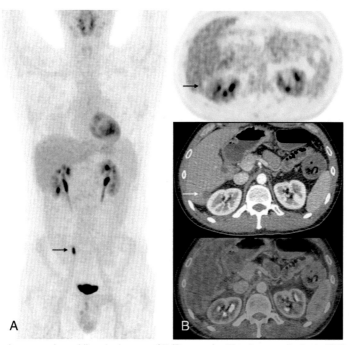

FIG. 6.11 Hypodense equivocal liver lesions on CT (B, *arrow*) without any pathologic FDG uptake. A, FDG PET MIP image.

REFERENCES

1. *Cancer Facts & Figures.* Atlanta: American Cancer Society; 2016.
2. Speights VO, Johnson MW, Stoltenberg PH, Rappaport ES, Helbert B, Riggs M. Colorectal cancer: current trends in initial clinical manifestations. *Southern Medical Journal.* 1991;84(5):575–578.
3. Hamilton W, Round A, Sharp D, Peters TJ. Clinical features of colorectal cancer before diagnosis: a population-based case-control study. *British Journal of Cancer.* 2005;93(4):399–405.
4. Rizk SN, Ryan JJ. Clinicopathologic review of 92 cases of colon cancer. *South Dakota Journal of Medicine.* 1994;47(3):89–93.
5. Majumdar SR, Fletcher RH, Evans AT. How does colorectal cancer present? Symptoms, duration, and clues to location. *The American Journal of Gastroenterology.* 1999;94(10):3039–3045.
6. Force USPST. Screening for colorectal cancer: U.S. Preventive Services Task Force recommendation statement. *Annals of Internal Medicine.* 2008;149(9):627–637.
7. McQuaid KR. Gastrointestinal disorders. In: Papadakis MA, McPhee SJ, Rabow MW, eds. *Current Medical Diagnosis & Treatment 2015.* New York: McGraw-Hill; 2014.
8. *Treatment of Colon Cancer, by Stage.* American Cancer Society; 2016.
9. Lansdorp-Vogelaar I, van Ballegooijen M, Zauber AG, Habbema JD, Kuipers EJ. Effect of rising chemotherapy costs on the cost savings of colorectal cancer screening. *Journal of the National Cancer Institute.* 2009;101(20):1412–1422.
10. Compton CC, Fielding LP, Burgart LJ, et al. Prognostic factors in colorectal cancer. College of American Pathologists Consensus Statement 1999. *Archives of Pathology & Laboratory Medicine.* 2000;124(7):979–994.
11. Hamilton SR, Bosman FT, Boffetta P. Carcinoma of the colon and rectum. In: Bosman FT, Carneiro F, Hruban RH, Theise ND, eds. *WHO Classification of Tumours of the Digestive System.* Lyon: IARC Press; 2010:134–146.
12. Borda F, Jimenez FJ, Borda A, et al. Endoscopic localization of colorectal cancer: study of its accuracy and possible error factors. *Revista espanola de enfermedades digestivas : organo oficial de la Sociedad Espanola de Patologia Digestiva.* 2012;104(10):512–517.
13. Siegel RL, Miller KD, Jemal A. Cancer statistics, 2016. *CA: A Cancer Journal for Clinicians.* 2016;66(1):7–30.
14. NCCN Clinical Practice Guidelines in Oncology, Colon Cancer. National Comprehensive Cancer Network. 2.2016.
15. NCCN Clinical Practice Guidelines in Oncology. Rectal Cancer. National Comprehensive Cancer Network. 2. 2016.
16. Schmoll HJ, Van Cutsem E, Stein A, et al. ESMO consensus guidelines for management of patients with colon and rectal cancer. a personalized approach to clinical decision making. *Annals of Oncology: Official Journal of the European Society for Medical Oncology.* 2012;23(10):2479–2516.
17. *Evidence-Based Indications for the Use of PET-CT in the UK.* London: The Royal College of Physicians and the Royal College of Radiologists; 2013.
18. Lejeune C, Bismuth MJ, Conroy T, et al. Use of a decision analysis model to assess the cost-effectiveness of 18F-FDG PET in the management of metachronous liver metastases of colorectal cancer. *Journal of Nuclear Medicine: Official Publication, Society of Nuclear Medicine.* 2005;46(12):2020–2028.
19. Valk PE, Pounds TR, Tesar RD, Hopkins DM, Haseman MK. Cost-effectiveness of PET imaging in clinical oncology. *Nuclear Medicine and Biology.* 1996;23(6):737–743.
20. Brush J, Boyd K, Chappell F, et al. The value of FDG positron emission tomography/computerised tomography (PET/CT) in pre-operative staging of colorectal cancer: a systematic review and economic evaluation. *Health Technology Assessment.* 2011;15(35): 1–192, iii–iv.
21. Long NM, Smith CS. Causes and imaging features of false positives and false negatives on F-PET/CT in oncologic imaging. *Insights Into Imaging.* 2011;2(6):679–698.
22. Gauthe M, Richard-Molard M, Cacheux W, et al. Role of fluorine 18 fluorodeoxyglucose positron emission tomography/computed tomography in gastrointestinal cancers. *Digestive and Liver Disease: Official Journal of the Italian Society of Gastroenterology and the Italian Association for the Study of the Liver.* 2015;47(6):443–454.
23. Meyerhardt JA, Mangu PB, Flynn PJ, et al. Follow-up care, surveillance protocol, and secondary prevention measures for survivors of colorectal cancer: American Society of Clinical Oncology clinical practice guideline endorsement. *Journal of Clinical Oncology: Official Journal of the American Society of Clinical Oncology.* 2013;31(35):4465–4470.
24. Ye Y, Liu T, Lu L, et al. Pre-operative TNM staging of primary colorectal cancer by (18)F-FDG PET-CT or PET: a meta-analysis including 2283 patients. *International Journal of Clinical and Experimental Medicine.* 2015;8(11):21773–21785.
25. Artiko V, Odalovic S, Sobic-Saranovic D, et al. Can (18)F-FDG PET/CT scan change treatment planning and be prognostic in recurrent colorectal carcinoma? A prospective and follow-up study. *Hellenic Society of Nuclear Medicine.* 2015;18(1):35–41.
26. Lu YY, Chen JH, Chien CR, et al. Use of FDG-PET or PET/CT to detect recurrent colorectal cancer in patients with elevated CEA: a systematic review and meta-analysis. *International Journal of Colorectal Disease.* 2013;28(8):1039–1047.
27. Niekel MC, Bipat S, Stoker J. Diagnostic imaging of colorectal liver metastases with CT, MR imaging, FDG PET, and/or FDG PET/CT: a meta-analysis of prospective studies including patients who have not previously undergone treatment. *Radiology.* 2010;257(3):674–684.
28. Kuehl H, Antoch G, Stergar H, et al. Comparison of FDG-PET, PET/CT and MRI for follow-up of colorectal liver metastases treated with radiofrequency ablation: initial results. *European Journal of Radiology.* 2008;67(2):362–371.

29. Gearhart SL, Frassica D, Rosen R, Choti M, Schulick R, Wahl R. Improved staging with pretreatment positron emission tomography/computed tomography in low rectal cancer. *Annals of Surgical Oncology*. 2006;13(3):397–404.

30. Petersen RK, Hess S, Alavi A, Hoilund-Carlsen PF. Clinical impact of FDG-PET/CT on colorectal cancer staging and treatment strategy. *American Journal of Nuclear Medicine and Molecular Imaging*. 2014;4(5):471–482.

31. Duffy MJ. Carcinoembryonic antigen as a marker for colorectal cancer: is it clinically useful? *Clinical Chemistry*. 2001;47(4):624–630.

32. Metser U, You J, McSweeney S, Freeman M, Hendler A. Assessment of tumor recurrence in patients with colorectal cancer and elevated carcinoembryonic antigen level: FDG PET/CT versus contrast-enhanced 64-MDCT of the chest and abdomen. *American Journal of Roentgenology*. 2010;194(3):766–771.

33. Patel DA, Chang ST, Goodman KA, et al. Impact of integrated PET/CT on variability of target volume delineation in rectal cancer. *Technology in Cancer Research & Treatment*. 2007;6(1):31–36.

34. Avallone A, Aloj L, Caraco C, et al. Early FDG PET response assessment of preoperative radiochemotherapy in locally advanced rectal cancer: correlation with long-term outcome. *European Journal of Nuclear Medicine and Molecular Imaging*. 2012;39(12):1848–1857.

35. Ogawa S, Itabashi M, Kondo C, Momose M, Sakai S, Kameoka S. Prognostic value of total lesion glycolysis measured by 18F-FDG-PET/CT in patients with colorectal cancer. *Anticancer Research*. 2015;35(6):3495–3500.

36. Xia Q, Liu J, Wu C, et al. Prognostic significance of (18) FDG PET/CT in colorectal cancer patients with liver metastases: a meta-analysis. *Cancer Imaging: The Official Publication of the International Cancer Imaging Society*. 2015;15:19.

37. de Geus-Oei LF, Wiering B, Krabbe PF, Ruers TJ, Punt CJ, Oyen WJ. FDG-PET for prediction of survival of patients with metastatic colorectal carcinoma. *Annals of Oncology: Official Journal of the European Society for Medical Oncology*. 2006;17(11):1650–1655.

38. Nakajo M, Nakajo M, Kajiya Y, et al. Diagnostic performance of (1)(8)F-fluorothymidine PET/CT for primary colorectal cancer and its lymph node metastasis: comparison with (1)(8)F-fluorodeoxyglucose PET/CT. *European Journal of Nuclear Medicine and Molecular Imaging*. 2013;40(8):1223–1232.

39. Yamamoto Y, Kameyama R, Izuishi K, et al. Detection of colorectal cancer using (1)(8)F-FLT PET: comparison with (1)(8)F-FDG PET. *Nuclear Medicine Communications*. 2009;30(11):841–845.

40. Dietz DW, Dehdashti F, Grigsby PW, et al. Tumor hypoxia detected by positron emission tomography with 60Cu-ATSM as a predictor of response and survival in patients undergoing Neoadjuvant chemoradiotherapy for rectal carcinoma: a pilot study. *Diseases of the Colon and Rectum*. 2008;51(11):1641–1648.

CHAPTER 7

Hepatobiliary Cancer

ALIREZA REZAEE • RATHAN M. SUBRAMANIAM • MARKUS RADERER •
WERNER LANGSTEGER • MOHSEN BEHESHTI

HEPATOCELLULAR CARCINOMA
Background
General[1-7]

- Hepatocellular carcinoma (HCC) is the sixth most common malignancy in Asia and Africa and constitutes 70% to 85% of primary liver cancers.
- HCC is the leading cause of death in cirrhotic patients.
- HCC is more prevalent among males.
- The risk factors are:
  - Cirrhosis
  - Hepatitis B virus (HBV) and hepatitis C virus (HCV) infection
  - Alcohol-related liver disease
  - Nonalcoholic fatty liver disease
  - Obesity
  - Diabetes
  - Number of metabolic syndrome components in an individual
  - Exposure to aflatoxin
  - Hereditary hemochromatosis
  - Autoimmune hepatitis
  - Glycogen storage diseases
  - α_1-Antitrypsin deficiency
  - Wilson disease
- It is prevented by HBV vaccination, anti-HCV treatment, diet modification to prevent obesity and to lose weight, and stopping alcohol and tobacco consumption.
- It rarely presents with extrahepatic metastases.

Early clinical symptoms[8]
- Right upper quadrant abdominal pain
- Jaundice
- Easy bleeding/bruising
- Weight loss

Primary diagnostic procedures
- Screening in cirrhotic patients[3,9]:
  - Liver ultrasonography
  - Serum α-fetoprotein level
- Noninvasive diagnosis[3,10]:

- Four-phase CT (unenhanced, arterial, venous, and delayed phases)
- Dynamic contrast MRI
- Image-guided biopsy confirms diagnosis (up to 30% false-negative rate).[3,11]

Standard treatment[3,7,12,13]
- Curative treatments
  - Tumor resection (single tumors with very-well-preserved liver function, Barcelona Clinic Liver Cancer [BCLC] stage 0)
  - Liver transplantation (single tumors ≤5 cm or three nodules ≤3 cm, BCLC stage A)
  - Tumor ablation (BCLC stage A)
    - Chemical (acetic acid, ethanol)
    - Thermal (radiofrequency, cryoablation, laser, microwave)
- Noncurative (palliative) treatments
  - Transarterial chemoembolization (TACE) (BCLC stage B)
  - Transarterial radioembolization
  - Systemic targeted molecular therapies (BCLC stage C) (sorafenib [Nexavar], oral tyrosine kinase inhibitor for advanced-stage disease)
  - Selected internal radionuclide therapy (SIRT) with yttrium-90
- Symptomatic therapy (BCLC stage D)

Prognostic factors[13]
- Tumor histology (better with fibrolamellar type)
- Tumor size and morphology (worse if >8 cm)
- Number of tumors and nodules (worse if higher)
- Vascular invasion
- Tumor markers (worse with higher α-fetoprotein)
- Symptoms and signs (worse if pain, hepatomegaly, hepatic failure exist)
- Stage/grade of malignancy (worse if higher)

Five-year survival[12,14]

- TNM stage I   55%
- TNM stage II   37%
- TNM stage III   16%

- BCLC stage 0, A   5-year survival = 50% to 70%
- BCLC stage B, C   3-year survival = 10% to 40%
- BCLC stage D   Survival <3 months

Tumor Characteristics and Typical Behavior

Histopathology[15]
- Fibrolamellar
- Scirrhous
- Sarcomatoid
- Lymphoepithelial-like carcinoma

Distribution and localization
T-primary
- Liver

N-lymph nodes[16]
- Regional nodes
  - Hilar
  - Periduodenal
  - Peripancreatic
  - Gastrohepatic
- Distant nodes
  - Celiac
  - Periaortic/caval

M-distant metastasis[17]. Most common sites of extrahepatic metastasis:
- Lung
- Lymph nodes
- Musculoskeletal
- Adrenal glands
- Peritoneum/omentum

TNM Classification[18]
The TNM classification is given in Table 7.1.

Primary tumor (T)
T1: Solitary tumor without vascular invasion
T2: Solitary tumor with vascular invasion or multiple tumors, none >5 cm
T3a: Multiple tumors >5 cm
T3b: Single tumor or multiple tumors of any size involving a major branch of the portal or hepatic vein

T4: Tumor(s) with direct invasion of adjacent organs other than gallbladder or with visceral peritoneum

Regional lymph nodes (N)
N0: No regional lymph node metastasis
N1: Regional lymph node metastasis

Distant metastasis (M)
M0: No distant metastasis
M1: Distant metastasis

BCLC Staging Classification[19]
The BCLC staging classification is given in Table 7.2.

Guidelines
The European Society for Medical Oncology (ESMO) and National Comprehensive Cancer Network (NCCN) guidelines are given in Table 7.3.

Evidence-based Viewpoints
- Fludeoxyglucose (FDG) PET/CT was useful in ruling in extrahepatic metastases and valuable for ruling out recurrent HCC.[21]
- Radiolabeled choline PET/CT could be a valuable tool in detecting HCC, and it is better than FDG PET/CT, especially in well- to moderately differentiated lesions.[22,23]
- Poorly differentiated and higher-stage HCC could be more accurately evaluated with FDG and dual-tracer imaging.[22,23]
- FDG PET/CT may help in determining the treatment modality for intermediate-to-advanced-stage HCC.[24]
- Pretreatment FDG PET/CT is a useful tool in predicting the prognosis of patients with HCC.[25]

Cost-effectiveness
- Recent estimates of costs for each year of life gained after liver transplantation for HCC range from $44,000 to $183,000.[26] In this setting the marginal costs associated with PET imaging become negligible.[27]

Clinical Point of View
HCC is a relatively rare disease in Western countries and is still characterized by a poor outcome. As surgery/transplantation remains the only curative procedure, defining the operability is the most important information for clinicians. Thus, assessment of intrahepatic spread, involvement of vascular structures, and diagnosis of distant metastasis are of utmost importance for decision making.

In the palliative setting, the options for oncologic management are relatively limited. Tyrosine kinase therapy (e.g., sorafenib) and transarterial bland embolization or chemoembolization or SIRT remain the

TABLE 7.1 Hepatocellular Carcinoma TNM Classification					
TNM	**T1**	**T2**	**T3a**	**T3b**	**T4**
N0	I	II	IIIA	IIIB	IIIC
N1	IVA	IVA	IVA	IVA	IVA
M1	IVB	IVB	IVB	IVB	IVB

TABLE 7.2
Barcelona Clinic Liver Cancer (BCLC) Staging Classification

BCLC Stage	Performance Status	Tumor Volume, Number, and Invasiveness	Child-Pugh
Very early 0	0	≤2 cm, vaguely nodular	A
Early A	0	Single <5 cm or 3 nodules <3 cm each	A and B
Intermediate B	0	Large/multinodular	A and B
Advanced C	1–2	Extrahepatic spread and/or vascular invasion	A and B
End stage D	3–4	Any of the above	C

TABLE 7.3
ESMO and NCCN Guidelines for Hepatocellular Carcinoma

Clinical Guidelines	Initial Diagnosis (Primary Tumor)	N-staging	M-staging
ESMO[20]	No statement	No statement	No statement
NCCN[18]	No statement	No statement	No statement

ESMO, European Society for Medical Oncology; *NCCN*, National Comprehensive Cancer Network.

only therapeutic approaches. In these settings, the classical response criteria using morphologic imaging and Response Evaluation Criteria in Solid Tumors (RECIST)-based strategies will not give a valid estimate of tumor response, as changes in size are not really expected. Thus, functional imaging seems to play an important role in the assessment of therapy response, which prevents unnecessary treatments particularly when using agents with multiple side effects.

Pitfalls[28,29]
False positive
- Postinterventional inflammation
- Reconstruction artifacts
- Misregistration of FDG-avid lung lesions caused by respiratory motion

False negative
- Infiltrative malignancy
- Well-differentiated carcinoma in FDG PET/CT
- Small lesions (<8 mm)
- Early-stage malignancy
- Hyperglycemic state

Discussion
¹⁸F-Fludeoxyglucose
FDG is a glucose analogue and the most widely used radiotracer for PET imaging. After transportation into the cells by glucose transporters (predominantly GLUT-1) and phosphorylation by active hexokinase bound to mitochondria, it is trapped in the cancerous cells in the form of FDG 6-phosphate.[30] However, in contrast to many malignancies with decreased expression of glucose-6-phosphatase, in the tumors such as HCC with high level of this enzyme, which catalyzes the reverse reaction, FDG 6-phosphate can be washed out after dephosphorylation.[31] Although FDG uptake is moderate to intense in poorly differentiated HCC compared with well-differentiated HCC,[29] the overall detection rate with FDG PET/CT is not promising, ranging from 50% to 65% in different studies.[29,32–35] The modality is not recommended by major clinical guidelines, such as ESMO and NCCN, as a diagnostic imaging method for primary HCC as well.[18,20]

According to a systematic review and meta-analysis, the modality is useful in the detection of HCC distant metastasis (pooled sensitivity and specificity of approximately 77% and 98%, respectively) and exclusion of malignancy recurrence (pooled sensitivity and specificity of approximately 82% and 89%, respectively).[21,36,37] It is reported in some studies that FDG PET/CT may change management in up to 30% of high-risk patients by detecting distant metastases.[35]

Since the standardized uptake value (SUV) is much higher in poorly differentiated HCC than in well-differentiated HCC, FDG PET/CT can play a prognostic role in well-differentiated HCC.[38] In addition, in a meta-analysis and multicenter cohort study, a high tumor to liver SUV ratio and tumor SUV were introduced as poor prognosis markers.[25,39] This is due to the higher avidity of high-grade tumors to FDG compared with low-grade malignancies. With this in mind, the method is valuable for guiding biopsy, leading to more accurate pathology reports.[40] It is also revealed that patients with high-FDG-avid tumors show more favorable survival, if treated with chemoradiation therapy (CCRT) rather than with TACE.[24]

Given the limitations of FDG PET/CT in the evaluation of HCC, the investigators tried other radiotracers for better assessment of this malignancy.

¹¹C-Acetate

Acetate is a precursor of acetyl-CoA, which is used by cells for the synthesis of fatty acids and cholesterol to build up the cell membrane.[41]

In contrast to FDG, ¹¹C-acetate PET/CT is able to detect well-differentiated HCC. In a study, it showed higher sensitivity than FDG PET/CT (87% vs 47%) for the detection of HCC and 34% of lesions had taken up both tracers.[42] This was confirmed in other investigations as well.[29] It is also superior to other nuclear medicine imaging methods, such as ⁶⁷Ga-scintigraphy, in the diagnosis of HCC.[43]

Owing to some false-positive results with ¹¹C-acetate (e.g., focal nodular hyperplasia), using a dual-tracer protocol helps clarify the liver masses more accurately.[29,44] If the mass is positive on both FDG and acetate PET/CT or only on the latter, it is highly suggestive of HCC. If it is only FDG avid, a liver malignancy other than HCC is suspected, and if it is negative on both studies, a benign lesion is more likely.[27] However, its short half-life of only 20 min requires an on-site cyclotron, which technically limits its commercial use.

¹¹C- and ¹⁸F-labeled choline

Choline is a quaternary ammonium salt and a precursor of phospholipids, such as sphingomyelin and phosphatidylcholine (lecithin), which are used to build the cell membrane during the cell proliferation process, the event that is augmented in malignant tissues.[45]

One of the limitations of scanning liver masses with choline is physiologic distribution of radiotracer in the healthy surrounding liver cells. However, ¹⁸F-fluorocholine (FCH) PET/CT seems to be a promising modality in the evaluation of HCC, with a sensitivity and specificity of 88% and 100%, respectively.[46-48] It is more sensitive than FDG PET/CT in the detection of this malignancy, particularly the well-differentiated type.[22,49] A sensitivity of 90% was calculated for HCC detection by ¹¹C-choline PET/CT as well.[50] It was shown to be superior to CT or MRI for the detection of extrahepatic HCC, with an accuracy of 99% versus 32%, respectively.[51] Similar to the disadvantage of ¹¹C-acetate, ¹¹C-choline needs an on-site cyclotron.[52]

¹⁸F-choline PET has indications for therapy evaluation of HCC because of its accuracy for the assessment of extrahepatic malignancy.[46,53]

Again, owing to the limited overall sensitivity of FDG PET/CT in the evaluation of HCC, its combination with choline-labeled PET/CT yields a higher sensitivity in the detection of this malignancy.[22,23,49,54,55]

Indeed, ¹¹C-acetate and choline-labeled PET/CT are potential imaging modalities to complement FDG PET/CT in the assessment of HCC.[56]

CHOLANGIOCARCINOMA

Background

General

- Cholangiocarcinoma is a relatively rare malignancy but prevalent in Eastern Asia, especially in Thailand.[57]
- It is the second most common primary hepatic malignancy, which accounts for 10% to 25% of all hepatobiliary cancers.[58]
- Risk factors[57-59]:
  - Parasitic infestation with liver flukes (*Clonorchis sinensis* and *Opisthorchis viverrini*)
  - Primary sclerosing cholangitis
  - Biliary duct cysts
  - Hepatolithiasis
  - Toxins
- Metastatic disease is seen at presentation in most cases.[60]

Early clinical symptoms

The early clinical symptoms are jaundice, pruritus, abdominal pain, weight loss, and fever.[61]

Primary diagnostic procedures[62]

- No screening test is available. The condition is often diagnosed at an advanced stage. The diagnosis is confirmed by biopsy.
- Diagnostic procedures:
  - Liver function test and tumor markers
  - Ultrasound
  - CT
  - MRI
  - Magnetic resonance cholangiopancreatography (MRCP)
  - Endoscopic retrograde cholangiopancreatography + tissue sampling (brush cytology, fine-needle aspiration, transpapillary biopsy)

Standard treatment[63-65]

- Surgery (partial hepatectomy for intrahepatic malignancy) is the main treatment strategy.
- CCRT and palliative care may be added in selected cases.

Prognostic factors[66–69]

- Bilirubin level (worse if >10 mg/dL)
- Histologic type (worse if mass-forming or periductal infiltrating type)
- Tumor diameter (worse in larger tumors)
- Carcinoembryonic antigen (CEA) and cancer antigen (CA) 19-9 levels (worse if higher)
- Lymph node metastases
- Vascular invasion
- Direct invasion and local metastasis
- Disease stage

Five-year survival[70]

The 5-year survival for intrahepatic and extrahepatic cancers is given in Table 7.4.

Tumor Characteristics and Typical Behavior

Histopathology[71]

- Adenocarcinoma   95%
- Squamous cell carcinoma   5%

Distribution and localization

T-primary[72]

- Hilum/proximal third of common bile duct (CBD)   50%
- Intrahepatic large ducts   15%
- Extrahepatic
  - Middle third CBD   17%
  - Distal third CBD   18%

N-lymph nodes. Intrahepatic cancer[16]:

- Regional lymph nodes (N1)
  - Right liver: hilar, periduodenal, peripancreatic
  - Left liver: hilar, gastrohepatic
- Distant lymph nodes (M1): celiac, periaortic, caval
  Perihilar cancer[18]:
- Regional lymph nodes (N1): cystic duct, CBD, perihepatic (artery), periportal (vein)
- Juxtaregional lymph nodes (N2): periaortic, pericaval, periceliac (artery), superior mesenteric (artery)
  Extrahepatic cancer[73]:

- Regional lymph nodes (N1): CBD, hepatic (artery), celiac trunk, pancreaticoduodenal, superior mesenteric (artery and vein)

M-distant metastasis[16]. Common:

- Liver
- Lymph nodes
- Peritoneum
  Uncommon:
- Lung
- Brain
- Bone

TNM Classification for Intrahepatic Subtype[18]

The TNM classification for intrahepatic subtype is given in Table 7.5.

Primary tumor (T)

T1: Solitary tumor without vascular invasion

T2: Solitary tumor with vascular invasion
- T2a: Solitary tumor with vascular invasion
- T2b: Multiple tumors, with or without vascular invasion

T3: Tumor perforating the visceral peritoneum or involving the local extrahepatic structures by direct invasion

T4: Tumor with periductal invasion
  Regional lymph nodes (N)

N0: No regional lymph node metastasis

N1: Regional lymph node metastasis present
  Distant metastasis (M)

M0: No distant metastasis

M1: Distant metastasis

Guidelines

The ESMO and NCCN guidelines are given in Table 7.6.

Evidence-based Viewpoints

- FDG PET/CT has been demonstrated to be an accurate diagnostic imaging method in the assessment of primary tumor in patients with cholangiocarcinoma, particularly the intrahepatic type. However,

---

TABLE 7.4
Five-year Survival

Stage	Intrahepatic	Extrahepatic
Localized disease	15%	30%
Regional lymph node involvement	6%	24%
Distant metastasis	2%	2%

TABLE 7.5
TNM Classification for Intrahepatic Subtype

TNM	T1	T2	T3	T4
N0	I	II	III	IVA
N1	IVA	IVA	IVA	IVA
M1	IVB	IVB	IVB	IVB

TABLE 7.6
ESMO and NCCN Guidelines for Cholangiocarcinoma

Clinical Guidelines	Initial Diagnosis (Primary Tumor)	N-staging	M-staging
ESMO[74]	No statement	No statement	No statement
NCCN[18]	Not recommended	FDG PET/CT is optional in patients with resectable disease	FDG PET/CT is optional in patients with resectable disease

ESMO, European Society for Medical Oncology; *FDG*, fludeoxyglucose; *NCCN*, National Comprehensive Cancer Network.

further studies are warranted to determine the accuracy for the hilar type.[75]

- FDG PET/CT is indicated for staging of potentially operable primary hepatobiliary malignancy (cholangiocarcinoma, gallbladder carcinoma, or HCC), in cases in which cross-sectional imaging is equivocal for metastatic disease, patients are fit for resection, and a positive PET/CT would lead to a decision not to operate.[76]
- There is a role for FDG PET/CT in the evaluation of abnormal lymph nodes seen on CT or MRI if a positive finding will change management. It is useful in detecting recurrent and metastatic disease in patients with abnormalities on CT or MRI.[77]

Cost-effectiveness

No large study has been performed yet to evaluate the cost-effectiveness of FDG PET/CT in cholangiocarcinoma.

Clinical Point of View

Cholangiocarcinoma is a silent malignancy that is non-resectable in 45% of patients at the time of diagnosis. Nonetheless, in another 45% of cases, the tumor is completely resectable, with no residual malignancy left behind after surgery. However, a very high incidence of local recurrence (up to 100%) is reported in this cancer. Therefore, imaging modalities have an important role in the diagnosis and localization of recurrent tumors. They are particularly beneficial for the optimization of therapy approach after surgical procedures. In this setting, metabolic imaging with FDG PET/CT seems to be superior to conventional imaging methods in the assessment of recurrent malignancy.

Pitfalls[62]

False positive

- Infectious lesions
- Inflammatory lesions
- Misregistration of FDG-avid lung lesions caused by respiratory motion

False negative

- Small lesions (<8 mm)
- Early-stage malignancy
- Mucin-producing cholangiocarcinoma
- Infiltrative cholangiocarcinoma
- Hyperglycemic state

Discussion

Cholangiocarcinoma is usually a silent malignancy that presents in the advanced unresectable stage, with an average survival of less than 1 year after diagnosis.[78] Thus, early detection of disease is really important for patients' survival.

Conventional imaging modalities, such as ultrasound, CT, MRI, and MRCP, are standard procedures in the evaluation of cholangiocarcinoma. Also, FDG PET/CT seems to be an accurate diagnostic method for the assessment of this malignancy, particularly the intrahepatic subtype.[62,75,79–81]

A meta-analysis of 23 studies and 1232 patients reported a pooled sensitivity and specificity of 95% and 83%, compared with 76% and 74%, for the intrahepatic and extrahepatic subtypes, respectively.[75]

Although FDG PET/CT has limited value for the assessment of regional lymph node metastases, it is still superior to stand-alone CT for this purpose.[82,83] In contrast, its detection rate for distant metastases is very high (>95%).[77,79,81,82,84,85]

Moreover, it led to change of patients' management in 16% to 30% of cases.[77,85–87]

The effectiveness of FDG PET/CT has also been shown in the detection of recurrent cholangiocarcinoma, with a sensitivity and specificity of approximately 94% and 100%, respectively.[77,84,87–89]

Furthermore, it seems to be a valuable technique for therapy monitoring in patients with this kind of cancer.[84]

In addition, tracer intensity on FDG PET/CT could be predictive of recurrent disease. A high SUV was found to be independently related to postoperative recurrence.[77] Also, the detection of involved lymph nodes on FDG PET/CT in patients with intrahepatic cholangiocarcinoma was associated with 1-year recurrence after surgical resection.[83]

GALLBLADDER CANCER
Background
General
- Gallbladder cancer is a rare malignancy in most Caucasian populations but prevalent in central and eastern Europe, Central and South America, northern India, and Japan.[90,91]
- Patients with gallstones have a four- to fivefold risk for gallbladder cancer. Female gender, obesity, high-fat and high-calorie diet, porcelain gallbladder, chronic typhoid, and increased parity are other risk factors.[91]
- About 70% of patients have liver metastases and 50% have regional lymph node metastases at presentation.[62]

Early Clinical Symptoms
The early clinical symptoms are right upper quadrant abdominal pain, icterus, and weight loss.[92]

Primary Diagnostic Procedures[18,60]
- No screening test is available. Elevated tumor markers (CEA > 4 ng/mL and CA 19-9 > 20 unit/mL) may be suggestive of gallbladder cancer. It is often diagnosed at an advanced stage. The diagnosis is confirmed by biopsy.
- Diagnostic procedures:
  - Ultrasound
  - CT
  - Endoscopic ultrasound
  - MRI
  - MRCP
  - Biopsy

Standard treatment[93,94]
- Cholecystectomy, partial hepatectomy, and lymph node dissection are the cornerstone of treatment.
- CCRT and palliative care may be added in selected cases.

Prognostic factors[95]
- Stage of the disease (worse with higher stages)
- Extent of resection (worse if more extended)
- Histologic differentiation
- Involvement of resection margin (worse prognosis)

Five-year survival[96]
- Stage 0   60%
- Stage I   39%
- Stage II   15%
- Stage III   5%
- Stage IV   1%

Tumor Characteristics and Typical Behavior
Histopathology[62,97]
- Adenocarcinoma   90%
- Squamous and adenosquamous cell carcinoma   5%
- Undifferentiated carcinoma   5%

Distribution and localization
T-primary[98]
- Fundus   60%
- Body   30%
- Neck   10%

N-lymph nodes[18]
- Regional lymph nodes (N1)
  - Cystic duct
  - Common bile duct
  - Hepatic (artery)
  - Portal (vein)
- Juxtaregional lymph nodes (N2)
  - Periaortic
  - Pericaval
  - Superior mesenteric (artery)
  - Celiac (artery)

M-distant metastasis[99]
- Liver   69%
- Regional lymph nodes   45%
- Lesser omentum   40%
- Greater omentum   22%
- Gastroduodenal area   16%

TNM Classification[18]

TNM	T1	T2	T3	T4
N0	IA	II	IIIA	IVA
N1	IIIB	IIIB	IIIB	IVA
N2	IVB	IVB	IVB	IVB
M1	IVB	IVB	IVB	IVB

Primary tumor (T)

T1: Tumor is only in the gallbladder and has only invaded the lamina propria or muscle layer.
- T1a: Tumor invades the lamina propria.
- T1b: Tumor invades the muscle layer.

T2: Tumor invades the perimuscular connective tissue; there is no extension beyond the serosa or into the liver.

T3: Tumor perforates the serosa (visceral peritoneum) and/or directly invades the liver and/or one other adjacent organ or structure, such as the stomach, duodenum, colon, pancreas, omentum, or extrahepatic bile ducts.

T4: Tumor invades the main portal vein or hepatic artery or invades two or more extrahepatic organs or structures.

Regional lymph nodes (N)

N0: No regional lymph node metastasis

N1: Metastases to nodes along the cystic duct, common bile duct, hepatic artery, and/or portal vein

N2: Metastases to periaortic, pericaval, superior mesenteric artery, and/or celiac artery lymph nodes

Distant metastasis (M)

M0: No distant metastasis

M1: Distant metastasis

Guidelines

ESMO and NCCN guidelines are given in Table 7.6.

Evidence-based Viewpoints

- FDG PET/CT demonstrated to be an accurate diagnostic imaging method in the assessment of primary tumor in patients with gallbladder cancer.[100]
- FDG PET/CT is indicated for staging of potentially operable primary hepatobiliary malignancy (cholangiocarcinoma, gallbladder carcinoma, or HCC) in cases in which cross-sectional imaging is equivocal for metastatic disease, patients are fit for resection, and a positive PET/CT would lead to a decision not to operate.[76]
- There is a role for FDG PET/CT in the evaluation of abnormal lymph nodes seen in CT or MRI if a positive finding will change management. It is useful in detecting recurrent and metastatic disease in patients with abnormalities in CT or MRI.[77]

Cost-effectiveness

No large study has been performed yet to evaluate the cost-effectiveness of FDG PET/CT in gallbladder cancer.

Clinical Point of View

Gallbladder cancer is a rare malignancy with a relatively high chance of hepatic and regional lymph node metastases at the time of diagnosis.

Cholecystectomy is the cornerstone of treatment. The data on adjuvant radiation or chemotherapy are anecdotal. Hepatic arterial infusion of chemotherapy agents may be beneficial in highly selected patients.

There is no definitive role for FDG PET/CT in preoperative staging. However, the method may be useful for the evaluation of metastatic disease in patients with equivocal findings on CT or MRI. For the assessment of recurrent disease, functional imaging may provide superior information compared with conventional imaging modalities.

Pitfalls[100,101]

False positive

- Cholecystitis
- Gallbladder adenomyomatosis

False negative

- Small lesions (<8 mm)
- Early-stage malignancy
- Mucin-producing adenocarcinoma
- Hyperglycemic state

Discussion

Gallbladder carcinoma is the most common cancer of the biliary system with a high mortality rate.[102] Although surgery is the cornerstone of treatment, precise evaluation and staging are essential to prevent futile surgical interventions.[88]

Among different diagnostic modalities, FDG PET/CT has been used to assess the disease extent in these patients.[103]

Several studies have investigated the diagnostic accuracy of FDG PET/CT in the staging of primary gallbladder cancer.[104,105] A meta-analysis that included 21 studies and 495 patients calculated a pooled sensitivity and specificity of 87% and 78%, respectively. It also introduced the method as accurate for the diagnosis of gallbladder cancer.[100] In a prospective study, the accuracy of FDG PET/CT was calculated as 96%, 86%, and 96% for primary gallbladder cancer, lymph node involvement, and distant metastases, respectively.[102] Thus, it is also a valuable method for the evaluation of regional lymph node involvement and particularly distant metastases.[82,85] Interestingly, the authors determined the SUV_{max} cutoff point of 3.65 for malignancy.[82,106] The use of delayed FDG PET/CT is also recommended to increase sensitivity for the detection of malignancy because of the increased uptake in the lesion, which leads to an increased lesion to background ratio.[107]

In addition, FDG PET/CT is also efficient in the evaluation of recurrent gallbladder cancer.[87] The corresponding calculated sensitivity, specificity, positive predictive value, negative predictive value, and accuracy were approximately 98%, 90%, 95%, 95%, and 95%, respectively. The modality is more specific than conventional imaging for this purpose.[108]

The role of FDG PET/CT in changing the subsequent management in patients with gallbladder cancer was also investigated.[108,109] Based on different studies, the management changed according to data from FDG PET/CT in about 15% to 23% of cases.[85,87,102,106]

FDG PET/CT has a prognostic value in patients with gallbladder cancer as well, and the SUV_{max} of the primary tumor is significantly related to survival.[110,111]

Teaching Cases
Case 1: Staging HCC—^{18}F-FCH PET/CT
Findings. An 81-year-old male with HCC. ^{18}F-FCH PET/CT shows tracer-avid hypodense primary tumor in the right liver lobe (yellow arrows). Small mildly ^{18}F-FCH-avid mediastinal lymph nodes are reactive in nature (arrowheads) (Fig. 7.1).

Teaching points
- ^{18}F-FCH PET/CT is a promising modality for the assessment of HCC with a sensitivity of 88% and specificity of 100%. It can differentiate HCC from other primary hepatic malignancies and is an accurate modality to rule out intrahepatic and extrahepatic metastases, which has a significant role in therapeutic decision making.
- It is more specific than FDG PET/CT for the detection of HCC, especially in well- to moderately differentiated lesions.
- Five-year survival in early-stage cancer reaches 55%.

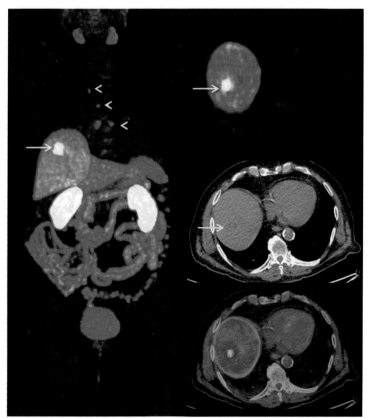

FIG. 7.1 ^{18}F-FCH PET/CT showing tracer-avid hypodense primary tumor in the right liver lobe (*yellow arrows*). Small mildly ^{18}F-FCH-avid mediastinal lymph nodes are reactive in nature *(arrowheads)*.

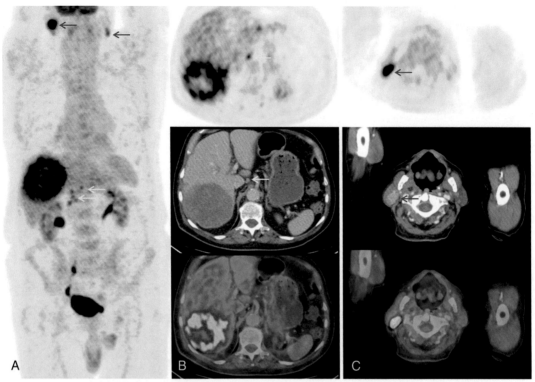

FIG. 7.2 FDG PET/CT showing a large tracer-avid primary malignancy (B) with multiple small regional lymph node metastases (A and B, *yellow arrows*). Intensely FDG-avid soft tissue nodules within the bilateral parotid glands are most likely benign in nature, such as Warthin tumor or pleomorphic adenoma (A and C, *red arrows*).

Pitfalls
- ^{18}F-FCH-avid mediastinal lymph nodes are reactive and should not be interpreted as metastatic disease.

Case 2: Staging cholangiocarcinoma
Findings. A 91-year-old male with cholangiocarcinoma. FDG PET/CT shows a large tracer-avid primary malignancy (Fig. 7.2B) with multiple small regional lymph node metastases (Fig. 7.2A and B, yellow arrows). Intensely FDG-avid soft tissue nodules within the bilateral parotid glands are most likely benign in nature, such as Warthin tumor or pleomorphic adenoma (Fig. 7.2A and C, red arrows).

Teaching points
- Cholangiocarcinoma is the second most common primary hepatic malignancy after HCC.
- Parasitic infestation with liver flukes and primary sclerosing cholangitis are among its risk factors.

- No screening test is available for this cancer, and it is often diagnosed at an advanced stage.
- FDG PET/CT is superior to stand-alone CT for small lymph node differentiation.

Pitfalls
- Warthin tumor is the second most common benign tumor of the parotid gland after pleomorphic adenoma and is also the most common bilateral or multifocal benign parotid neoplasm. Such benign tumors usually show intensive FDG uptake. They should not be misinterpreted as metastatic disease.

Case 3: Staging HCC — ^{18}F-FCH PET/CT
Findings. A 66-year-old male with HCC. ^{18}F-FCH PET/CT shows disseminated tracer-avid liver tumors (Fig. 7.3A and B). There are multiple ^{18}F-FCH-avid skeletal metastases within the cervical spine, right clavicle, sternum, left femur, and left pubic bone (Fig. 7.3C, arrow, ^{18}F-FCH-avid lytic lesion in the cervical spine).

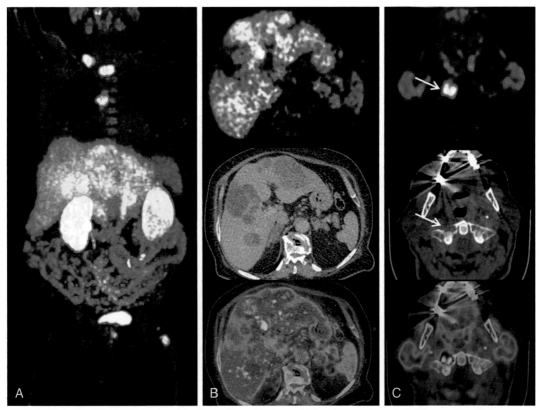

FIG. 7.3 ^{18}F-FCH PET/CT showing disseminated tracer-avid liver tumors (A and B). There are multiple ^{18}F-FCH-avid skeletal metastases within the cervical spine, right clavicle, sternum, left femur, and left pubic bone (C, *arrow*, ^{18}F-FCH-avid lytic lesion in the cervical spine).

Teaching points
- Choline is a precursor of cell membrane phospholipids, such as sphingomyelin and phosphatidylcholine (lecithin), and represents cell proliferation.
- ^{18}F-FCH PET/CT can differentiate necrotic tissue from viable malignancy in the liver, which could be useful in guiding biopsy.
- ^{18}F-FCH PET/CT is superior to CT or MRI for the detection of extrahepatic HCC, with an accuracy of 99% versus 32%, respectively.
- ^{18}F-FCH physiologically distributes in the liver, pancreas, duodenum, stomach, kidneys, urinary bladder, and salivary and parotid glands, as well as in the lacrimal glands, nasal mucosa, thyroid, tonsils, adrenal glands, large bowel, bone marrow, and spleen. Low-grade-to-moderate uptake was present in the pituitary, choroid plexus, pharynx, soft palate, lungs, myocardium, mediastinal blood pool, testicles, and muscles.

Pitfalls
- A high physiologic ^{18}F-FCH uptake in the liver may limit its diagnostic accuracy for the assessment of intrahepatic lesions. However, it seems that ^{18}F-FCH PET/CT is more accurate for extrahepatic metastases.

Case 4: Recurrent HCC
Findings. A 61-year-old female with HCC, status post–left hemihepatectomy. There is a mild FDG uptake around the cystic lesion at the resection margin, which is most likely inflammatory in nature (Fig. 7.4A, arrow). FDG PET/CT shows tracer-avid recurrent HCC within the liver (Fig. 7.4B, arrow). A focal FDG uptake in the left sixth rib with no corresponding morphologic lesion on CT is consistent with bone marrow metastasis (Fig. 7.4C, arrow).

Teaching points
- FDG PET/CT is able to exclude HCC recurrence with a sensitivity of 82% and specificity of 89%.

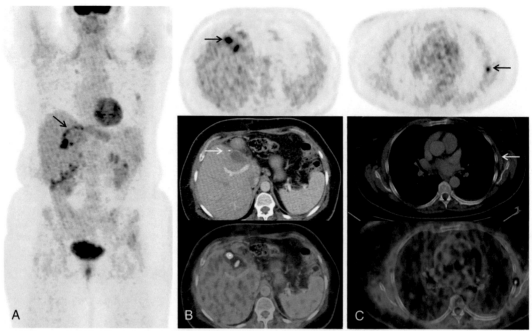

FIG. 7.4 Mild FDG uptake around the cystic lesion at the resection margin, which is most likely inflammatory in nature (A, *arrow*). FDG PET/CT shows tracer-avid recurrent HCC within the liver (B, *arrows*). Focal FDG uptake in the left sixth rib with no corresponding morphologic lesion on CT is consistent with bone marrow metastasis (C, *arrows*).

- The modality could be useful in the evaluation of HCC (detection rate of 50% to 65%) if specific radiotracers (e.g., [11]C- or ^{18}F-choline) are not available.
- Reduced sensitivity is due to tumoral overexpression of glucose-6-phosphatase, which enhances the tracer washout from the tumor.

Pitfalls
- Postoperative inflammatory uptakes are the common pitfalls on FDG PET/CT and should be interpreted with caution.
- There is nonspecific bilateral cervical muscles uptake.
- Focal uptake in bilateral sternoclavicular joints is secondary to degenerative changes.

Case 5: Recurrent cholangiocarcinoma (dual-time liver imaging)
Findings. A 77-year-old male with recurrent cholangiocarcinoma. FDG PET/CT shows focal tracer accumulations in the liver, with no corresponding morphologic lesion on CT, consistent with metastatic disease (Fig. 7.5A and B). There is a focal tracer uptake in liver segment VIII (Fig. 7.5C, arrow). A delayed scan (i.e., 120 min p.i.) depicts the tumor much better (Fig. 7.5D, arrow) because of washout of the physiologic tracer uptake, which leads to an increased tumor to background ratio.

Teaching points
- Cholangiocarcinoma accounts for 10% to 25% of all hepatobiliary cancers and presents at the advanced unresectable stage in the vast majority of cases, with an average survival of less than 1 year after diagnosis.
- FDG PET/CT is superior to stand-alone CT in N- and M-staging for cholangiocarcinoma, with a detection rate of >95% for distant metastases.
- FDG PET/CT could be predictive of recurrent disease.
- Dual-time scanning with additional delayed acquisition (i.e., 100 to 120 min p.i.) is useful for better detection of small hepatic lesions and increases the diagnostic accuracy. The sensitivity of FDG PET/CT for the detection of HCC improves from 56% on standard to 63% on delayed images. It may also provide additional prognostic data, because opposite to less aggressive tumors and inflammatory lesions, more aggressive cancers show increased uptake on delayed scan.

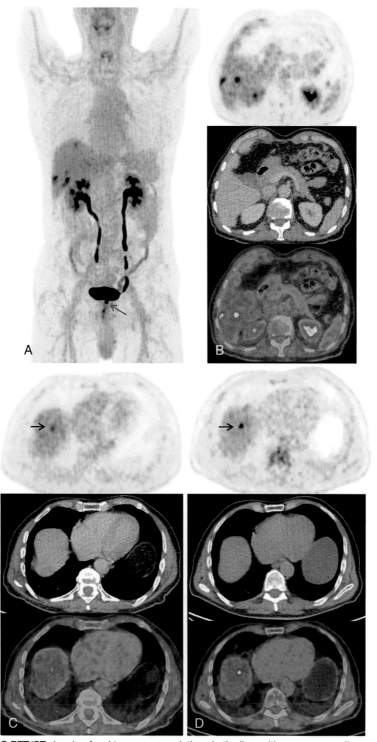

FIG. 7.5 FDG PET/CT showing focal tracer accumulations in the liver with no corresponding morphologic lesion on CT, consistent with metastatic disease (A and B). There is a focal tracer uptake in liver segment VIII (C, *arrow*). A delayed scan (i.e., 120 min p.i.) depicts the tumor much better (D, *arrow*) because of washout of the physiologic tracer uptake, which leads to an increased tumor to background ratio. A, FDG PET MIP image.

Pitfalls
- Focal uptake in the prostate area is a urinary accumulation after transurethral prostatectomy (Fig. 7.5A, red arrow).

Case 6: Recurrent cholangiocarcinoma

Findings. A 77-year-old male with recurrent cholangiocarcinoma. FDG PET/CT shows tracer-avid recurrent malignancy in the liver without significant changes on CT (Fig. 7.6B, red arrows). There are several FDG-avid bone metastases within the rib (Fig. 7.6A, arrow) and the spine (Fig. 7.6C, arrows). FDG uptake of the small and large intestines is nonspecific (Fig. 7.6).

Teaching points
- FDG PET/CT is superior to stand-alone CT in the evaluation of recurrent cholangiocarcinoma, with a sensitivity of 94% and specificity of 100%.
- It is also a promising method for the assessment of metastatic disease.

Pitfalls
- Physiologic FDG uptake in the bowels can limit the evaluation of intraabdominal malignant lesions.

Case 7: 18F-FCH and FDG PET/CT in recurrent HCC

Findings. A 79-year-old male with HCC, status post–liver resection. FDG PET/CT shows no or faintly tracer-avid lesion without any morphologic change on CT (Fig. 7.7A and D). 18F-FCH PET/CT few days later shows multiple intensely tracer-avid metastatic lesions within the pericardium (Fig. 7.7B, white arrow), abdominal wall (Fig. 7.7C, arrows), rib (Fig. 7.7A, yellow arrow), and vertebral body (Fig. 7.7E, arrows). The heterogeneous 18F-FCH uptake in the liver is physiologic (Fig. 7.7).

Teaching points
- HCC comprises 70% to 85% of primary liver cancers and is the leading cause of death in cirrhotic patients.

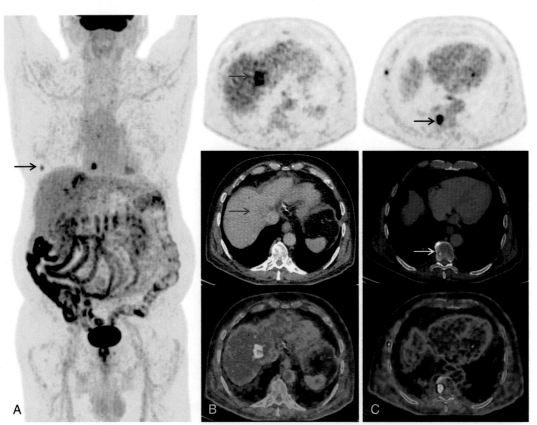

FIG. 7.6 FDG PET/CT showing tracer-avid recurrent malignancy in the liver without significant changes on CT (B, *red arrows*). There are several FDG-avid bone metastases within the rib (A, *arrow*) and the spine (C, *arrows*).

- In spite of the physiologic uptake of the radiotracer in the liver, ^{18}F-FCH PET/CT still seems to be a promising modality in the evaluation of primary HCC.
- ^{18}F-FCH PET/CT is superior to FDG PET/CT in the evaluation of HCC primary and metastatic lesions, par-

ticularly for the well-differentiated type. It revealed a sensitivity of >88% vs <65% for FDG PET/CT.

- Poorly differentiated and higher-stage HCC could be more accurately evaluated with PET/CT using FDG or dual-tracer imaging.

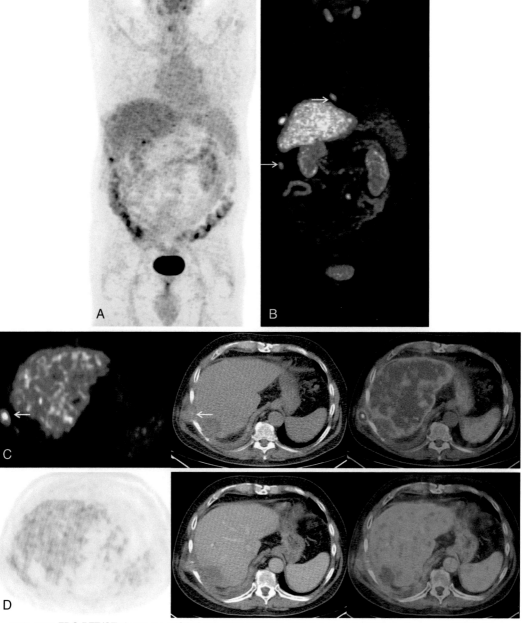

FIG. 7.7 FDG PET/CT shows no or faintly tracer-avid lesion without any morphologic change on CT (A, D, and F). ^{18}F-FCH PET/CT a few days later shows multiple intensely tracer-avid metastatic lesions within the pericardium (B, *white arrow*), abdominal wall (C, *arrows*), rib (B, *yellow arrow*), and vertebral body (E, *arrows*).

Continued

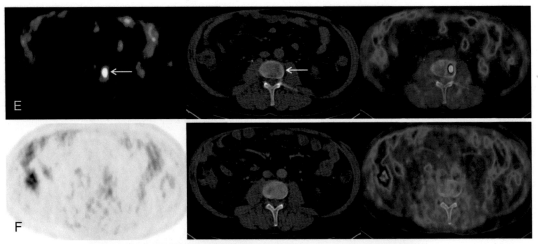

FIG. 7.7, cont'd

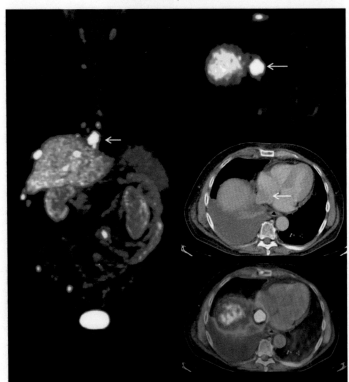

FIG. 7.8 ¹⁸F-FCH PET/CT showing multiple tracer-avid intrahepatic and osseous metastatic lesions. Of incidental note is an ¹⁸F-FCH-avid tumor thrombosis in the inferior vena cava, extending to the right atrium (*arrows*).

- ¹⁸F-FCH PET/CT is superior in staging and restaging of HCC to stand-alone CT.

Case 8: HCC — tumor thrombosis
Findings. A 79-year-old male with HCC, status post–liver transplantation. ¹⁸F-FCH PET/CT shows multiple tracer-avid intrahepatic and osseous metastatic lesions.

Of incidental note is an ¹⁸F-FCH-avid tumor thrombosis in the inferior vena cava, extending to the right atrium (arrows) (Fig. 7.8).

Teaching point
- The tumor thrombosis contains malignant cells and accordingly is ¹⁸F-FCH positive in HCC.

REFERENCES

1. Ahmed F, Perz JF, Kwong S, Jamison PM, Friedman C, Bell BP. National trends and disparities in the incidence of hepatocellular carcinoma, 1998–2003. *Preventing Chronic Disease.* July 2008;5(3):A74.
2. Alazawi W, Cunningham M, Dearden J, Foster GR. Systematic review: outcome of compensated cirrhosis due to chronic hepatitis C infection. *Alimentary Pharmacology & Therapeutics.* August 2010;32(3):344–355.
3. El-Serag HB. Hepatocellular carcinoma. *The New England Journal of Medicine.* September 22, 2011;365(12):1118–1127.
4. Howlader N, Noone A, Krapcho M, et al. *SEER Cancer Statistics Review, 1975–2009 (Vintage 2009 Populations).* Bethesda, MD: National Cancer Institute; 2012. based on November 2011 SEER data submission, posted to the SEER web site, 2012.
5. Kanda M, Tateishi R, Yoshida H, et al. Extrahepatic metastasis of hepatocellular carcinoma: incidence and risk factors. *Liver International: Official Journal of the International Association for the Study of the Liver.* November 2008;28(9):1256–1263.
6. Poon D, Anderson BO, Chen LT, et al. Management of hepatocellular carcinoma in Asia: consensus statement from the Asian Oncology Summit 2009. *The Lancet. Oncology.* November 2009;10(11):1111–1118.
7. Waghray A, Murali AR, Menon KN. Hepatocellular carcinoma: from diagnosis to treatment. *World Journal of Hepatology.* May 18, 2015;7(8):1020–1029.
8. Di Bisceglie A, Befeler A. Hepatic tumors and cysts. In: Feldman M, Friedman L, Brandt L, eds. *Sleisenger and Fordtran's Gastrointestinal and Liver Disease: Pathophysiology/Diagnosis/Management.* 10th ed. Philadelphia, PA: Elsevier Saunders; 2016.
9. Singal A, Volk ML, Waljee A, et al. Meta-analysis: surveillance with ultrasound for early-stage hepatocellular carcinoma in patients with cirrhosis. *Alimentary Pharmacology & Therapeutics.* July 2009;30(1):37–47.
10. Bruix J, Sherman M, American Association for the Study of Liver Diseases. Management of hepatocellular carcinoma: an update. *Hepatology.* March 2011;53(3):1020–1022.
11. Forner A, Vilana R, Ayuso C, et al. Diagnosis of hepatic nodules 20 mm or smaller in cirrhosis: prospective validation of the noninvasive diagnostic criteria for hepatocellular carcinoma. *Hepatology.* January 2008;47(1):97–104.
12. Llovet JM, Bru C, Bruix J. Prognosis of hepatocellular carcinoma: the BCLC staging classification. *Seminars in Liver Disease.* 1999;19(3):329–338.
13. Pons F, Varela M, Llovet JM. Staging systems in hepatocellular carcinoma. *HPB: The Official Journal of the International Hepato Pancreato Biliary Association.* 2005;7(1):35–41.
14. Vauthey JN, Lauwers GY, Esnaola NF, et al. Simplified staging for hepatocellular carcinoma. *Journal of Clinical Oncology: Official Journal of the American Society of Clinical Oncology.* March 15, 2002;20(6):1527–1536.
15. Theise N, Curado M, Franceschi S, Hytiroglou P, Kudo M, Park Y. Hepatocellular carcinoma. In: Bosman F, Carneiro F, Hruban R, Theise N, eds. *WHO Classification of Tumours of the Digestive System.* 4th ed. Lyon, France: International Agency for Research on Cancer; 2010:205–216.
16. Liver and intrahepatic bile ducts. In: Robin P, Hansen JT, eds. *TNM Staging Atlas With Oncoanatomy.* 2nd ed. Philadelphia, USA: Wolters Kluwer/LWW; 2012:276–287.
17. Katyal S, Oliver 3rd JH, Peterson MS, Ferris JV, Carr BS, Baron RL. Extrahepatic metastases of hepatocellular carcinoma. *Radiology.* September 2000;216(3):698–703.
18. Version 1. *NCCN Clinical Practice Guidelines in Oncology. Hepatobiliary Cancers;* 2016. www.NCCN.org.
19. Forner A, Reig ME, de Lope CR, Bruix J. Current strategy for staging and treatment: the BCLC update and future prospects. *Seminars in Liver Disease.* February 2010;30(1):61–74.
20. Verslype C, Rosmorduc O, Rougier P, Group EGW. Hepatocellular carcinoma: ESMO-ESDO Clinical Practice Guidelines for diagnosis, treatment and follow-up. *Annals of Oncology: Official Journal of the European Society for Medical Oncology/ESMO.* October 2012;23(suppl 7):vii41–48.
21. Lin CY, Chen JH, Liang JA, Lin CC, Jeng LB, Kao CH. ^{18}F-FDG PET or PET/CT for detecting extrahepatic metastases or recurrent hepatocellular carcinoma: a systematic review and meta-analysis. *European Journal of Radiology.* September 2012;81(9):2417–2422.
22. Bertagna F, Bertoli M, Bosio G, et al. Diagnostic role of radiolabelled choline PET or PET/CT in hepatocellular carcinoma: a systematic review and meta-analysis. *Hepatology International.* October 2014;8(4):493–500.
23. Treglia G, Giovannini E, Di Franco D, et al. The role of positron emission tomography using carbon-11 and fluorine-18 choline in tumors other than prostate cancer: a systematic review. *Annals of Nuclear Medicine.* 2012;26(6):451–461.
24. Lee JW, Oh JK, Chung YA, et al. Prognostic Significance of ^{18}F-FDG Uptake in Hepatocellular Carcinoma Treated with Transarterial Chemoembolization or Concurrent Chemoradiotherapy: A Multicenter Retrospective Cohort Study. *Journal of Nuclear Medicine: Official Publication, Society of Nuclear Medicine.* April 2016;57(4):509–516.
25. Sun DW, An L, Wei F, et al. Prognostic significance of parameters from pretreatment ^{18}F-FDG PET in hepatocellular carcinoma: a meta-analysis. *Abdominal Radiology.* January 2016;41(1):33–41.
26. Sarasin F, Giostra E, Mentha G, Hadengue A. Partial hepatectomy or orthotopic liver transplantation for the treatment of respectable hepatocellular carcinoma? A cost-effectiveness perspective. *Hepatology.* 1998;28:436–442.
27. Delbeke D, Pinson CW. ^{11}C-acetate: a new tracer for the evaluation of hepatocellular carcinoma. *Journal of Nuclear Medicine: Official Publication, Society of Nuclear Medicine.* February 2003;44(2):222–223.

28. Blechacz B, Gores GJ. Positron emission tomography scan for a hepatic mass. *Hepatology.* December 2010; 52(6):2186–2191.

29. Park JW, Kim JH, Kim SK, et al. A prospective evaluation of ^{18}F-FDG and ^{11}C-acetate PET/CT for detection of primary and metastatic hepatocellular carcinoma. *Journal of Nuclear Medicine: Official Publication, Society of Nuclear Medicine.* December 2008;49(12):1912–1921.

30. Pauwels EK, Ribeiro MJ, Stoot JH, McCready VR, Bourguignon M, Maziere B. FDG accumulation and tumor biology. *Nuclear Medicine and Biology.* May 1998;25(4):317–322.

31. Izuishi K, Yamamoto Y, Mori H, et al. Molecular mechanisms of [^{18}F]fluorodeoxyglucose accumulation in liver cancer. *Oncology Reports.* February 2014;31(2):701–706.

32. Delbeke D, Martin WH, Sandler MP, Chapman WC, Wright Jr JK, Pinson CW. Evaluation of benign vs malignant hepatic lesions with positron emission tomography. *Archives of Surgery.* May 1998;133(5):510–515. discussion 515–516.

33. Khan MA, Combs CS, Brunt EM, et al. Positron emission tomography scanning in the evaluation of hepatocellular carcinoma. *Journal of Hepatology.* May 2000;32(5):792–797.

34. Trojan J, Schroeder O, Raedle J, et al. Fluorine-18 FDG positron emission tomography for imaging of hepatocellular carcinoma. *The American Journal of Gastroenterology.* November 1999;94(11):3314–3319.

35. Wudel Jr LJ, Delbeke D, Morris D, et al. The role of [^{18}F] fluorodeoxyglucose positron emission tomography imaging in the evaluation of hepatocellular carcinoma. *The American Surgeon.* February 2003;69(2):117–124. discussion 124–116.

36. Shiomi S, Kawabe J. Clinical applications of positron emission tomography in hepatic tumors. *Hepatology Research: The Official Journal of the Japan Society of Hepatology.* July 2011;41(7):611–617.

37. Wolfort RM, Papillion PW, Turnage RH, Lillien DL, Ramaswamy MR, Zibari GB. Role of FDG-PET in the evaluation and staging of hepatocellular carcinoma with comparison of tumor size, AFP level, and histologic grade. *International Surgery.* January-March 2010;95(1):67–75.

38. Seo S, Hatano E, Higashi T, et al. Fluorine-18 fluorodeoxyglucose positron emission tomography predicts tumor differentiation, P-glycoprotein expression, and outcome after resection in hepatocellular carcinoma. *Clinical Cancer Research: An Official Journal of the American Association for Cancer Research.* January 15, 2007;13(2 pt 1):427–433.

39. Hyun SH, Eo JS, Lee JW, et al. Prognostic value of ^{18}F-fluorodeoxyglucose positron emission tomography/computed tomography in patients with Barcelona Clinic Liver Cancer stages 0 and a hepatocellular carcinomas: a multicenter retrospective cohort study. *European Journal of Nuclear Medicine and Molecular Imaging.* March 2, 2016.

40. Dong A, Yu H, Wang Y, Dong H, Zuo C. FDG PET/CT and enhanced CT imaging of tumor heterogeneity in hepatocellular carcinoma: imaging-pathologic correlation. *Clinical Nuclear Medicine.* September 2014;39(9):808–810.

41. Howard BV, Howard WJ. Lipids in normal and tumor cells in culture. *Progress in Biochemical Pharmacology.* 1975;10:135–166.

42. Ho CL, Yu SC, Yeung DW. ^{11}C-acetate PET imaging in hepatocellular carcinoma and other liver masses. *Journal of Nuclear Medicine: Official Publication, Society of Nuclear Medicine.* February 2003;44(2):213–221.

43. Li S, Beheshti M, Peck-Radosavljevic M, et al. Comparison of ^{11}C-acetate positron emission tomography and [67]Gallium citrate scintigraphy in patients with hepatocellular carcinoma. *Liver International: Official Journal of the International Association for the Study of the Liver.* October 2006;26(8):920–927.

44. Larsson P, Arvidsson D, Björnstedt M, et al. Adding ^{11}C-acetate to ^{18}F-FDG at PET Examination Has an Incremental Value in the Diagnosis of Hepatocellular Carcinoma. *Molecular Imaging and Radionuclide Therapy.* 2012;21(1):6–12.

45. Zeisel SH, da Costa KA. Choline: an essential nutrient for public health. *Nutrition Reviews.* November 2009;67(11):615–623.

46. Bieze M, Klumpen HJ, Verheij J, et al. Diagnostic accuracy of ^{18}F-methylcholine positron emission tomography/computed tomography for intra- and extrahepatic hepatocellular carcinoma. *Hepatology.* March 2014;59(3):996–1006.

47. Kwee SA, Wong LL, Hernandez BY, Chan OT, Sato MM, Tsai N. Chronic Liver Disease and the Detection of Hepatocellular Carcinoma by [^{18}F]fluorocholine PET/CT. *Diagnostics.* 2015;5(2):189–199.

48. Mertens K, Slaets D, Lambert B, Acou M, De Vos F, Goethals I. PET with ^{18}F-labelled choline-based tracers for tumour imaging: a review of the literature. *European Journal of Nuclear Medicine and Molecular Imaging.* November 2010;37(11):2188–2193.

49. Talbot JN, Fartoux L, Balogova S, et al. Detection of hepatocellular carcinoma with PET/CT: a prospective comparison of ^{18}F-fluorocholine and ^{18}F-FDG in patients with cirrhosis or chronic liver disease. *Journal of Nuclear Medicine: Official Publication, Society of Nuclear Medicine.* November 2010;51(11):1699–1706.

50. Kuang Y, Salem N, Tian H, et al. Imaging lipid synthesis in hepatocellular carcinoma with [methyl-^{11}C]choline: correlation with in vivo metabolic studies. *Journal of Nuclear Medicine: Official Publication, Society of Nuclear Medicine.* January 2011;52(1):98–106.

51. Lopci E, Torzilli G, Poretti D, et al. Diagnostic accuracy of ^{11}C-choline PET/CT in comparison with CT and/or MRI in patients with hepatocellular carcinoma. *European Journal of Nuclear Medicine and Molecular Imaging.* August 2015;42(9):1399–1407.

52. Kirienko M, Sollini M, Lopci E, Versari A, Chiti A. Applications of PET imaging with radiolabelled choline (^{11}C/^{18}F-choline). *The Quarterly Journal of Nuclear Medicine and Molecular Imaging: Official Publication of the Italian Association of Nuclear Medicine.* March 2015;59(1):83–94.

53. Hartenbach M, Weber S, Albert NL, et al. Evaluating Treatment Response of Radioembolization in Intermediate-Stage Hepatocellular Carcinoma Patients Using ^{18}F-Fluoroethylcholine PET/CT. *Journal of Nuclear Medicine: Official Publication, Society of Nuclear Medicine.* November 2015;56(11):1661–1666.

54. Castilla-Lievre MA, Franco D, Gervais P, et al. Diagnostic value of combining ^{11}C-choline and ^{18}F-FDG PET/CT in hepatocellular carcinoma. *European Journal of Nuclear Medicine and Molecular Imaging.* May 2016;43(5):852–859.

55. Wu HB, Wang QS, Li BY, Li HS, Zhou WL, Wang QY. F-18 FDG in conjunction with ^{11}C-choline PET/CT in the diagnosis of hepatocellular carcinoma. *Clinical Nuclear Medicine.* December 2011;36(12):1092–1097.

56. Talbot N, Michaud L, Grange J, Rosmorduc O, Balogova S. Use of choline PET for studying hepatocellular carcinoma. *Clinical and Translational Imaging.* 2014;2:103–113.

57. Shin HR, Oh JK, Masuyer E, et al. Epidemiology of cholangiocarcinoma: an update focusing on risk factors. *Cancer Science.* March 2010;101(3):579–585.

58. Tyson GL, El-Serag HB. Risk factors for cholangiocarcinoma. *Hepatology.* July 2011;54(1):173–184.

59. Tsaitas C, Semertzidou A, Sinakos E. Update on inflammatory bowel disease in patients with primary sclerosing cholangitis. *World Journal of Hepatology.* April 27, 2014;6(4):178–187.

60. Vabi BW, Carter J, Rong R, Wang M, Corasanti JG, Gibbs JF. Metastatic colon cancer from extrahepatic cholangiocarcinoma presenting as painless jaundice: case report and literature review. *Journal of Gastrointestinal Oncology.* April 2016;7(2):E25–E30.

61. Signs and Symptoms of Bile Duct Cancer. http://www.cancer.org/cancer/bileductcancer/detailedguide/bile-duct-cancer-signs-symptoms.

62. Van Beers BE. Diagnosis of cholangiocarcinoma. *HPB: The Official Journal of the International Hepato Pancreato Biliary Association.* 2008;10(2):87–93.

63. Farges O, Fuks D, Boleslawski E, et al. Influence of surgical margins on outcome in patients with intrahepatic cholangiocarcinoma: a multicenter study by the AFC-IHCC-2009 study group. *Annals of Surgery.* November 2011;254(5):824–829. discussion 830.

64. Tan JC, Coburn NG, Baxter NN, Kiss A, Law CH. Surgical management of intrahepatic cholangiocarcinoma–a population-based study. *Annals of Surgical Oncology.* February 2008;15(2):600–608.

65. Khan SA, Davidson BR, Goldin R, et al. Guidelines for the diagnosis and treatment of cholangiocarcinoma: consensus document. *Gut.* November 2002;51(suppl 6): VI1–9.

66. Dhanasekaran R, Hemming AW, Zendejas I, et al. Treatment outcomes and prognostic factors of intrahepatic cholangiocarcinoma. *Oncology Reports.* April 2013;29(4):1259–1267.

67. Farhat MH, Shamseddine AI, Tawil AN, et al. Prognostic factors in patients with advanced cholangiocarcinoma: role of surgery, chemotherapy and body mass index. *World Journal of Gastroenterology.* May 28, 2008;14(20):3224–3230.

68. Guglielmi A, Ruzzenente A, Campagnaro T, et al. Intrahepatic cholangiocarcinoma: prognostic factors after surgical resection. *World Journal of Surgery.* June 2009;33(6):1247–1254.

69. Wang Y, Li J, Xia Y, et al. Prognostic nomogram for intrahepatic cholangiocarcinoma after partial hepatectomy. *Journal of Clinical Oncology: Official Journal of the American Society of Clinical Oncology.* March 20, 2013;31(9):1188–1195.

70. Survival Statistics for Bile Duct Cancers. http://www.cancer.org/cancer/bileductcancer/detailedguide/bile-duct-cancer-survival-by-stage.

71. Alberts S, Goldberg R. Gastrointestinal tract cancers. In: Casciato D, ed. *Manual of Clinical Oncology.* 5th ed. Philadelphia, USA: LWW; 2004:185–232.

72. Han JK, Choi BI, Kim AY, et al. Cholangiocarcinoma: pictorial essay of CT and cholangiographic findings. *Radiographics: A Review Publication of the Radiological Society of North America, Inc.* January-February 2002;22(1):173–187.

73. Extrahepatic bile ducts. In: Robin P, Hansen JT, eds. *TNM Staging Atlas With Oncoanatomy.* 2nd ed. Philadelphia, USA: Wolters Kluwer/LWW; 2012:276–287.

74. Eckel F, Brunner T, Jelic S, Group EGW. Biliary cancer: ESMO Clinical Practice Guidelines for diagnosis, treatment and follow-up. *Annals of Oncology: Official Journal of the European Society for Medical Oncology/ESMO.* September 2011;22(suppl 6): vi40–44.

75. Annunziata S, Caldarella C, Pizzuto DA, et al. Diagnostic accuracy of fluorine-18-fluorodeoxyglucose positron emission tomography in the evaluation of the primary tumor in patients with cholangiocarcinoma: a meta-analysis. *BioMed Research International.* 2014;2014:247693.

76. The Royal College of Physicians and the Royal College of Radiologists. *Evidence-based Indications for the Usage of PET-CT in the UK.* London: RCP, RCR; 2013.

77. Srinivasa S, McEntee B, Koea J. The role of PET scans in the management of Cholangiocarcinoma and Gallbladder Cancer: a systematic review for surgeons. *International Journal of Diagnostic Imaging.* 2015;2(1):1–9.

78. Anderson CD, Pinson CW, Berlin J, Chari RS. Diagnosis and treatment of cholangiocarcinoma. *The Oncologist.* 2004;9(1):43–57.

79. Breitenstein S, Apestegui C, Clavien PA. Positron emission tomography (PET) for cholangiocarcinoma. *HPB: The Official Journal of the International Hepato Pancreato Biliary Association.* 2008;10(2):120–121.

80. Kim YJ, Yun M, Lee WJ, Kim KS, Lee JD. Usefulness of ^{18}F-FDG PET in intrahepatic cholangiocarcinoma. *European Journal of Nuclear Medicine and Molecular Imaging.* November 2003;30(11):1467–1472.

81. Kluge R, Schmidt F, Caca K, et al. Positron emission tomography with [^{18}F]fluoro-2-deoxy-D-glucose for diagnosis and staging of bile duct cancer. *Hepatology.* May 2001;33(5):1029–1035.

82. Lee SW, Kim HJ, Park JH, et al. Clinical usefulness of ^{18}F-FDG PET-CT for patients with gallbladder cancer and cholangiocarcinoma. *Journal of Gastroenterology.* May 2010;45(5):560–566.

83. Park TG, Yu YD, Park BJ, et al. Implication of lymph node metastasis detected on ^{18}F-FDG PET/CT for surgical planning in patients with peripheral intrahepatic cholangiocarcinoma. *Clinical Nuclear Medicine.* January 2014;39(1):1–7.

84. Jadvar H, Henderson RW, Conti PS. [F-18]fluorodeoxyglucose positron emission tomography and positron emission tomography: computed tomography in recurrent and metastatic cholangiocarcinoma. *Journal of Computer Assisted Tomography.* March-April 2007;31(2):223–228.

85. Petrowsky H, Wildbrett P, Husarik DB, et al. Impact of integrated positron emission tomography and computed tomography on staging and management of gallbladder cancer and cholangiocarcinoma. *Journal of Hepatology.* July 2006;45(1):43–50.

86. Anderson CD, Rice MH, Pinson CW, Chapman WC, Chari RS, Delbeke D. Fluorodeoxyglucose PET imaging in the evaluation of gallbladder carcinoma and cholangiocarcinoma. *Journal of Gastrointestinal Surgery: Official Journal of the Society for Surgery of the Alimentary Tract.* January 2004;8(1):90–97.

87. Corvera CU, Blumgart LH, Akhurst T, et al. ^{18}F-fluorodeoxyglucose positron emission tomography influences management decisions in patients with biliary cancer. *Journal of the American College of Surgeons.* January 2008;206(1):57–65.

88. Albazaz R, Patel CN, Chowdhury FU, Scarsbrook AF. Clinical impact of FDG PET-CT on management decisions for patients with primary biliary tumours. *Insights Into Imaging.* October 2013;4(5):691–700.

89. Cameron K, Golan S, Simpson W, et al. Recurrent pancreatic carcinoma and cholangiocarcinoma: ^{18}F-fluorodeoxyglucose positron emission tomography/computed tomography (PET/CT). *Abdominal Imaging.* August 2011; 36(4):463–471.

90. Kapoor VK, McMichael AJ. Gallbladder cancer: an 'Indian' disease. *The National Medical Journal of India.* July-August 2003;16(4):209–213.

91. Lowenfels AB, Maisonneuve P, Boyle P, Zatonski WA. Epidemiology of gallbladder cancer. *Hepato-gastroenterology.* May-June 1999;46(27):1529–1532.

92. Chao TC, Greager JA. Primary carcinoma of the gallbladder. *Journal of Surgical Oncology.* April 1991;46(4):215–221.

93. Sasson AR, Hoffman JP, Ross E, et al. Trimodality therapy for advanced gallbladder cancer. *The American Surgeon.* March 2001;67(3):277–283. discussion 284.

94. Shoup M, Fong Y. Surgical indications and extent of resection in gallbladder cancer. *Surgical Oncology Clinics of North America.* October 2002;11(4):985–994.

95. Lim H, Seo DW, Park do H, et al. Prognostic factors in patients with gallbladder cancer after surgical resection: analysis of 279 operated patients. *Journal of Clinical Gastroenterology.* May-June 2013;47(5):443–448.

96. Donohue JH, Stewart AK, Menck HR. The National Cancer Data Base report on carcinoma of the gallbladder, 1989–1995. *Cancer.* December 15, 1998;83(12):2618–2628.

97. Yadav R, Jain D, Mathur SR, Sharma A, Iyer VK. Gallbladder carcinoma: an attempt of WHO histological classification on fine needle aspiration material. *CytoJournal.* 2013;10:12.

98. Albores-Saavedra J, Henson D. *Tumors of the Gallbladder and Extrahepatic Bile Ducts. Atlas of Tumor Pathology.* Washington, DC: Armed Forces Institute of Pathology; 1986.

99. Piehler JM, Crichlow RW. Primary carcinoma of the gallbladder. *Surgery, Gynecology & Obstetrics.* December 1978;147(6):929–942.

100. Annunziata S, Pizzuto DA, Caldarella C, Galiandro F, Sadeghi R, Treglia G. Diagnostic accuracy of fluorine-18-fluorodeoxyglucose positron emission tomography in gallbladder cancer: a meta-analysis. *World Journal of Gastroenterology.* October 28, 2015;21(40):11481–11488.

101. Maldjian PD, Ghesani N, Ahmed S, Liu Y. Adenomyomatosis of the gallbladder: another cause for a "hot" gallbladder on ^{18}F-FDG PET. *AJR. American Journal of Roentgenology.* July 2007;189(1):W36–W38.

102. Ramos-Font C, Gomez-Rio M, Rodriguez-Fernandez A, Jimenez-Heffernan A, Sanchez Sanchez R, Llamas-Elvira JM. Ability of FDG-PET/CT in the detection of gallbladder cancer. *Journal of Surgical Oncology.* March 2014;109(3):218–224.

103. Treglia G, Cason E, Fagioli G. Recent applications of nuclear medicine in diagnostics (first part). *Italian Journal of Medicne.* 2010;4:84–91.

104. Koh T, Taniguchi H, Yamaguchi A, Kunishima S, Yamagishi H. Differential diagnosis of gallbladder cancer using positron emission tomography with fluorine-18-labeled fluoro-deoxyglucose (FDG-PET). *Journal of Surgical Oncology.* October 2003;84(2):74–81.

105. Rodriguez-Fernandez A, Gomez-Rio M, Medina-Benitez A, et al. Application of modern imaging methods in diagnosis of gallbladder cancer. *Journal of Surgical Oncology.* June 15, 2006;93(8):650–664.

106. Ramos-Font C, Gomez Rio M, Rodriguez-Fernandez A, Sanchez Sanchez R, Llamas Elvira JM. Positron tomography with ^{18}F-fluorodeoxyglucose in the preoperative evaluation of gall bladder lesions suspicious of malignancy. Diagnostic utility and clinical impact. *Revista espanola de medicina nuclear.* September-October 2011;30(5):267–275.

107. Nishiyama Y, Yamamoto Y, Fukunaga K, et al. Dual-time-point ^{18}F-FDG PET for the evaluation of gallbladder carcinoma. *Journal of Nuclear Medicine: Official Publication, Society of Nuclear Medicine*. April 2006;47(4):633–638.

108. Kumar R, Sharma P, Kumari A, Halanaik D, Malhotra A. Role of ^{18}F-FDG PET/CT in detecting recurrent gallbladder carcinoma. *Clinical Nuclear Medicine*. May 2012;37(5):431–435.

109. Butte JM, Redondo F, Waugh E, et al. The role of PET-CT in patients with incidental gallbladder cancer. *HPB: The Official Journal of the International Hepato Pancreato Biliary Association*. November 2009;11(7):585–591.

110. Hwang JP, Lim I, Na II , et al. Prognostic Value of SUVmax Measured by Fluorine-18 Fluorodeoxyglucose Positron Emission Tomography with Computed Tomography in Patients with Gallbladder Cancer. *Nuclear Medicine and Molecular Imaging*. June 2014;48(2):114–120.

111. Lee JY, Kim HJ, Yim SH, et al. Primary tumor maximum standardized uptake value measured on ^{18}F-fluorodeoxyglucose positron emission tomography-computed tomography is a prognostic value for survival in bile duct and gallbladder cancer. *The Korean Journal of Gastroenterology [Taehan Sohwagi Hakhoe chi]*. October 2013;62(4):227–233.

CHAPTER 8

Lymphoma

ALIREZA REZAEE • HEIKO SCHÖDER • MARKUS RADERER • WERNER LANGSTEGER • MOHSEN BEHESHTI

BACKGROUND
General[1]
- Neoplasms of the hematopoietic and lymphoid tissues are histologically highly diverse and encompass 145 entities according to the recent World Health Organization (WHO) classification, with the number increasing.
- In clinical practice, mature lymphoid neoplasms are simply divided into Hodgkin lymphoma (HL, consisting of six subtypes) and non-Hodgkin lymphomas (NHLs), including B-cell lymphomas (39 histologically defined entities) and T-cell lymphomas (22 entities). The oversimplified subdivision into "high-grade" and "low-grade" lymphomas should no longer be used, because histology and clinical course are included into the defined entities as put forward in the WHO classification.
- Incidence 2016: Non-HL is the sixth most common cancer and the ninth leading cause of death among US men and women.
- Main risk factors:
  - Advanced age (HL shows a peak in early adulthood as well)
  - Posttransplant immunosuppression
  - Chronic immune stimulation, including infections (Epstein-Barr virus, human immunodeficiency virus [HIV], hepatitis C virus, human T-lymphotropic virus, *Helicobacter pylori*) and autoimmune diseases (including Sjögren syndrome, chronic autoimmune thyroiditis, rheumatoid arthritis)
  - Positive family history of lymphoma
- Currently no screening test is available.

Early Clinical Symptoms[1]
- Painless lymphadenopathy (may cause chest or abdominal pain or dyspnea)
- Anorexia
- Night sweating
- Fatigue
- Unintentional weight loss
- Fever
- Body itching

Primary Diagnostic Procedure[2]
- History and physical examination
- Tissue biopsy—definition of any malignant lymphoma is based on histopathologic assessment

Standard Treatment[1]
Owing to the highly diverse nature, it is beyond the scope of this short overview to provide the reader with an in-depth assessment of therapeutic choices.
- Therapeutic choices might range from wait and see, antibiotic therapy (mucosa-associated lymphoid tissue [MALT] lymphoma), and radiation therapy only (patients with localized follicular lymphoma [FL] or marginal zone lymphoma) to chemoimmunotherapies with or without stem cell transplantation.

Prognostic Factors[3,4]
For the different subtypes of lymphomas, various prognostic scores, including the International Prognostic Index (see later discussion as an example), Follicular Lymphoma International Prognostic Index (versions 1 and 2), Mantle Cell International Prognostic Index, and Cumulative Illness Rating Scale score, have been defined.

Most of these prognostic indices include simple clinical parameters for pretherapeutic stratification of patients, e.g.:

Risk factors (diffuse large B-cell lymphoma)
- Age >60 years
- Abnormal serum lactate dehydrogenase level
- Performance status score 2–4
- Stage III or IV disease
- Extranodal involvement >1 site
International prognostic index
- Low risk: 0 or 1
- Low-intermediate risk: 2
- High-intermediate risk: 3
- High risk: 4 or 5

Five-Year Survival[1]

Survival differs according to the subtype and stage of the disease.

- NHL: 70%
- HL: 86%

TUMOR CHARACTERISTICS AND TYPICAL BEHAVIOR

Histopathology[5,6]

Histopathologic findings for NHL are given in Table 8.1.

Non-Hodgkin lymphoma

- High-grade or aggressive (including diffuse large B-cell lymphoma): 60%
- Low-grade or indolent (including FL): 40%

The two most common subtypes diagnosed from lymph node biopsies are diffuse large B-cell lymphoma and FL (accounting for roughly 50% of all newly diagnosed lymphomas), followed by mantle cell lymphoma and extranodal marginal zone B-cell lymphoma of the MALT (MALT lymphoma), accounting for 8% each.

These statistics, however, fail to take into account that the most common neoplasm is chronic lymphocytic leukemia (CLL), because they refer only to tissue or lymph node biopsies.

Hodgkin lymphoma

- Classic: 95%
  - Nodular sclerosis: 60% to 70%
  - Mixed cellularity: 25%
  - Lymphocyte depleted: 4%
  - Lymphocyte-rich classic: rare
- Nodular lymphocyte predominant: 5%

CLINICAL CLASSIFICATION AND STAGING: ANN ARBOR STAGING SYSTEM[8]

- *Stage I*: Localized disease, limited to one lymph node
- *Stage II*: Involvement of two separate lymph node stations on one side of the diaphragm
- *Stage III*: Spread to both sides of the diaphragm, involving lymph nodes, spleen, tonsils, and Waldeyer ring
- *Stage IV*: Extralymphatic dissemination (bone marrow, liver, lung, bone, skin, pleura)

The Ann Arbor System is still the most commonly applied staging system, although specific staging systems for distinct histologic subtypes (e.g., MALT lymphoma: Lugano Staging System, Paris Staging System) have been developed as a result of various shortcomings of the Ann Arbor Staging System, especially in primary extranodal lymphomas.

GUIDELINES

The European Society for Medical Oncology (ESMO) and National Comprehensive Cancer Network (NCCN) guidelines are given in Table 8.2.

Evidence-based Viewpoints

- Fludeoxyglucose (FDG) PET/CT is recommended for[11,12]:
  - Staging and restaging of HL and most NHLs
  - Early-stage FL
  - Posttransplant lymphoproliferative disorders
  - Interim and end-of-therapy response assessment
  - Before bone marrow transplantation and in cases of low-grade lymphoma, suspicious for transformation
- FDG PET/CT could be a useful method to replace bone marrow biopsy in patients with newly diagnosed Hodgkin lymphoma and also in diffuse large B-cell lymphomas.[13]

TABLE 8.1 Histopathology		
NHL Type[7]	**Aggressive/High Grade**	**Indolent/Low Grade**
B-cell	Diffuse large B-cell lymphoma Follicular lymphoma (grade 3) Mantle cell lymphoma Burkitt lymphoma	Chronic lymphocytic leukemia Small lymphocytic lymphoma Follicular lymphoma (grades 1 & 2) Splenic and nodal marginal zone lymphoma Mucosa-associated lymphoid tissue lymphoma
T-cell	Adult T-cell leukemia/lymphoma	Cutaneous T-cell lymphoma (mycosis fungoides and Sézary syndrome)
Others	AIDS-related lymphoma Primary central nervous system lymphoma Posttransplant lymphoproliferative disorder	Hairy cell leukemia

TABLE 8.2 Guidelines	
Clinical Guidelines	**Recommendations Regarding FDG PET/CT**
ESMO[9]	• Gold standard for staging and restaging in DLBCL • Therapy monitoring after 3 to 4 cycles of chemotherapy in DLBCL • May be considered in addition to stand-alone CT in staging of HL
NCCN	
HL[10]	• Essential for initial staging • Restaging and evaluation of response after completion of chemotherapy • Follow-up after completion of therapy up to 5 years only if last FDG PET was Deauville 4 or 5, to confirm complete response. Thus, it is not recommended for routine posttherapy surveillance • Making decision about the chemotherapy regimen after 2 cycles of therapy if FDG PET is positive or negative

NHL[4]	• *Essential for initial staging*
	  • DLBCL
	  • AIDS-related B-cell lymphoma
	  • Extranodal NK/T-cell lymphoma, nasal type
	  • Peripheral T-cell lymphoma[a]
	• *Useful in selected cases (initial staging)*
	  • FL grade 1 to 2
	  • Nongastric MALT lymphoma
	  • Nodal and splenic MZL
	  • MCL[b]
	  • BL
	  • LL
	  • Primary cutaneous BCL
	  • MF/SS
	  • ATLL
	  • PTLD
	  • T-cell prolymphocytic leukemia
	• *Not useful*
	  • CLL/SLL[c]
	  • HCL

ATLL, adult T-cell leukemia/lymphoma; *BCL*, B-cell lymphoma; *BL*, Burkitt lymphoma; *CLL*, chronic lymphocytic leukemia; *DLBCL*, diffuse large B-cell lymphoma; *ESMO*, European Society for Medical Oncology; *FDG*, fludeoxyglucose; *FL*, follicular lymphoma; *HCL*, hairy cell leukemia; *HL*, Hodgkin lymphoma; *MALT*, mucosa-associated lymphoid tissue; *MCL*, mantle cell lymphoma; *MF*, mycosis fungoides; *MZL*, marginal zone lymphoma; *NCCN*, National Comprehensive Cancer Network; *NHL*, non-Hodgkin lymphoma; *NK*, natural killer; *PTLD*, posttransplant lymphoproliferative disorder; *SLL*, small lymphocytic lymphoma; *SS*, Sézary syndrome.
[a]Chest/abdomen/pelvic contrast-enhanced CT and/or FDG PET/CT.
[b]Useful under certain circumstances.
[c]FDG PET/CT can assist indirectly nodal biopsy if Richter transformation is suspected.

Cost-effectiveness
• FDG PET/CT is highly cost-effective in patients with HL. The PET/CT expenses before and after treatment would increase the total costs of HL staging and initial therapy by only 2%.[14,15]
• FDG PET/CT is a cost-effective modality for staging or restaging, as well as treatment monitoring, of lymphoma in selected histologies.[16–18]

Clinical Point of View
Accurate staging of the lymphoma is of great importance before determining the therapeutic approach. However, it is closely related to the histopathology of the lymphoma, which could be different for the various subtypes. Therefore, only selected types of lymphoma have been covered in this chapter.

Hodgkin lymphoma: Initial staging (including non-invasive assessment of bone marrow involvement) is imperative for the choice of therapy (i.e., abbreviated chemotherapy plus involved field radiotherapy versus prolonged systemic therapy). In addition, in HL, interim functional imaging has become widely accepted as the standard of care with pronounced influence on ongoing therapy. In the case of bulky disease, functional imaging by means of FDG PET/CT after systemic therapy plays a crucial role for defining additional radiotherapy (in case of viable tumor remnants) versus no radiation in patients with complete metabolic remission (i.e., no abnormal FDG uptake).

NHL (mostly diffuse large B-cell lymphoma [DLBCL]): Because systemic therapy has become the universally accepted standard, staging is less important for the selection of treatment (i.e., radiation versus systemic therapy) than in indolent lymphomas. However, as the stage is an integral part of prognostic scoring systems, correct staging is still of importance to the clinicians. In addition, data revealed that bone marrow biopsy can be skipped if there are negative findings on functional imaging modalities (e.g., FDG PET/CT).

In selected patients and histologies (e.g., enteropathy-associated T-cell lymphoma or DLBCL of the small bowel), surgery may still be indicated in cases with localized disease to prevent complications (perforation, bleeding) following chemotherapy. In such patients, primary staging with functional imaging modalities (e.g., FDG PET/CT) seems to be helpful to differentiate localized versus disseminated disease.

Indolent NHL (mostly FL): Initial staging is mandatory to define the small percentage of patients with localized disease in follicular and nodal marginal zone lymphoma. Although the percentage of patients with stage I/II disease is below 10%, these patients are still candidates for potentially curative radiotherapy. In addition, FDG PET/CT might also be suggestive of transformation in case of a markedly elevated standardized uptake value (SUV) in selected locations with a potential to guide rebiopsy for correct histopathologic assessment. It may also be able to define the lymphoma subtypes with the potential for transformation at recurrence (FL, small lymphocytic lymphoma [SLL]/CLL, to a much lesser extent nodal marginal zone lymphoma or splenic marginal zone lymphoma). However, the current clinical recommendations do not support the application of ^{18}F-FDG-PET/CT in patients with extranodal marginal zone B-cell lymphoma of MALT type (irrespective of stage) or follicular duodenal lymphoma.

In patients with stage III or IV disease, FDG PET/CT may have no impact on clinical management because these cases receive systemic immunochemotherapy irrespective of additional sites of the disease.

PITFALLS[6,19–22]

False Positive

- Sarcoidosis
- HIV lymphadenopathy
- Reactive lymph nodes
- Chemotherapy-induced thymic hyperplasia (rebound phenomenon)
- Infection (pneumonia, tonsillitis)
- Granulocyte-colony stimulating factor (G-CSF)-induced bone marrow reactivation
- Drug toxicity (bleomycin)
- Postradiation, postsurgical, or biopsy changes
- FDG-avid benign tumors
- Talc pleurodesis
- Physiologic FDG uptake (brown fat, bone marrow, urinary and gastrointestinal tracts)
- Nodular fasciitis

False Negative

- Low-grade lymphoma: SLL, FL (grades 1 and 2), splenic and nodal marginal zone lymphoma, MALT lymphoma, cutaneous T-cell lymphoma (mycosis fungoides and Sézary syndrome)
- Common false-negative results for all cancers: Early-stage malignancy, hyperglycemic state, small lesions (<8 mm)

DISCUSSION

Primary Staging or Restaging

There are abundant articles in the literature discussing the outstanding role of FDG PET/CT in staging and restaging of HL and NHL.[17,23–29] However, the exceptions are low-grade NHLs, which show little FDG uptake, such as small lymphocytic, MALT, splenic marginal zone, and cutaneous T-cell lymphomas.[6] This is concordant with the major clinical and procedure guidelines, such as ESMO and NCCN, as well as recommendations from the Society of Nuclear Medicine and Molecular Imaging (SNMMI).[4,9,10,12] It is also more sensitive and accurate than stand-alone CT scan in staging lymphoma.[30] In a retrospective study in staging of 210 patients with HL, the sensitivity of FDG PET/CT was higher than that of CT alone (98% vs. 87%). The former was more sensitive than bone marrow biopsy (94% vs. 71%) as well.[14]

FDG PET/CT is capable of detecting metabolic before morphologic changes in the involved organ, such as bone marrow, bone, spleen, and gastrointestinal (GI) tract, which could be missed in the early phases on conventional imaging modalities, such as CT alone.[23,31]

Another potential of FDG PET/CT is the assessment of lymphomatous bone marrow involvement. In a study, the authors calculated a sensitivity, specificity, and negative predictive value (NPV) of 100%, 90%, and 100%, respectively. With an NPV of 100%, they suggested that bone marrow biopsy can be safely omitted in patients with lymphoma with unremarkable homogeneous pattern of marrow uptake on FDG PET/CT.[13,31] This is also accepted by the NCCN guideline. On the other hand, the NCCN and ESMO guidelines clearly indicate that if there are multifocal (≥3) skeletal FDG PET/CT lesions, the marrow may be assumed to be involved.[4,9,10]

Therapy Monitoring

With a large variety in treatment options for patients with lymphoma, it is crucial to optimize management to achieve the best disease control with least side effects to patients. FDG PET/CT is superior to conventional methods in the early assessment of response to treatment.[25] It is a pivotal method to distinguish responders from nonresponders and decide about continuation of ongoing therapy. The interim FDG PET/CT can be successfully utilized for risk-adapted treatment.[25,26,30,32,33]

It is noteworthy that in the workshop at the 12th International Conference on Malignant Lymphoma, FDG PET/CT was not only formally incorporated in standard staging for FDG-avid lymphomas but also was recommended as a method to evaluate response to therapy using the five-point scale/Deauville criteria[30,34] (Table 8.3).

In addition, semiquantitative analysis by means of SUV provides accurate information regarding treatment response and may reduce false-positive interim PET interpretations at two cycles after chemotherapy.[35]

TABLE 8.3
Deauville Criteria

Deauville Score	PET/CT Results
1	No uptake
2	Lesion uptake < mediastinum
3	Mediastinum < lesion uptake ≤ liver
4	Lesion uptake moderately higher than liver
5	Lesion uptake markedly higher[a] than liver and/or new lesions
X	New area of uptake unlikely to be related to lymphoma

[a]2 to 3 times the SUV_{max} of normal liver.

This modality is also capable of differentiating posttherapeutic fibrotic scar tissue from residual malignancy.[36]

Prognostic Value and Change of Management

Similar to other roles of FDG PET/CT in the assessment of lymphoma, its ability to predict prognosis in these patients is also well addressed in the medical literature. A retrospective, international, multicenter study revealed that the patients with interim negative FDG PET/CT had a 95% 3-year progression-free survival rate, compared with only 28% for patients with interim positive images. Also, the sensitivity, specificity, positive predictive value, and NPV of the modality for prediction of therapy outcome was 73%, 94%, 73%, and 94%, respectively.[37]

Some authors believe that interim and/or end-of-therapy FDG PET/CT have a prognostic role in the evaluation of lymphoma.[23,29,38,39] This is accepted by the UK Royal College of Radiologists and SNMMI guidelines but has not been universally incorporated into guidelines put forward by hematooncologic societies.[11,12]

Based on semiquantitative analysis, Ngeow and colleagues realized that among the 122 enrolled patients, an SUV >10 may predict an aggressive histology for lymphoma. The disease was upstaged in 17% of the patients by FDG PET/CT.[31] In another study of 210 patients, FDG PET/CT led to upstaging in 24%, downstaging in 17%, and a change of treatment in 15% of cases.[14]

In addition, a 65.7% reduction in the SUV_{max} after two cycles of chemotherapy can better predict event-free survival (EFS).[35] It could also be used for the prediction of prognosis in DLBCL. The early FDG PET predicts EFS with an accuracy of approximately 65%.

The 2-year EFS was 51% and 79% in PET-positive and PET-negative groups, respectively.[40]

TEACHING CASES
Case 1: Staging—DLBCL
Findings

A 61-year-old male with DLBCL, Ann Arbor stage IIIS. FDG PET/CT shows tracer-avid cervical, axillary, mediastinal, supradiaphragmatic, subpleural, upper abdominal, peritoneal, mesenterial, retroperitoneal, paraaortic, iliac, and inguinal lymph nodes; multifocal tracer uptakes throughout the spleen (Fig. 8.1A and B, black arrows); and FDG-avid lymph node within the right arm muscles (Fig. 8.1A and C, red arrow), consistent with lymphomatous involvement.

Teaching points

- Lymphoma is usually FDG avid, except for the indolent or low-grade types.
- Lymphoma may present with an atypical pattern, such as involvement of subpleural and intermuscular lymph nodes (Fig. 8.1C, red arrow, and Fig. 8.1D, arrows).
- Although fine-needle aspiration (FNA) is the standard diagnostic procedure in the assessment of bone marrow involvement, with an NPV of about 100% for FDG PET/CT, the bone marrow biopsy can be safely omitted in patients with lymphoma with unremarkable homogeneous pattern of marrow FDG uptake. The histopathologic result for FNA was negative in this patient.
- FDG PET/CT is superior to stand-alone CT for the assessment of small and morphologically nonsuspicious lymph nodes.

Pitfalls

- Sarcoidosis, which may cause FDG-avid lymphadenopathy, is a differential diagnosis for lymphoma on FDG PET/CT. However, lack of metabolically active bilateral hilar lymph nodes is not typical for sarcoidosis in this patient.

Case 2: Restaging—DLBCL
Findings

A 59-year-old male with gastric diffuse large B-cell lymphoma, status post–chemotherapy with rituximab-cyclophosphamide, doxorubicin, vincristine, and prednisone. Staging FDG PET/CT shows tracer-avid bilateral pulmonary masses (Fig. 8.2A, black arrow) and mediastinal and abdominal lymph nodes. Heterogeneous multifocal increased FDG uptake in liver (Fig. 8.2A and C, blue arrows) and stomach (Fig. 8.2C, red arrow) represents

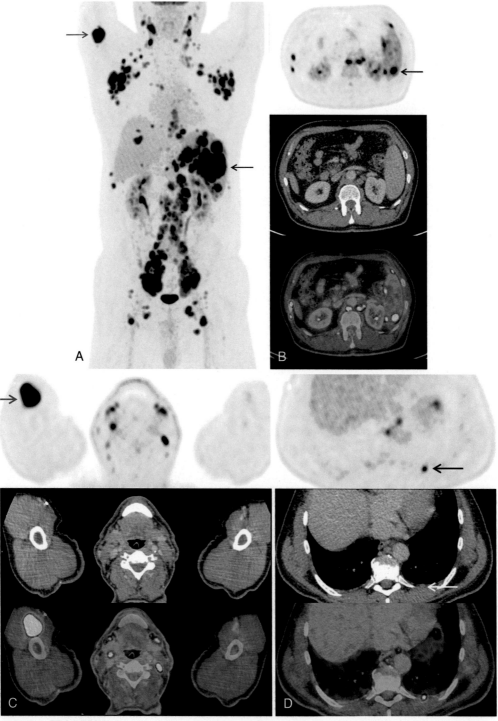

FIG. 8.1 FDG PET/CT showing tracer-avid cervical, axillary, mediastinal, supradiaphragmatic, subpleural, (D), upper abdominal, peritoneal, mesenterial, retroperitoneal, paraaortic, iliac, and inguinal lymph nodes, and multifocal tracer uptakes throughout the spleen (A and B, *black arrows*), as well as an FDG-avid lymph node within the right arm muscles (A and C, *red arrow*), consistent with lymphomatous involvement.

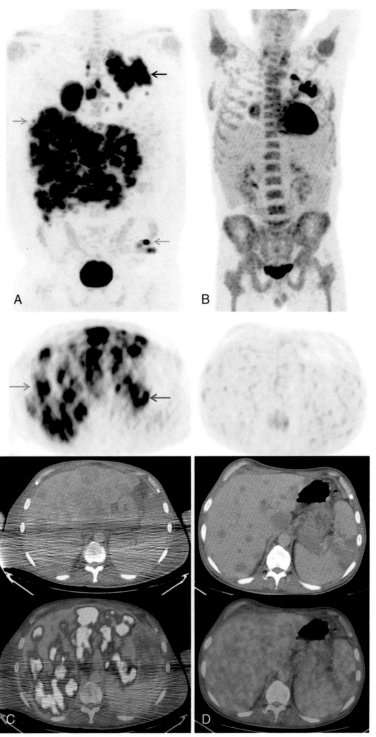

FIG. 8.2 Staging FDG PET/CT (A) showing tracer-avid bilateral pulmonary masses (A, *black arrow*) and mediastinal and abdominal lymph nodes. Heterogeneous multifocal increased FDG uptake in the liver (A and C, *blue arrows*) and stomach (C, *red arrow*) represents lymphomatous involvement. Interim study after three cycles of chemotherapy (B) shows partial metabolic response to therapy.

lymphomatous involvement. Interim study after three cycles of chemotherapy (Fig. 8.2B) shows partial metabolic response to therapy. Of note are non-FDG-avid morphologic changes in the liver, representing a favorable metabolic response. Diffuse bone marrow uptake is caused by chemotherapy and resultant bone marrow reactivation (Fig. 8.2).

Teaching points
- FDG PET/CT is capable of assessing therapy response after two cycles of chemotherapy.
- It is superior to morphologic imaging modalities and able to detect metabolic response before morphologic changes in the involved organs, such as bone marrow, bone, spleen, and GI tract, appear.

Pitfalls
- Diffuse bone marrow uptake after chemotherapy is a physiologic reaction and should not be interpreted as disseminated bone marrow involvement with lymphoma. The histopathology result of bone marrow aspiration was negative in this patient.
- The patient was imaged with the arms down by the sides, and FDG uptake at the site of tracer injection on the left hand is seen on the lower left abdomen (Fig. 8.2A, green arrow). Also, beam-hardening artifact is evident on CT because of the arms-down position, which affects the quality of CT images.

Case 3: Therapy Monitoring—Hodgkin Lymphoma
Findings
A 28-year-old male with nodular sclerosis classical HL, Ann Arbor classification IIB. Staging FDG PET/CT demonstrates tracer-avid bulky mediastinal lymphadenopathy (Fig. 8.3A and C, black arrow) with small bilateral metabolically active supraclavicular lymph nodes (Fig. 8.3A, red arrows), consistent with known primary lymphoma. Follow-up images show a favorable complete metabolic response to chemotherapy in spite of faint FDG uptake in the residual mass (Fig. 8.3B and D, arrow), which is less than mediastinal blood pool uptake (Deauville score: 2).

Teaching points
- Residual soft tissue mass with very faint FDG uptake (less than mediastinal), which represents an excellent metabolic response of lymphoma to chemotherapy, is indicative of stand-alone CT limitations for the evaluation of lymphoma.
- The sensitivity of FDG PET/CT is higher than that of CT alone (98% vs. 87%) and bone marrow biopsy (94% vs. 71%).

Pitfalls
- A mild increased FDG uptake in the thymic tissue is known as "rebound thymic hyperplasia" caused by chemotherapy and should not be interpreted as lymphomatous involvement.
- A mild to moderate increased testicular FDG uptake in young patients is physiologic.

Case 4: DLBCL—Atypical Presentation in Genitourinary Tract
Findings
A 73-year-old male with DLBCL. FDG PET/CT shows tracer-avid lymphomatous involvement of the left cervical lymph nodes, right kidney (Fig. 8.4A and B, red arrows), and left testis (Fig. 8.4A and C, yellow arrows) and generalized bone marrow involvement. Of incidental note is mildly FDG-avid bilateral paraspinal brown fat tissue, which is physiologic (Fig. 8.4).

Teaching points
- Renal and testicular involvement with lymphoma is not a common presentation.
- FDG PET/CT is superior to stand-alone CT for the evaluation of bone marrow lymphomatous involvement, which could be missed on CT images.
- FDG PET/CT has a sensitivity, specificity, and NPV of 100%, 90%, and 100% for the detection of bone marrow involvement, respectively.

Pitfalls
- Renal parenchymal lymphomatous involvement should not be interpreted as physiologic radioactive urine in the renal collecting system. Correlation with CT is pivotal in correct diagnosis.
- Usually, physiologically active brown fat tissue has a typical pattern on PET and should not be misinterpreted as nodal lymphomatous involvement. Pattern and localization of tracer uptake and CT correlation are helpful for correct interpretation.
- The normal testis shows physiologic FDG uptake that declines with age. It should be differentiated with pathologic accumulation as in this case. An SUV_{max} >5.0 should be further evaluated to rule out malignancy.

Case 5: Burkitt Lymphoma—Atypical Presentation
Findings
A 46-year-old female with DLBCL/Burkitt lymphoma. FDG PET/CT shows tracer-avid tumors of the body and tail of the pancreas (yellow arrows) and spleen (red arrow). A faintly FDG-avid right cervical lymph node is most likely reactive in nature (Fig. 8.5A, blue arrow).

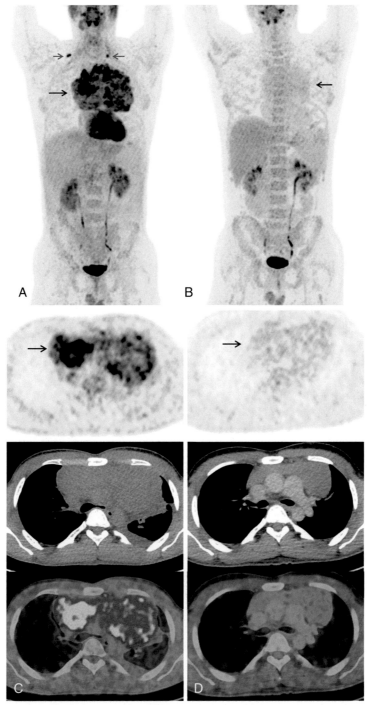

FIG. 8.3 Staging FDG PET/CT (A and C) demonstrating tracer-avid bulky mediastinal lymphadenopathy (A and C, *black arrow*) with small bilateral metabolically active supraclavicular lymph nodes (A, *red arrows*), consistent with known primary lymphoma. Follow-up images (B and D) show a favorable complete metabolic response to chemotherapy in spite of faint FDG uptake in residual mass (B and D, *arrow*), which is less than mediastinal blood pool uptake (Deauville score: 2).

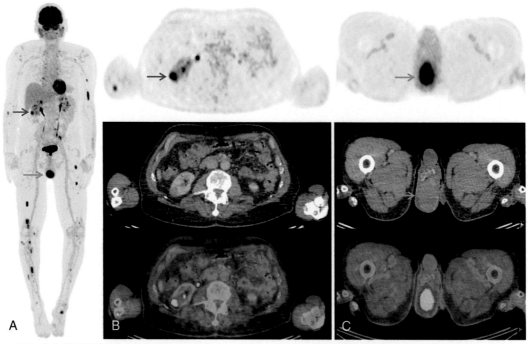

FIG. 8.4 FDG PET/CT showing tracer-avid lymphomatous involvement of left cervical lymph nodes, right kidney (A and B, *red arrows*), and left testis (A and C, *blue arrows*) and generalized bone marrow involvement.

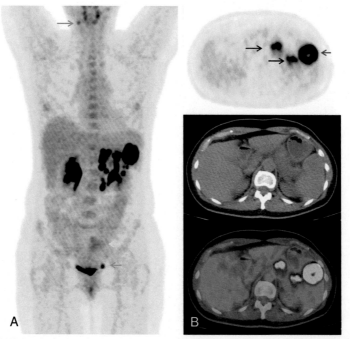

FIG. 8.5 FDG PET/CT showing tracer-avid tumors of the body and tail of the pancreas (*yellow arrows*) and spleen (*red arrow*). A faintly FDG-avid right cervical lymph node is most likely reactive in nature (A, *blue arrow*). A focal uptake in the left distal ureter is accumulation of radioactive urine (A, *green arrow*). A faint FDG uptake in the uterus is most likely physiologic, related to the hormonal cycle in this premenopausal woman (A, *yellow arrow*). B, Axial FDG PET, CT, and fused images.

A focal uptake in the left distal ureter is accumulation of radioactive urine (Fig. 8.5A, green arrow). The faint FDG uptake in the uterus is most likely physiologic, related to the hormonal cycle in this premenopausal woman (Fig. 8.5A, yellow arrow).

Teaching points
- In this case, the lesions on anatomic imaging can be misinterpreted as pancreatic adenocarcinoma with splenic metastases. Correlation with tissue diagnosis is strongly recommended to prevent unnecessary surgeries in the case of lymphoma.
- The intensity of FDG uptake is usually higher in most types of lymphoma (except for the indolent type) compared with adenocarcinoma.

Pitfalls
- Radioactive urine accumulation in ureters, a urinary bladder diverticulum, or atypical tracer accumulation in the bladder after gynecologic surgical procedures may be misinterpreted as malignancy on PET alone. Correlation with CT improves specificity.
- Reactive lymph nodes may falsely be interpreted as positive. Comparison of tracer intensity with the primary tumor is crucial for clarification.
- A mild uterine FDG uptake in premenopausal age could be physiologic.

Case 6: DLBCL—Prominent Bone Marrow Infiltration
Findings
A 58-year-old male with DLBCL, status post four cycles of chemotherapy. FDG PET/CT shows generalized, multifocal tracer-avid bone marrow lymphomatous involvement, with no corresponding anatomic changes on CT (Fig. 8.6C). There are numerous FDG-avid mediastinal, axillary, and abdominal lymph nodes, as well as a focal increased uptake in the spleen (Fig. 8.6A and E), compatible with the primary diagnosis of lymphoma. A follow-up scan demonstrates a favorable metabolic response to therapy (Fig. 8.6B,D, and F).

Teaching points
- FDG PET/CT is superior to stand-alone CT for the early detection of bone marrow involvement.
- There is significant correlation between positive PET and the result of FNA.
- FDG PET/CT can successfully be used for guiding bone marrow biopsy to increase accuracy.

- Major clinical guidelines indicate that if there are multifocal (≥3) skeletal FDG PET/CT lesions, the marrow may be assumed to be involved in patients with lymphoma.

Pitfalls
- The uptake in the floor of the mouth is caused by inflammation after chemotherapy (Fig. 8.6B).

Case 7: Hodgkin Lymphoma—Therapy Evaluation (Deauville Criteria)
Findings
A 55-year-old male with HL. Staging FDG PET/CT shows tracer-avid left inguinal, bilateral iliac, left supraclavicular, right axillary, and left cervical lymph nodes (Fig. 8.7A and C, arrows), consistent with lymphomatous involvement. A follow-up scan (Fig. 8.7B and D) shows an excellent response to chemotherapy, with faintly FDG-avid residual left inguinal lymph node (Fig. 8.7D, arrows).

Teaching points
- According to Deauville criteria, this patient is in complete remission. A low uptake in the residual left inguinal lymph node is less than that in the liver.
- Owing to residual soft tissue, clinical and imaging follow-up is recommended.
- Patients with interim negative FDG PET/CT have a 95% 3-year progression-free survival rate, compared with only 28% for patients with interim positive images.

Pitfalls
- FDG PET has a poorer quality in obese patients.
- Bilateral cervical muscles uptake in the follow-up image is nonspecific.

Case 8: DLBCL—Disease Progression
Findings
A 79-year-old female with DLBCL. FDG PET/CT shows tracer-avid right meningeal lesions (Fig. 8.8A and B, arrows). There are numerous FDG-avid skeletal and left parotid involvement and retroperitoneal, iliac, and inguinal lymph nodes, compatible with lymphomatous involvement. A metabolically active tumor within the right iliac bone with infiltration to the adjacent abdominal wall is also malignant in nature. Follow-up PET/CT demonstrates progression based on an increased intensity in the old metastatic disease and development of new FDG-avid lesions (Fig. 8.8).

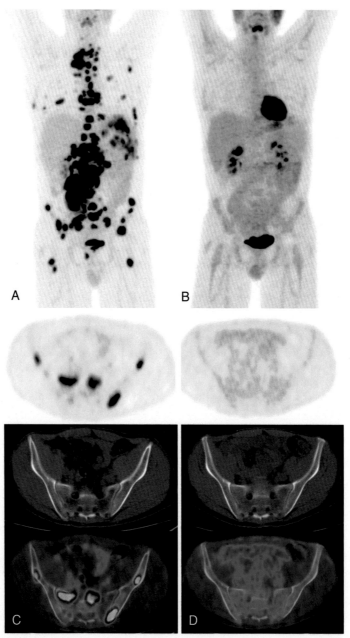

FIG. 8.6 FDG PET/CT showing generalized multifocal tracer-avid bone marrow lymphomatous involvement, with no corresponding anatomic changes on CT (C). There are numerous FDG-avid mediastinal,
axillary, and abdominal lymph nodes, as well as a focal increased uptake in the spleen (A; E, arrow),
compatible with the primary diagnosis of lymphoma. A follow-up scan demonstrates a favorable metabolic
response to therapy (B,D, and F).

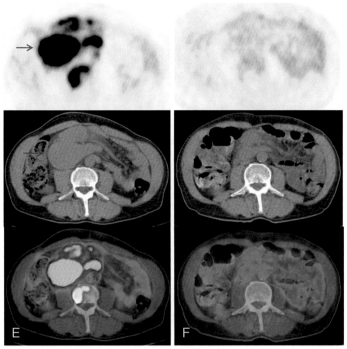

FIG. 8.6, cont'd

Teaching points
- PET/CT is more accurate for the assessment of the status of disease compared with stand-alone CT.
- Although brain tissue shows a markedly increased physiologic FDG uptake, metabolically active intracranial lesions could be depicted by this modality.
- The modality is also capable of differentiating posttherapeutic fibrotic scar tissue from residual malignancy.

Pitfalls
- Radiotracer extravasation and contamination at the site of injection make the SUVs unreliable, which should be considered when using delta-SUV for the assessment of treatment response.

Case 9: Staging and Restaging Burkitt Lymphoma
Findings
A 23-year-old male with Burkitt lymphoma. FDG PET/CT shows diffuse tracer-avid omental lymphomatous involvement (Fig. 8.9A, arrows), numerous FDG-avid liver lesions (Fig. 8.9C, black arrows), disseminated bone involvement with prominent lytic lesions and cortical defects (Fig. 8.9C, red arrows), and FDG-avid bilateral internal mammary, supradiaphragmatic, and abdominal lymph nodes, all compatible with the primary diagnosis of lymphoma. There is diffuse nonhomogeneous FDG-avid bone marrow involvement and multifocal lytic bony uptakes, prominently within the appendicular skeleton. Follow-up FDG PET/CT 1 month after chemotherapy (Fig. 8.9B) demonstrates excellent metabolic response to treatment. Of incidental note is a focal FDG uptake in midabdomen on follow-up scan (Fig. 8.9B, arrow), corresponding to a foreign body inflammation (Fig. 8.9).

Teaching points
- Burkitt lymphoma has poor prognosis.
- Diffuse abdominal involvement may not correlate on CT.
- FDG PET/CT is superior to stand-alone CT for the evaluation of bone metastases in lymphoma.

Pitfalls
- Reactive or hyperplastic bone marrow should be differentiated from diffuse bone marrow lymphomatous involvement by interpreters. The pattern of uptake is homogeneous for reactive and heterogeneous for bone marrow infiltration.

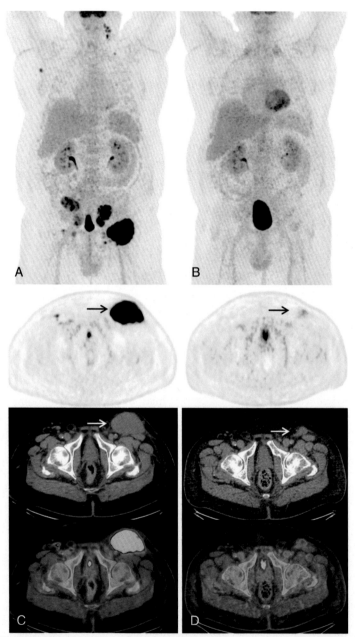

FIG. 8.7 Staging FDG PET/CT showing tracer-avid left inguinal, bilateral iliac, left supraclavicular, right axillary, and left cervical lymph nodes (A; C, *arrows*), consistent with lymphomatous involvement. A follow-up scan (B and D) shows excellent response to chemotherapy with faintly FDG-avid residual left inguinal lymph node (D, *arrows*).

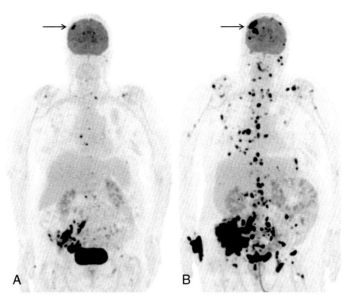

FIG. 8.8 FDG PET/CT showing tracer-avid right meningeal lesions (A and B, *arrows*). There are numerous FDG-avid skeletal and left parotid involvement and retroperitoneal, iliac, and inguinal lymph nodes, compatible with lymphomatous involvement.

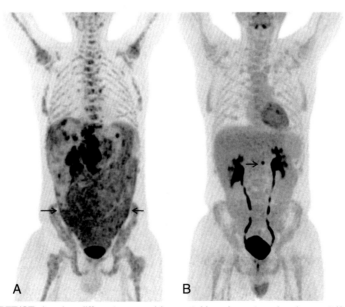

FIG. 8.9 FDG PET/CT showing diffuse tracer-avid omental lymphomatous involvement (A, *arrows*), numerous FDG-avid liver lesions (C, *black arrows*), disseminated bone involvement with prominent lytic lesions and cortical defects (C, *red arrows*), and FDG-avid bilateral internal mammary, supradiaphragmatic, and abdominal lymph nodes, all compatible with the primary diagnosis of lymphoma. Follow-up FDG PET/CT 1 month after chemotherapy (B) demonstrates excellent metabolic response to treatment. Of incidental note is a focal FDG uptake in midabdomen on follow-up scan (B, *arrow*), corresponding to a foreign body inflammation. Image D also demonstrates excellent response to therapy.

Continued

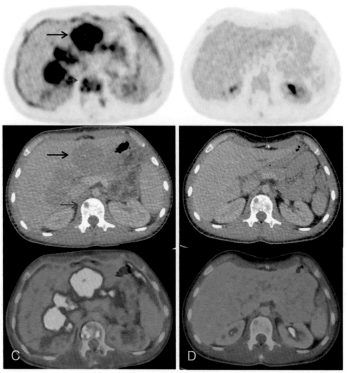

FIG. 8.9, cont'd

Case 10: Meningeal Lymphomatosis
Findings

A 71-year-old male with DLBCL referred for follow-up imaging. An incidental finding is that FDG PET/CT shows lumbar leptomeningeal uptake, consistent with leptomeningeal lymphomatosis (red arrows). There is FDG uptake within the left subclavian vein (blue arrow), most likely inflammatory, secondary to prior vascular intervention/catheterization. A focal FDG uptake on the right thyroid lobe is suggestive of thyroid adenoma (green arrow). A focal uptake in the dorsal right hand is the site of tracer injection (arrowhead) (Fig. 8.10).

Teaching points
- PET/CT is superior to stand-alone CT in the evaluation of leptomeningeal lymphomatosis.
- In patients with DLBCL, the 2-year event-free survival is 51% versus 79% in PET-positive and PET-negative groups, respectively.

Pitfalls
- Every FDG-positive thyroid nodule should be further evaluated clinically and histologically.
- FDG uptake in bilateral cervical muscles is nonspecific.

- The CT images show beam-hardening artifact from the arm-down position at the time of acquisition.

Case 11: Marrow Uptake After Therapy Using G-CSF
Findings

A 36-year-old male with DLBCL, status post–G-CSF therapy. FDG PET/CT shows a diffuse FDG uptake throughout the axial and proximal appendicular skeleton after G-CSF treatment. The bone marrow FNA was negative in this patient. FDG uptake is moderately increased in the spleen compared with that in the liver, also a consequence of recent therapy (Fig. 8.11).

Teaching points
- G-CSF can increase marrow uptake because of bone marrow hyperplasia, even shortly after therapy. It should not be interpreted as marrow infiltration by malignant cells.

Case 12: Hodgkin Lymphoma—Treatment Monitoring
Findings

A 67-year-old female with HL, status postchemotherapy. FDG PET/CT shows multiple tracer-avid thoracic

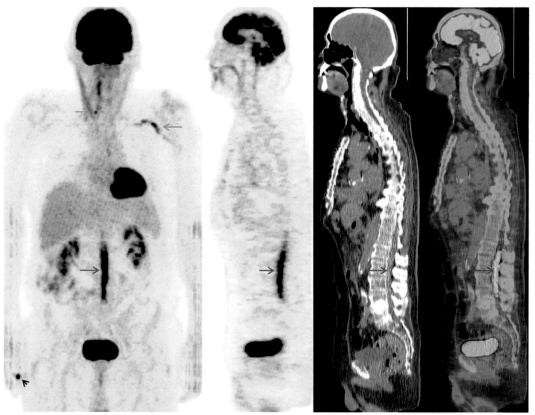

FIG. 8.10 FDG PET/CT showing lumbar leptomeningeal uptake, consistent with leptomeningeal lymphomatosis (*red arrows*). There is FDG uptake within the left subclavian vein (*blue arrow*), most likely inflammatory, secondary to prior vascular intervention/catheterization. A focal FDG uptake on the right thyroid lobe is suggestive of thyroid adenoma (*green arrow*). A focal uptake in the dorsal right hand is the site of tracer injection (*arrowhead*).

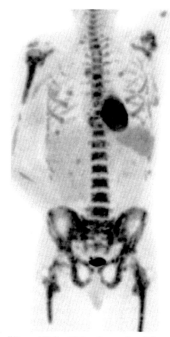

FIG. 8.11 FDG PET/CT showing diffuse FDG uptake throughout the axial and proximal appendicular skeleton after granulocyte-colony stimulating factor treatment.

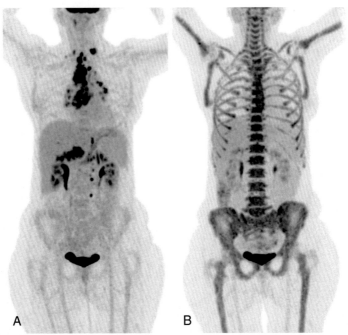

FIG. 8.12 FDG PET/CT showing multiple tracer-avid thoracic and abdominal lymph nodes, compatible with the known diagnosis of lymphoma (A). A follow-up scan demonstrates a favorable complete metabolic response to chemotherapy (B). A diffuse FDG uptake throughout the axial and proximal appendicular skeleton on the follow-up scan is caused by bone marrow hyperplasia secondary to chemotherapy (B).

and abdominal lymph nodes, compatible with the known diagnosis of lymphoma (Fig. 8.12A). A follow-up scan demonstrates a favorable complete metabolic response to chemotherapy (Fig. 8.12B). A diffuse FDG uptake throughout the axial and proximal appendicular skeleton on the follow-up scan is caused by bone marrow hyperplasia secondary to chemotherapy (Fig. 8.12B).

Teaching points

- Marrow hyperplasia is in the differential diagnosis of lymphomatous infiltration. History of recent chemotherapy and favorable metabolic response in primary lesions on surveillance scan are the key points for correct interpretation.
- Complete remission after first-line therapy has a higher rate for progression-free survival than partial remission.
- An average of 10% and 25% of patients with HL and NHL have bone marrow infiltration on initial presentation, respectively. These patients and those with liver or splenic involvement have poor prognosis compared with those with isolated nodal malignancy.

REFERENCES

1. American Cancer Society. *Cancer Facts & Figures*; 2016. Available at: www.cancer.org/acs/groups/content/@editorial/documents/document/acspc-044552.pdf.
2. Diagnostic Procedure. www.cancer.net.
3. Prognostic Factors. www.cancer.org.
4. Version 3. *NCCN Clinical Practice Guidelines in Oncology. Non-Hodgkin's Lymphomas*; 2016. www.NCCN.org.
5. Leukemia & Lymphoma Society. www.lls.org/lymphoma.
6. D'Souza MM, Jaimini A, Bansal A, et al. FDG-PET/CT in lymphoma. *The Indian Journal of Radiology & Imaging*. October 2013;23(4):354–365.
7. www.cancer.ca/en/cancer-information/cancer-type/non-hodgkin-ymphoma/grading.
8. Carbone PP, Kaplan HS, Musshoff K, Smithers DW, Tubiana M. Report of the Committee on Hodgkin's Disease Staging Classification. *Cancer Research*. November 1971;31(11):1860–1861.
9. Tilly H, Gomes da Silva M, Vitolo U, et al. Diffuse large B-cell lymphoma (DLBCL): ESMO Clinical Practice Guidelines for diagnosis, treatment and follow-up. *Annals of Oncology: Official Journal of the European Society for Medical Oncology/ESMO*. September 2015;26(suppl 5): v116–v125.
10. Version 2. *NCCN Clinical Practice Guidelines in Oncology. Hodgkin Lymphoma*; 2016. www.NCCN.org.

11. The Royal College of Physicians and the Royal College of Radiologists. *Evidence-based Indications for the Usage of PET-CT in the UK.* London: RCP, RCR; 2013.

12. Fletcher JW, Djulbegovic B, Soares HP, et al. Recommendations on the use of ^{18}F-FDG PET in oncology. *Journal of Nuclear Medicine: Official Publication, Society of Nuclear Medicine.* March 2008;49(3):480–508.

13. Adams HJ, Kwee TC, de Keizer B, et al. Systematic review and meta-analysis on the diagnostic performance of FDG-PET/CT in detecting bone marrow involvement in newly diagnosed Hodgkin lymphoma: is bone marrow biopsy still necessary? *Annals of Oncology: Official Journal of the European Society for Medical Oncology/ESMO.* May 2014;25(5):921–927.

14. Cerci JJ, Trindade E, Buccheri V, et al. Consistency of FDG-PET accuracy and cost-effectiveness in initial staging of patients with Hodgkin lymphoma across jurisdictions. *Clinical Lymphoma, Myeloma & Leukemia.* August 2011;11(4):314–320.

15. Cerci JJ, Trindade E, Pracchia LF, et al. Cost effectiveness of positron emission tomography in patients with Hodgkin's lymphoma in unconfirmed complete remission or partial remission after first-line therapy. *Journal of Clinical Oncology: Official Journal of the American Society of Clinical Oncology.* March 10, 2010;28(8):1415–1421.

16. Buck AK, Herrmann K, Stargardt T, Dechow T, Krause BJ, Schreyogg J. Economic evaluation of PET and PET/CT in oncology: evidence and methodologic approaches. *Journal of Nuclear Medicine: Official Publication, Society of Nuclear Medicine.* March 2010;51(3):401–412.

17. Hoh CK, Glaspy J, Rosen P, et al. Whole-body FDG-PET imaging for staging of Hodgkin's disease and lymphoma. *Journal of Nuclear Medicine: Official Publication, Society of Nuclear Medicine.* March 1997;38(3):343–348.

18. Annunziata S, Caldarella C, Treglia G. Cost-effectiveness of Fluorine-18-Fluorodeoxyglucose positron emission tomography in tumours other than lung cancer: a systematic review. *World Journal of Radiology.* March 28, 2014;6(3):48–55.

19. Carter K, Kotlyarov E. Common causes of false positive F18 FDG PET/CT scans in oncology. *Brazilian Archives of Biology and Technology.* 2007;50:29–35.

20. Kazama T, Faria SC, Varavithya V, Phongkitkarun S, Ito H, Macapinlac HA. FDG PET in the evaluation of treatment for lymphoma: clinical usefulness and pitfalls. *Radiographics: A Review Publication of the Radiological Society of North America, Inc.* January-February 2005;25(1):191–207.

21. Rezaee A, Chen W, Dilsizian V, Chen Q, Kimball AS. Giant Cell Tumor of the Tendon Sheath With Discordant Metabolism as a False Positive on Staging of Mantle Cell Lymphoma. *Clinical Nuclear Medicine.* October 2015;40(10):814–815.

22. Zhou Q, Young D, Vingan H. Nodular fasciitis mimicking recurrent lymphoma on positron emission tomography-computed tomography. *Radiology Case Reports.* June 2016;11(2):110–112.

23. Friedberg JW, Chengazi V. PET scans in the staging of lymphoma: current status. *The Oncologist.* 2003;8(5):438–447.

24. Herrmann K, Queiroz M, Huellner MW, et al. Diagnostic performance of FDG-PET/MRI and WB-DW-MRI in the evaluation of lymphoma: a prospective comparison to standard FDG-PET/CT. *BMC Cancer.* 2015;15:1002.

25. Kostakoglu L, Cheson BD. Current role of FDG PET/CT in lymphoma. *European Journal of Nuclear Medicine and Molecular Imaging.* May 2014;41(5):1004–1027.

26. Mylam KJ, Nielsen AL, Pedersen LM, Hutchings M. Fluorine-18-fluorodeoxyglucose Positron Emission Tomography in Diffuse Large B-cell Lymphoma. *PET Clinics.* October 2014;9(4):443–455, vi.

27. Perry C, Lerman H, Joffe E, et al. The Value of PET/CT in Detecting Bone Marrow Involvement in Patients With Follicular Lymphoma. *Medicine.* March 2016;95(9):e2910.

28. Thanarajasingam G, Bennani-Baiti N, Thompson CA. PET-CT in Staging, Response Evaluation, and Surveillance of Lymphoma. *Current Treatment Options in Oncology.* May 2016;17(5):24.

29. Tirumani SH, LaCasce AS, Jacene HA. Role of 2-Deoxy-2-[^{18}F]-fluoro-D-glucose-PET/Computed Tomography in Lymphoma. *PET Clinics.* April 2015;10(2):207–225.

30. Barrington SF, Mikhaeel NG, Kostakoglu L, et al. Role of imaging in the staging and response assessment of lymphoma: consensus of the International Conference on Malignant Lymphomas Imaging Working Group. *Journal of Clinical Oncology: Official Journal of the American Society of Clinical Oncology.* September 20, 2014;32(27):3048–3058.

31. Ngeow JY, Quek RH, Ng DC, et al. High SUV uptake on FDG-PET/CT predicts for an aggressive B-cell lymphoma in a prospective study of primary FDG-PET/CT staging in lymphoma. *Annals of Oncology: Official Journal of the European Society for Medical Oncology/ESMO.* September 2009;20(9):1543–1547.

32. Barrington SF, Mikhaeel NG. When should FDG-PET be used in the modern management of lymphoma? *British Journal of Haematology.* February 2014;164(3):315–328.

33. Lynch RC, Advani RH. Risk-Adapted Treatment of Advanced Hodgkin Lymphoma With PET-CT. *American Society of Clinical Oncology Educational Book/ASCO. American Society of Clinical Oncology. Meeting.* 2016;35:e376–e385.

34. Cheson BD, Fisher RI, Barrington SF, et al. Recommendations for initial evaluation, staging, and response assessment of Hodgkin and non-Hodgkin lymphoma: the Lugano classification. *Journal of Clinical Oncology: Official Journal of the American Society of Clinical Oncology.* September 20, 2014;32(27):3059–3068.

35. Itti E, Lin C, Dupuis J, et al. Prognostic value of interim ^{18}F-FDG PET in patients with diffuse large B-Cell lymphoma: SUV-based assessment at 4 cycles of chemotherapy. *Journal of Nuclear Medicine: Official Publication, Society of Nuclear Medicine.* April 2009;50(4):527–533.

36. Cronin CG, Swords R, Truong MT, et al. Clinical utility of PET/CT in lymphoma. *AJR. American Journal of Roentgenology.* January 2010;194(1):W91–W103.

37. Gallamini A, Barrington SF, Biggi A, et al. The predictive role of interim positron emission tomography for Hodg-

kin lymphoma treatment outcome is confirmed using the interpretation criteria of the Deauville five-point scale. *Haematologica.* June 2014;99(6):1107–1113.

38. Martelli M, Ceriani L, Zucca E, et al. [18F]fluorodeoxyglucose positron emission tomography predicts survival after chemoimmunotherapy for primary mediastinal large B-cell lymphoma: results of the International Extranodal Lymphoma Study Group IELSG-26 Study. *Journal of Clinical Oncology: Official Journal of the American Society of Clinical Oncology.* June 10, 2014;32(17):1769–1775.

39. Radford J, Illidge T, Counsell N, et al. Results of a trial of PET-directed therapy for early-stage Hodgkin's lymphoma. *The New England Journal of Medicine.* April 23, 2015;372(17):1598–1607.

40. Lin C, Itti E, Haioun C, et al. Early 18F-FDG PET for prediction of prognosis in patients with diffuse large B-cell lymphoma: SUV-based assessment versus visual analysis. *Journal of Nuclear Medicine: Official Publication, Society of Nuclear Medicine.* October 2007;48(10):1626–1632.

CHAPTER 9

Gynecologic Cancers

ALIREZA REZAEE • NIKLAUS SCHÄFER • NORBERT AVRIL •
LUKAS HEFLER • WERNER LANGSTEGER • MOHSEN BEHESHTI

CERVICAL CANCER

Background

General

- Chronic high-risk human papillomavirus (HPV) infection is the cardinal cause of squamous cell carcinoma (SCC) of the cervix.[1]
- Pap smear and HPV DNA testing are the two major screening methods for cervical cancer.[2]
- Widespread use of the Papanicolaou test (Pap smear) has led to early detection of cervical cancer and decline by more than 80% in death rate in developed countries in the last century. However, it is the second leading cause of cancer-related death in American females of 20–39 years.[3]
- Main risk factors[4]:
  - HPV
  - Smoking
  - Human immunodeficiency virus (HIV)
  - Using oral contraceptive pills for ≥5 years
  - Multiparity of ≥3
  - Having multiple sex partners

Early clinical symptoms[5]

- Could be asymptomatic
- Watery vaginal discharge
- Postcoital bleeding
- Intermittent spotting

Primary diagnostic procedures[5]

- Physical examination with colposcopy, Pap testing, and biopsy
- Cone biopsy (conization) in the case of inadequate cervical biopsy to define invasiveness

Standard treatment[6]

- Surgery and radiation therapy are the backbones of management.
- Chemotherapy is used in selected cases.

Prognostic factors[7,8]

- Lymph node status (worse if positive and most important prognostic factor)
- Clinical stage (worse if higher)
- Cancer histology (worse with adenocarcinoma and adenosquamous carcinoma)
- HIV status (worse if positive)
- HPV-18 DNA (worse if present)
- C-*myc* oncogene status (worse if overexpressed)
- Polymorphism in the γ-glutamyl hydrolase enzyme (worse if present)

Five-year survival[9]

- Stage IA: 93%
- Stage IB: 80%
- Stage IIA: 63%
- Stage IIB: 58%
- Stage IIIA: 35%
- Stage IIIB: 32%
- Stage IVA: 16%
- Stage IVB: 15%

Tumor Characteristics and Typical Behavior

Histopathology[10]

- SCC 80%–85%
- Adenocarcinoma and adenosquamous carcinoma 15%–20%

Distribution and localization

T-primary

- Uterine cervix

N-lymph nodes[11]

- Iliac (internal, external, and common)
- Presacral and sacral
- Obturator

M-distant metastasis[11]

- Lungs: 21%
- Paraaortic nodes: 11%
- Peritoneum: 8%
- Supraclavicular nodes: 7%
- Spine: 7%
- Gastrointestinal tract: 4%
- Liver: 4%
- Inguinal nodes: 3%

TABLE 9.1
Cervical Cancer TNM Classification

TNM	T1a1	T1a2	T1b	T2a	T2b	T3a	T3b	T4
N0	IA1	IA2	IB	IIA	IIB	IIIA	IIIB	IVA
N1	IIIB	IIIB	IIIB	IIIB	IIIB	IIIB	IIIB	IVA
M1	IVB	IVB	IVB	IVB	IVB	IVB	IVB	IVB

TNM and International Federation of Gynecology and Obstetrics Classification[5]

The TNM and International Federation of Gynecology and Obstetrics (FIGO) classifications are provided in Tables 9.1 and 9.2.

Guidelines

The European Society for Medical Oncology (ESMO), National Comprehensive Cancer Network (NCCN), and Society of Gynecologic Oncology (SGO) guidelines for cervical cancer are given in Table 9.3.

Evidence-Based Viewpoints

- Fludeoxyglucose positron emission tomography/computed tomography (FDG PET/CT) is recommended for staging or restaging of patients considered for exenterative surgery or radical chemoradiotherapy, response assessment of locally advanced cancer after chemoradiotherapy, and equivocal conventional imaging in suspected recurrent cervical cancers.[13]
- FDG PET/CT is recommended for women with recurrent disease who are candidates for pelvic exenteration or chemoradiation with curative intent.[14]
- FDG PET/CT is a valuable modality in detecting recurrent cancer of the cervix.[15,16]
- FDG PET/CT is an effective pretreatment imaging modality in patients with cervical cancer treated by radiotherapy.[17]

Cost-Effectiveness

The use of FDG PET/CT for routine surveillance and follow-up is not cost-effective.[18] However, large studies with specific patient selection are warranted to evaluate the cost-effectiveness of FDG PET/CT in cervical carcinoma.

Clinical Point of View

Cervical cancer is currently the third most common cancer in women and presents in advanced stages in a vast majority of cases, particularly in developing countries.[19] However, an estimated protection rate of about 70% will be achieved by early vaccination in the future.[20]

As with many other malignancies, staging is an essential step in the evaluation of cervical cancer. Only the IA1 stages (maximum 7 mm of horizontal spread, maximum 3 mm depth) are treated by conization only. All other cases need more aggressive surgery and if risk factors such as G3 histology or positive margins are detected, further adjuvant treatments are necessary. The Federation of Gynecology and Obstetrics (FIGO) classification, which is mainly a clinical- and surgical- but not an imaging-based staging system, is usually applied. However, because surgical lymph node assessment may not be available in all centers in developing countries, it is not per se mandatory.[21] In the current ESMO guidelines, only an intravenous pyelogram and a chest x-ray are recommended.[12] The roles of magnetic resonance imaging (MRI), CT, and FDG PET/CT are well evaluated in the current medical literature. Although CT and MRI may detect local lymph node involvement and local invasion, respectively, the impact of data from these imaging modalities on patients' treatment is unclear because local invasion is defined in FIGO stages I–IV. In stage IV, which is identified with infiltration of either rectum or bladder, a histologic verification is needed and imaging plays a complementary rather than diagnostic role. Also, the identification of patients amenable for adjuvant therapy (IB2 tumors, >4 cm in greatest dimension) is based on local parameters. Adjuvant treatment, usually platinum-based chemoradiation, is the current standard choice and yields a local tumor control rate of around 40%–90% according to the tumor stages in patients beyond IA stages.[22,23] Those with IA stage malignancy could receive adjuvant chemoradiation if risk factors are identified.[24] The role of neoadjuvant treatment is not yet established, although it may be effective in locally advanced disease. Currently, in these cases, palliative care with platinum-based chemotherapy is the standard strategy.

Pitfalls[25–27]

False positive

- Uterine fibroids
- Functional ovarian cysts
- Menstruating endometrium

TABLE 9.2
International Federation of Gynecology and Obstetrics (FIGO) Classification for Cervical Cancer

PRIMARY TUMOR (T)

TNM	FIGO	Description
T1	I	Cervical carcinoma confined to the cervix (disregard extension to the corpus)
T1a	IA	Invasive carcinoma diagnosed only by microscopy; stromal invasion with a maximum depth of 5.0 mm measured from the base of the epithelium and a horizontal spread of 7.0 mm or less; vascular space involvement, venous or lymphatic, does not affect classification
T1a1	IA1	Measured stromal invasion ≤3.0 mm in depth and ≤7.0 mm in horizontal spread
T1a2	IA2	Measured stromal invasion >3.0 mm and ≤5.0 mm with a horizontal spread ≤7.0 mm
T1b	IB	Clinically visible lesion confined to the cervix or microscopic lesion greater than T1a/IA2
T1b1	IB1	Clinically visible lesion ≤4.0 cm in greatest dimension
T1b2	IB2	Clinically visible lesion >4.0 cm in greatest dimension
T2	II	Cervical carcinoma invades beyond uterus but not to pelvic wall or to lower third of vagina
T2a	IIA	Tumor without parametrial invasion
T2a1	IIA1	Clinically visible lesion ≤4.0 cm in greatest dimension
T2a2	IIA2	Clinically visible lesion >4.0 cm in greatest dimension
T2b	IIB	Tumor with parametrial invasion
T3	III	Tumor extends to pelvic wall and/or involves lower third of vagina and/or causes hydronephrosis or nonfunctional kidney
T3a	IIIA	Tumor involves lower third of vagina, no extension to pelvic wall
T3b	IIIB	Tumor extends to pelvic wall and/or causes hydronephrosis or nonfunctional kidney
T4	IV	Tumor invades mucosa of bladder or rectum and/or extends beyond true pelvis (bullous edema is not sufficient to classify a tumor as T4)
T4a	IVA	Tumor invades mucosa of bladder or rectum (bullous edema is not sufficient to classify a tumor as T4)
T4b	IVB	Tumor extends beyond true pelvis

REGIONAL LYMPH NODES (N)

TNM	FIGO	Description
N0	–	No regional lymph node metastasis
N1	–	Regional lymph node metastasis

DISTANT METASTASIS (M)

TNM	FIGO	Description
M0	–	No distant metastasis
M1	–	Distant metastasis (including peritoneal spread; involvement of supraclavicular, mediastinal, or paraaortic lymph nodes; and lung, liver, or bone)

- Hyperplastic lymph nodes
- Reactive lymph nodes
- Physiologic activity in the bowel or urinary tract
- Pelvic inflammatory/infectious disease
- Mucinous malignant lesions
- Low-grade malignancy
- Hyperglycemic patients
- Small-sized lesions (<8 mm)

False negative
- Small or necrotic metastatic lymph nodes
- Early nodal involvement

Discussion

Most cervical cancers are hypermetabolic on FDG PET/CT; however, the indication for the assessment

TABLE 9.3
ESMO, NCCN, and SGO Guidelines for Cervical Cancer

Clinical Guidelines	Initial Diagnosis (Primary Tumor)	N-staging	M-staging
ESMO[12]	• No statement for initial diagnosis • Response evaluation and follow-up if clinically indicated	• Optional if equivocal finding on CT	• No statement
NCCN[5]	Recommended • Stage IB2, IIA2, or advanced stage • If suspicious for recurrence • Follow-up in patients at high risk for locoregional failure • To rule out gross residual disease Advantageous to CT • Stage IA1 with LVSI (lymphovascular space invasion) or ≥ stage IA2	Recommended • Stage IB2, IIA2, or advanced-stage tumors • If paraaortic nodes involved in surgery • To define the nodal volume of coverage for radiation therapy if not surgically staged	Recommended • Advanced stages
SGO	No statement		

CT, computed tomography; ESMO, European Society for Medical Oncology; NCCN, National Comprehensive Cancer Network; SGO, Society of Gynecologic Oncology.

of primary tumor stage seems not to be clinically relevant. This is mainly due to surgical staging of primary malignancy.

Different investigations revealed that based on very low chance of nodal metastases in stage IA-IIA cervical cancers the value of FDG PET/CT is limited in the evaluation of such patients, especially if CT or MRI is negative for lymph node involvement.[28–30] In contrast, it is a valuable method in the assessment of pelvic, paraaortic, and distant lymph node metastases in advanced-stage malignancies and is superior to stand-alone CT and MRI for this purpose.[31–33] In early stage disease, FDG PET/CT has a sensitivity and specificity of 53%–73% and 90%–97%, respectively, for the evaluation of lymph node metastases, which will be increased in sensitivity in advanced stages.[32]

FDG PET/CT is an accurate and specifically sensitive modality superior to conventional methods for detection of distant metastases in patients with advanced cervical cancer.[32]

The effective role of FDG PET/CT in the assessment of recurrent cervical cancer is well documented in the medical literature, and the technique has been shown to be superior to conventional imaging.[15,16,27,32,34,35] An analysis of 431 patients showed a pooled sensitivity, specificity, and accuracy of 95%, 84%, and 88%, respectively.[36]

In addition, FDG PET/CT is a promising modality for monitoring response to therapy in cervical cancers.[37] Sensitivity, specificity, negative predictive value

(NPV), and positive predictive value (PPV) of 92%, 94%, 99%, and 61%, respectively, are reported for diagnosis of residual tumor at a cutoff maximum standardized uptake value (SUV_{max}) of 4.0 on postchemoradiotherapy examination.[38]

Moreover, metabolic tumor volume (MTV) and total lesion glycolysis (TLG) parameters are considered as early prognostic factors during treatment of patients with locally advanced cervical cancer.[39] A high FDG uptake of primary tumor is a predictor of disease-free survival, and patients with higher metabolic activity may need more aggressive initial radiation therapy.[40] Also, patients with positive lymph nodes on FDG PET/CT have significantly shorter disease-specific survival than those with negative lymph nodes. Moreover, the metabolic activity of metastatic lymph nodes can predict response to therapy as well as risk of recurrence in the pelvis.[41–43]

FDG PET/CT also showed a significant role in the management of cervical carcinoma and was able to change treatment approach in up to two-thirds of patients.[44]

Currently, novel imaging by FDG PET/MRI showed promising results in the assessment of cervical cancers. One study revealed that, with an accuracy of approximately 83% vs 53%, the modality is superior to FDG PET/CT for primary cervical cancer staging. However, for the detection of lymph node metastasis, the sensitivity, specificity, and accuracy were comparable in both techniques (92%, 88%, and 90%, respectively).[45]

ENDOMETRIAL CANCER
Background
General
- The fourth most common cancer and the sixth leading cause of cancer-related death among US females.[3]
- The most common cancer of the female reproductive system in Western population.[46]
- Risk factors[47,48]:
  - Long-term exposure to estrogen but inadequate progesterone
  - Obesity and high-fat diet
  - Nulliparity
  - Early menarche
  - Late menopause (after the age of 55 years)
  - Diabetes
  - Hypertension
  - Older age
  - Family history of endometrial or colorectal cancer (Lynch syndrome or hereditary nonpolyposis colon cancer)
  - Past medical history of ovarian cancer (particularly granulosa cell tumor), breast cancer, or endometrial hyperplasia
  - History of pelvic radiation therapy
- Protective factors against endometrial cancer[47]:
  - Pregnancy
  - Oral contraceptive pills
  - Intrauterine device
  - Exercise
  - Confined to the uterus in 70%–75% of cases (stage I) at the time of diagnosis[6]

Early clinical symptoms[47]
- Abnormal uterine bleeding (90%) or abnormal nonbloody vaginal discharge (10%)
- Pelvic pain
- Unintentional weight loss (not in early stages)

Primary diagnostic procedures[49,50]
- Endometrial biopsy or sampling during dilation and curettage

Standard treatment[51]
- Total abdominal hysterectomy + bilateral salpingo-oophorectomy (TAH + BSO) is the cornerstone of treatment.
- Chemotherapy, radiotherapy, or hormone therapy is applied for selected cases with more advanced disease.

Prognostic factors[52]
- Subtype (worse with serous and small cell carcinoma)
- Older age (worse prognosis)
- Advanced-stage disease (worse prognosis)
- Lymph node status (worse if positive)
- High-grade malignancy (worse prognosis)
- Tumor size (worse prognosis if larger)
- Lymphovascular invasion (worse prognosis)
- Tumors of the inferior uterine segments (worse prognosis)
- Depth of myometrial invasion (worse prognosis if deeper)

Five-year survival[53]
- Stage 0: 90%
- Stage IA: 88%
- Stage IB: 75%
- Stage II: 69%
- Stage IIIA: 58%
- Stage IIIB: 50%
- Stage IIIC: 47%
- Stage IVA: 17%
- Stage IVB: 15%

Tumor Characteristics and Typical Behavior
Histopathology[54]
- Endometrioid: 75%–80%
- Papillary serous carcinoma: <10%
- Clear cell carcinoma: 4%
- Squamous cell carcinoma: <1%
- Mixed: 10%

Distribution and localization
T-primary
- Uterine endometrium

N-lymph nodes[53]
- Regional lymph nodes
  - Pelvic (N1)
  - Paraaortic (N2)
- Distant lymph nodes
  - Inguinal
  - Abdominal and beyond

M-distant metastasis[53]
- Peritoneal
- Lung
- Liver
- Bone

TNM and International Federation of Gynecology and Obstetrics Classification[52]
The TNM and FIGO classifications are provided in Tables 9.4 and 9.5.

TABLE 9.4
TNM Classification for Endometrial Cancer

TNM	T1a	T1b	T2	T3a	T3b	T4
N0	IA	IB	II	IIIA	IIIB	IVA
N1	IIIC1	IIIC1	IIIC1	IIIC1	IIIC1	IVA
N2	IIIC2	IIIC2	IIIC2	IIIC2	IIIC2	IVA
M1	IVB	IVB	IVB	IVB	IVB	IVB

TABLE 9.5
International Federation of Gynecology and Obstetrics (FIGO)[a] Classification for Endometrial Cancer

PRIMARY TUMOR (T)		
TNM	*FIGO*	*Description*
T1	I	Tumor confined to corpus uteri
T1a	IA	Tumor limited to endometrium or invades less than one half of the myometrium
T1b	IB	Tumor invades one half or more of the myometrium
T2	II	Tumor invades stromal connective tissue of the cervix but does not extend beyond uterus
T3a	IIIA	Tumor involves serosa and/or adnexa (direct extension or metastasis)
T3b	IIIB IIIC IV	Vaginal involvement (direct extension or metastasis) or parametrial involvement Metastases to pelvic and/or paraaortic lymph nodes Tumor invades bladder mucosa and/or bowel mucosa, and/or distant metastases
T4	IVA	Tumor invades bladder mucosa and/or bowel mucosa (bullous edema is not sufficient to classify a tumor as T4)
REGIONAL LYMPH NODES (N)		
TNM	*FIGO*	*Description*
N0	–	No regional lymph node metastasis
N1	IIIC1	Regional lymph node metastasis to pelvic lymph nodes
N2	IIIC2	Regional lymph node metastasis to paraaortic lymph nodes, with or without positive pelvic lymph nodes
DISTANT METASTASIS (M)		
TNM	*FIGO*	*Description*
M0	–	No distant metastasis
M1	IVB	Distant metastasis (includes metastasis to inguinal lymph nodes, peritoneal disease, or lung, liver, or bone metastases; it excludes metastasis to paraaortic lymph nodes, vagina, pelvic serosa, or adnexa)

[a]FIGO (Fédération Internationale de Gynécologie et d'Obstétrique) system is most commonly used for staging uterine cancer.[52]

Guidelines

The ESMO, NCCN, and SGO guidelines for endometrial cancer are provided in Table 9.6.

Evidence-Based Viewpoints

- FDG PET/CT is indicated for staging or restaging of patients with endometrial carcinoma considered for pelvic exenteration (evisceration) surgery as well as for the evaluation of suspected recurrence of endometrial carcinoma when other imaging is equivocal.[13]
- FDG PET/CT has an excellent diagnostic performance for preoperative detection of lymph node metastases and malignancy recurrence in patients with endometrial cancer.[57]

TABLE 9.6
ESMO, NCCN, and SGO Guidelines for Endometrial Cancer

Clinical Guidelines	Initial Diagnosis (Primary Tumor), N-staging, and M-staging
ESMO[55]	• More accurate than CT alone for assessment of recurrence • Optional for assessment of distant metastasis
NCCN[52]	• Evaluation of suspected extrauterine endometrioid-type cancer if clinically indicated by symptoms, physical or laboratory examinations • Evaluation of serous or clear cell carcinoma or uterine sarcoma if clinically indicated
SGO[56]	• Optional in patients with intermediate to high risk for extrauterine disease or disease recurrence if they were not good candidate for surgery • Useful for suspected recurrent disease

CT, computed tomography; *ESMO*, European Society for Medical Oncology; *NCCN*, National Comprehensive Cancer Network; *SGO*, Society of Gynecologic Oncology.

• FDG PET/CT has been reported to be of particular value in the detection of occult metastatic disease, in the prediction of response to therapy, and as a prognostic factor.[58]
• FDG PET/CT is an accurate modality for detecting endometrial cancer recurrence and changing therapy planning in these patients.[59]
• In patients with untreated endometrial cancer, a positive FDG PET/CT is extremely helpful to detect pelvic and paraaortic lymph nodes metastasis.[60]

Cost-Effectiveness
No large study has been performed yet to evaluate the cost-effectiveness of FDG PET/CT in endometrial carcinoma.

Clinical Point of View
Similar to cervical cancer, endometrial carcinoma is more prevalent in developing countries, where it ranks as the fourth most common cancer in women. In contrast to cervical cancer, endometrial carcinomas are diagnosed in lower stages due to the postmenopausal vaginal bleeding as the first symptom. This early detection results in better overall 5-year survival of over 75%.[61] Due to the high likelihood of early disease, local staging methods such as ultrasound and endometrial biopsy play a major role.[62] Like cervical cancer, FIGO classification is used for staging.[52] The burden of malignancy is a very important factor to determine the extent of surgery from hysterectomy with bilateral salpingo-oophorectomy to extensive anterior and posterior pelvic exenteration. In this setting, the imaging modalities such as MRI, CT, and FDG PET/CT play an essential role. In a nutshell, CT is indicated to assess the extrapelvic disease and MRI is able to depict cervical involvement.[63,64] Although MRI is not

an operator-dependent method, the local ultrasound is superior for this purpose.[65] Adjuvant therapy is used for patients with G3 stage I or higher stages, and chemoradiotherapy is superior to radiotherapy alone.[55,66] Moreover, the management is different in hormonal- versus nonhormonal-dependent metastatic endometrioid-type cancer. Antihormonal treatment such as tamoxifen or aromatase inhibitors may be used for the former, whereas platinum-based chemotherapy, combined with taxanes, is the standard regimen for the latter.

Pitfalls[67,68]
False positive
• Normal premenopausal endometrial or ovarian physiologic activity
• Uterine fibroids
• Menstruation
• An inflammatory/infectious process
• Recent curettage
• Endometrial polyps

False negative
• Well-differentiated carcinoma
• Early stage malignancy
• Small lesions (<8 mm)
• Hyperglycemic patients

Discussion
Although primary endometrial cancers show increased FDG uptake, it has limited value in defining the depth of myometrial invasion. Therefore, FDG PET/CT has not been shown to be of value in T-staging of most patients with endometrial cancer.[33] Nevertheless, combined FDG-PET/MRI is an accurate (80%) modality for T-staging compared with PET/CT (60%).[69]

Imaging modalities play an important role in N- and M-staging of endometrial cancers and will diminish both the costs and complications, guiding treatment policy.[70]

Although FDG PET/CT showed limited value (sensitivity of 17%) for the detection of micrometastases to small lymph nodes (<5 mm), it revealed satisfactory results (sensitivity of 93%) in lymph nodes ≥10 mm.[71]

Nevertheless, FDG PET/CT seems to be superior to conventional imaging modalities for assessing lymph node involvement.[57,60] In preoperative imaging for N-staging of 287 patients with FDG PET/CT and MRI, the calculated per-patient sensitivity and specificity were 70% and 95% versus 34% and 95%, respectively.[46,72]

Based on a very high NPV of FDG PET/CT (approximately 100%), the method could be helpful in the selection of patients for lymphadenectomy and prevent unnecessary surgical interventions.[46,73]

For M-staging, FDG PET/CT showed a sensitivity, specificity, NPV, PPV, and accuracy of approximately 93%, 99%, 100%, 81%, and 99%, respectively.[46] It was found to be superior to conventional imaging in discovering distant metastases to the abdomen and thorax.[73]

Moreover, the modality is highly effective in the differentiation of true recurrence in patients with endometrial cancer,[59,74,75] with sensitivity and specificity of about 95% and 91%, respectively.[57] It seems that its overall performance is superior to conventional imaging methods (contrast-enhanced CT or MRI), with a much better specificity (96% vs 62%) and accuracy (92% vs 76%) as well as comparable sensitivity (90% vs 85%).[76]

Although more clinical studies are warranted to determine the role of FDG PET/CT in the evaluation of response to therapy among patients with endometrial cancers,[58] its prognostic value is established in the medical literature. In fact, a better progression-free survival is expected for patients with endometrial cancer with a negative FDG PET/CT.[77] In addition, preoperative metabolic activity (SUV) of endometrial primary tumor seems to be an independent prognostic factor for malignancy recurrence and mortality,[78] as well as for both disease-free and overall survival.[79]

In addition, the modality may affect therapeutic plans.[73] Some authors shared the point that the management planning was changed in approximately 23% of patients, according to FDG PET/CT data.[75,77]

OVARIAN CANCER
Background
General
- Although not a very common malignancy among women, it is the fifth leading cause of cancer-relat-

ed death in the United States, causing more deaths than any other female reproductive system cancers.[3]
- Risk factors[80,81]:
  - Older age at pregnancy and first delivery (>30 years)
  - Infertility
  - Nulliparity
  - Menstruation starting before the age of 12 years
  - Late menopause after the age of 55 years
  - Postmenopausal hormone replacement therapy
  - Pelvic inflammatory disease
  - Ovarian stimulation during in vitro fertilization (for borderline epithelial tumors)
  - Positive family history of ovarian (including linkage with BRCA1 and BRCA2), breast, or colorectal cancers
  - Obesity
- Protective factors (30%–60% reduced risk) against ovarian cancer[81,82]:
  - Younger age at pregnancy and first delivery (≤25 years)
  - Oral contraceptive pill consumption
  - Breast-feeding
- No routine screening test is recommended.[81]
- About 75% of patients present with advanced stage disease.[83]

Early clinical symptoms[a,84]
- Bloating
- Pelvic/abdominal pain
- Early satiety
- Urinary symptoms (frequency, urgency)

Primary diagnostic procedures[b,6]
- Transvaginal ultrasound
- Biopsy of ovary or any other abdominal masses

Standard treatment[6]
- Surgery and chemotherapy are the backbone of treatment.
- Radiation therapy is used in selected cases.

Prognostic factors[85–87]
- Initial and residual tumor volume after surgery (worse if larger; most important factor)
- Tumor stage (worse if advanced)
- Grade and stage of the tumor (worse if advanced)
- Rate of tumor response to therapy (worse if slow)

---

[a] Particularly if new and frequent (more than 12 days/month).
[b] Any pelvic mass in a woman who is more than 1 year postmenopausal is suspicious for ovarian cancer.

- Tumor histologic type (worse in serous cystadeno-carcinoma, anaplastic and clear cell carcinoma)
- Performance status (worse if poor)
- Age (worse with older age)

Five-year survival[c,88]
- Stage I: 90%
  - IA: 94%
  - IB: 92%
  - IC: 85%
- Stage II: 70%
  - IIA: 78%
  - IIB: 73%
- Stage III: 39%
  - IIIA: 59%
  - IIIB: 52%
  - IIIC: 39%
- Stage IV: 17%

Tumor Characteristics and Typical Behavior
Histopathology[89–91]
- Epithelial cancer: >90%
  - Serous: 30%–70%
  - Endometrioid: 10%–20%
  - Mucinous: 5%–20%
  - Clear cell: 3%–10%
  - Undifferentiated: 1%
- Germ cell, sex cord-stromal, and other cancers <10%

---

[c] Exclusively for invasive epithelial ovarian cancer. For other subtypes of ovarian cancer, refer to the same reference.

Distribution and localization
T-primary
- Ovary

N-lymph nodes[92]
- Regional
  - Iliac (internal, external, and common)
  - Paraaortic
- Nonregional
  - Inguinal

M-distant metastasis[d,93]
- Lung: 71%
- Subcutaneous nodules: 3.5%
- Brain: 2%
- Bone: 1.6%

TNM and International Federation of Gynecology and Obstetrics Classification[81,94]
TNM and FIGO classifications for ovarian cancer are given in Tables 9.7 and 9.8.

Guidelines
ESMO, NCCN, and SGO guidelines for ovarian cancer are given in Table 9.9.

---

[d] Except for peritoneal seeding involving peritoneum, omentum, liver, and diaphragm, as well as metastasis to fallopian tubes or contralateral ovary.

TABLE 9.7
TNM Classification for Ovarian Cancer

TNM	T1a	T1b	T1c	T2a	T2b	T2c	T3a	T3b	T3c
N0	IA	IB	IC	IIA	IIB	IIC	IIIA	IIIB	IIIC
N1	IIIC	IIIC	IIIC	IIIC	IIIC	IIIC	IIIC	IIIC	IIIC
M1	IV	IV	IV	IV	IV	IV	IV	IV	IV

TABLE 9.8
International Federation of Gynecology and Obstetrics (FIGO) Classification For Ovarian Cancer

PRIMARY TUMOR (T)

TNM	FIGO	Description
T1	I	Tumor confined to ovaries or fallopian tubes
T1a	IA	Tumor limited to one ovary (capsule intact) or fallopian tube; no tumor on ovarian or fallopian tube surface; no malignant cells in ascites or peritoneal washings
T1b	IB	Tumor limited to both ovaries (capsules intact) or fallopian tubes; no tumor on ovarian or fallopian tube surface; no malignant cells in ascites or peritoneal washings
T1c	IC IC1 IC2 IC3	Tumor limited to one or both ovaries or fallopian tubes, with any of the following: Surgical spill Capsule ruptured before surgery or tumor on ovarian or tube surface Malignant cells in the ascites or peritoneal washings
T2	II	Tumor involves one or both ovaries or fallopian tubes with pelvic extension (below pelvic brim) or peritoneal cancer
T2a	IIA	Extension and/or implants on uterus and/or tube(s) and/or ovaries
T2b	IIB	Extension to other pelvic intraperitoneal tissues
T2c	IIC	Pelvic extension and/or implants (T2a or T2b) with malignant cells in ascites or peritoneal washings
T3	III	Tumor involves one or both ovaries or fallopian tubes, or peritoneal cancer, with cytologically or histologically confirmed spread to the peritoneum outside the pelvis and/or metastasis to the retroperitoneal lymph nodes
T3a	IIIA IIIA1 IIIA1 (i) IIIA1 (ii) IIIA2	Positive retroperitoneal lymph nodes and/or microscopic metastasis beyond pelvis Positive retroperitoneal lymph nodes only (cytologically or histologically proven) Metastasis up to 10 mm in greatest dimension Metastasis more than 10 mm in greatest dimension Microscopic extrapelvic (above the pelvic brim) peritoneal involvement, with or without positive retroperitoneal lymph nodes
T3b	IIIB	Macroscopic peritoneal metastasis beyond pelvis up to 2 cm in greatest dimension, with or without positive retroperitoneal lymph nodes
T3c	IIIC	Macroscopic peritoneal metastasis beyond pelvis more than 2 cm in greatest dimension (includes extension of tumor to capsule of liver and spleen without parenchymal involvement of either organ), with or without positive retroperitoneal lymph nodes

REGIONAL LYMPH NODES (N)

TNM	FIGO	Description
N0	–	No regional lymph node metastasis
N1	III	Regional lymph node metastasis

DISTANT METASTASIS (M)

TNM	FIGO	Description
M0	–	No distant metastasis
M1	IV IVA IVB	Distant metastasis (excludes peritoneal metastasis) Pleural effusion with positive cytology Parenchymal metastases and metastases to extraabdominal organs (including inguinal lymph nodes and lymph nodes outside the abdominal cavity)

The presence of ascites does not affect staging unless malignant cells are present.
Liver capsule metastasis is T3/stage III; liver parenchymal metastasis is M1/stage IV.
Pleural effusion must have positive cytology for M1/stage IV.

TABLE 9.9
ESMO, NCCN, and SGO Guidelines for Ovarian Cancer

Clinical Guidelines	Initial Diagnosis (Primary Tumor), N-staging, and M-staging
ESMO[95,96]	• Recommended in epithelial cancer before secondary debulking surgery if no evidence of M1 on CT
NCCN[81]	Recommended • Staging of advanced epithelial cancers in case of equivocal findings on CT • Follow-up and restaging of epithelial cancers' recurrence or post primary treatment if clinically indicated • Restaging of germ cell tumors after surgery, if incompletely staged and after chemotherapy • Surveillance of germ cell and sex-cord tumors
SGO[97]	Recommended • Staging of advanced epithelial cancers in case of equivocal findings on CT

CT, computed tomography; *ESMO*, European Society for Medical Oncology; *NCCN*, National Comprehensive Cancer Network; *SGO*, Society of Gynecologic Oncology.

Evidence-Based Viewpoints

- In staging of ovarian cancer, there is no significant difference between FDG PET/CT, stand-alone CT, and MRI; however, FDG PET/CT is more accurate for the detection of supradiaphragmatic metastases.[98]
- FDG PET/CT is superior to stand-alone CT or MRI in the assessment of recurrent ovarian cancer, with sensitivity of 91%, 79%, and 75% and specificity of 88%, 84%, and 78%, respectively.[99]
- FDG PET/CT may discover the site of recurrence in patients with CA-125 relapse but equivocal or negative conventional imaging.[13,33]
- FDG-PET/CT has a high sensitivity with few false-negative results, which could make it an effective method for evaluating recurrent ovarian cancer.[100,101]

Cost-Effectiveness

- FDG PET/CT is cost-effective and redirects the management of patients with recurrent ovarian cancer toward more appropriate therapies.[102]
- By replacing the second-look laparotomy in the surveillance of patients with advanced ovarian carcinoma, FDG PET/CT can prevent unnecessary surgical procedures and save healthcare costs.[37,103,104]

Clinical Point of View

Ovarian cancer is a disease of older women (80% of the patients are >50 years). Since the symptoms such as pain, constipation, loose stools, or bleeding develop late in the course of disease, it is still the fourth common cause of cancer related to females. Ascites and pleural effusion are more common in patients with advanced malignancy. Abdominal ultrasonography could be the first step to assess suspected cases, supplemented with the transvaginal method to identify malignant phenotypes.[105] Classical staging is performed using CT/ultrasound and relies on the FIGO staging classification. However, the surgical approach is favored in operable cases because the suspected imaging findings need histologic verification, and the treatment plan commonly relies on surgical and histologic rather than imaging findings. Overall, surgery plays an essential role in primary ovarian cancer, and a complete cytoreduction is an important parameter to provide better prognosis in these patients.[106] The value of cytoreduction in recurrent disease is less clear. Adjuvant chemotherapy is highly recommended in early ovarian carcinoma with high-risk parameters (FIGO stages of IB/C grade 2/3, any grade 3 or clear-cell histology).[107] All patients with pelvic extension (FIGO II) need postsurgical chemotherapy (usually carboplatin area under curve six combined with paclitaxel 175 mg/m^2, every 3 weeks). Targeted treatments have been tested and ICON-7 showed benefit of adding bevacizumab in high-risk patients.[108] Despite these treatments, the recurrent rate is approximately 70%. Second-line options are either a repeat of carboplatin/paclitaxel if patients are platinum sensitive (>12 months duration of response) or administration of gemcitabine/pegylated doxorubicin or topotecan. Targeted treatments in the recurrent setting have been evaluated. The OCEANS trial showed that in patients in remission >6 months, adding bevacizumab to the chemotherapy regimen will prolong progression-free survival.[109] The AURELIA trial proved the benefit of bevacizumab in combination with second-line chemotherapy in platinum-resistant ovarian carcinoma.[110] In addition to clinical parameters, CA-125 plays an essential role in patient follow-up, and rising levels after surgery may warrant further evaluation with FDG PET/CT. However, there is currently no evidence that CA-125 plays a role in overall survival compared with onset of clinical symptoms.[111]

Pitfalls[33,68,112–117]
False positive
- Hydrosalpinx
- Pedunculated fibroids
- Endometriosis
- Premenopausal late follicular to early luteal cyst
- Inflammatory/infectious process such as tuboovarian abscess and postsurgical changes
- Benign cystadenoma, teratoma, schwannoma, and endometrioma
- Misregistration of physiologic uptake in bowel and bladder

False negative
- Borderline tumors (low-malignant potential tumors)
- Low-grade/early adenocarcinomas
- Large cystic tumors
- Mucinous tumors
- Peritoneal carcinomatosis <5 mm
- Hyperglycemic patients
- Small-sized lesions (<8 mm)

Discussion
The role of FDG PET/CT in the assessment of primary ovarian cancer is controversial. Although FDG PET/CT is not recommended by major clinical guidelines and some investigators due to its limited sensitivity and specificity (52%–58% and 76%–78%, respectively),[114,118] other investigators showed a promising role for the technique. When compared with stand-alone CT, it is more accurate (69%–75% vs 53%–55%) in pretreatment staging of patients with ovarian cancer.[119,120] Specifically, it is valuable in differentiating patients with stages IIIC-IV from I-IIIB cancers, with sensitivity, specificity, and accuracy of 100%, 91%, and 98% versus 97%, 64%, and 88% for stand-alone CT, respectively.[116,120] Reviewing the literature shows that FDG PET/CT is a promising modality in staging of ovarian cancer. However, it is not established as a standard procedure in routine clinical practice yet.[121]

FDG PET/CT is an accurate modality with high NPV for the detection of lymph node involvement from ovarian cancer and prevention of systematic pelvic and aortic lymphadenectomy in most of the patients, leading to fewer surgery-related complications.[122] It is also superior to stand-alone CT in the detection of supradiaphragmatic nodal metastases (67% vs 33%).[123] Moreover, the method is highly sensitive for the detection of peritoneal deposits >10 mm and lymph nodes >7 mm in size.[119]

In addition, FDG PET/CT is a useful modality in the evaluation of distant metastases.[119,120,124] It has sensitivity, specificity, PPV, NPV, and accuracy of 63%, 98%, 88%, 93%, and 93% for the detection of extrapelvic metastatic disease.[125]

Nearly 60%–70% of patients who favorably respond to first-line therapy will experience disease relapse.[126] Early detection and anatomic localization of metastatic disease are very important in planning optimal therapy in patients with biochemical recurrence.[116] FDG PET/CT is the most accurate technique to evaluate suspected recurrent ovarian cancer,[100,125,127–129] particularly in the case of equivocal conventional imaging.[119,120,130] Also, it is found to be a powerful tool with a sensitivity >90% in the assessment of patients with suspected ovarian cancer recurrence who have elevated CA-125 but inconclusive or negative conventional imaging studies.[37,99,131,132]

There is a correlation between metabolic response to therapy on FDG PET/CT and better survival in patients with advanced ovarian cancer.[133] FDG PET/CT plays an important role in therapy monitoring, which helps optimizing neoadjuvant treatment protocols and prevents futile therapy in nonresponders early on.[134] A vast majority of metabolic responders defined by interim FDG PET/CT showed complete histologic response after termination of chemotherapy.[135]

In addition, the method has been shown to have prognostic value after neoadjuvant chemotherapy.[133,136,137] A multicenter study on 168 patients revealed that a negative FDG PET/CT after neoadjuvant therapy is significantly correlated with longer progression-free and overall survivals.[138] Heterogeneous FDG uptake of epithelial ovarian tumors on baseline FDG PET/CT could be a potential predictor of recurrence.[139] Furthermore, the whole-body MTV and TLG were both prognostic factors for postrelapse survival.[140] Also, a high SUV may be an ominous sign for a higher rate of malignancy recurrence in the future.[141,142]

Moreover, FDG PET/CT affects the patients' clinical management in 30%–58% of cases based on different studies.[37,143–145]

TEACHING CASES
Case 1: Staging and Restaging Cervical Cancer
Findings
A 58-year-old female with SCC of the cervix. FDG PET/CT shows tracer-avid primary tumor (Fig. 9.1A

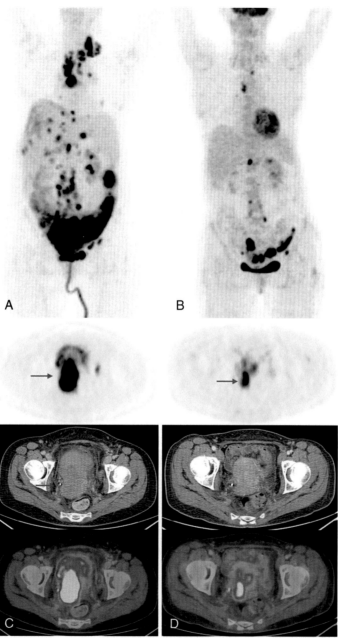

FIG. 9.1 Fludeoxyglucose positron emission tomography/computed tomography (FDG PET/CT) showing tracer-avid primary tumor (A, C; *arrows*) with peritoneal carcinomatosis (A, E; *arrows*) and multiple distant metastases in liver and lungs, as well as in left supraclavicular, mediastinal, and retroperitoneal lymph nodes (A). Interim FDG PET/CT after three cycles of chemotherapy (B) demonstrates partial response in the primary tumor (D, *arrows*) as well as peritoneal (F, *arrows*), retroperitoneal, and mediastinal lymph node metastases (B).

Continued

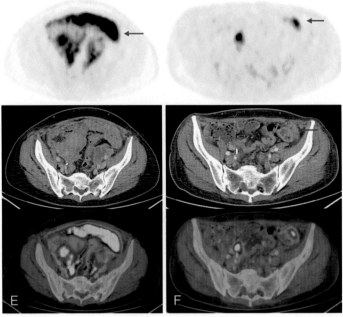

FIG. 9.1, cont'd

and C; arrows) with peritoneal carcinomatosis (Fig. 9.1A and E; arrows) and multiple distant metastases in liver and lungs as well as in left supraclavicular, mediastinal, and retroperitoneal lymph nodes (Fig. 9.1A). Interim FDG PET/CT after three cycles of chemotherapy (Fig. 9.1B) demonstrates partial response in the primary tumor (Fig. 9.1D, arrows) as well as in peritoneal (Fig. 9.1F, arrows), retroperitoneal, and mediastinal lymph node metastases (Fig. 9.1B).

Teaching points
• FDG PET/CT is an accurate method for T-, N-, and M-staging of uterine cervix carcinoma.
• The left supraclavicular region (Virchow node) is a common site of distant lymph node metastasis from gynecologic cancers.
• Cervical cancer metastasizes to the lungs, paraaortic lymph nodes, peritoneum, and supraclavicular lymph nodes in 21%, 11%, 8%, and 7% of cases, respectively.
• FDG PET/CT is an accurate and specifically sensitive modality superior to conventional methods for the detection of distant metastases in patients with advanced cervical cancer.
• A high FDG uptake of primary tumor is a predictor of disease-free survival, and patients with higher

metabolic activity may need more aggressive initial radiation therapy.

Case 2: Staging and Restaging Vulvar Cancer
Findings
An 83-year-old female with well-differentiated vulvar SCC. FDG PET/CT shows tracer-avid primary tumor (Fig. 9.2A, black arrow) with bilateral inguinal lymph node metastases (Fig. 9.2A, red arrows). Physiologic cardiac uptake is noted as well (Fig. 9.2A–C, arrowheads). The restaging scan demonstrates a large right pleural effusion with multiple FDG-avid pleural metastases (Fig. 9.2D, arrows).

Teaching points
• FDG PET/CT is a promising modality to guide biopsy.
• FDG PET can differentiate viable from necrotic tissues.
• It is a useful method for the assessment of vulvar cancer and can differentiate lymph node metastases that are within the normal size on CT.

Pitfalls
• FDG uptake in intercostal muscles is due to patient's respiratory distress and overuse of respiratory muscles.

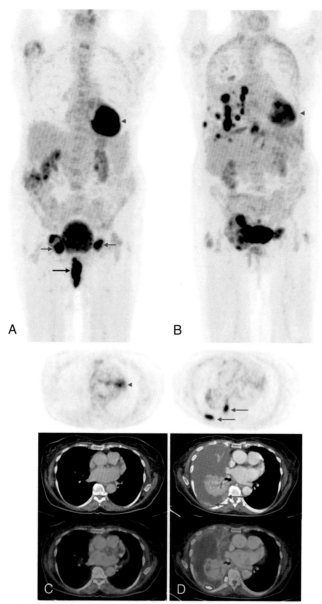

FIG. 9.2 Fludeoxyglucose (FDG) positron emission tomography/computed tomography showing tracer-avid primary tumor (A, *black arrow*) with bilateral inguinal lymph node metastases (A, *red arrows*). Physiologic cardiac uptake is noted as well (A–C, *arrowheads*). Restaging scan demonstrates a large right pleural effusion with multiple FDG-avid pleural metastases (D, *arrows*).

Case 3: Staging Cervical Cancer
Findings
A 57-year-old female with invasive nonkeratinized basaloid cell cervical SCC. FDG PET/CT shows a tracer-avid primary tumor (Fig. 9.3B, red arrows) with presacral soft tissue (Fig. 9.3B, yellow arrows), as well as paraaortic, iliac, and inguinal lymph node metastases (Fig. 9.3A). An FDG-avid right retrocrural lymph node is too small to be suspicious on CT (Fig. 9.3C, arrows). A mildly diffuse relatively homogenous FDG uptake in axial skeleton is secondary to tumor reaction (Fig. 9.3A).

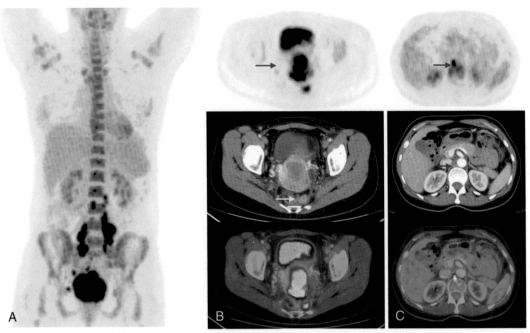

FIG. 9.3 Fludeoxyglucose (FDG) positron emission tomography/computed tomography (CT) showing a tracer-avid primary tumor (B, *red arrows*) with presacral soft tissue (B, *yellow arrows*) as well as paraaortic, iliac, and inguinal lymph node metastases (A). An FDG-avid right retrocrural lymph node is too small to be suspicious on CT (C, *arrows*). Mildly diffuse relatively homogenous FDG uptake in axial skeleton is secondary to tumor reaction (A).

Teaching points

- Lymph node involvement above the renal arteries is crucial for planning treatment, which may change treatment approach from lymphadenectomy to additional systemic therapy.
- Aggressive tumors may cause nonmalignant reactive diffuse mild to moderate increased symmetric bone marrow uptake.
- FDG PET/CT is superior to stand-alone CT in N- and M-staging of cervical cancers.
- Patients with positive lymph nodes on FDG PET/CT have a significantly shorter disease-specific survival than those with negative lymph nodes.
- The metabolic activity of metastatic lymph nodes can predict response to therapy as well as risk of recurrence in the pelvis.

Pitfalls

- A mild FDG uptake in the breast tissue is physiologic and could be more prominent in breastfeeding.

Case 4: Staging and Restaging Cervical Cancer

Findings

A 68-year-old female with cervical cancer. FDG PET/CT shows tracer-avid primary tumor with infiltration to uterus (Fig. 9.4C, arrows). There is an FDG-avid right paracolic soft tissue metastasis (Fig. 9.4E, arrows). Multiple FDG-avid cervical, thoracic, axillary, abdominal, and pelvic lymph nodes have been determined to be due to sarcoidosis (Fig. 9.4A and B). Restaging FDG PET/CT demonstrates a major metabolic response in primary tumor (Fig. 9.4D, arrows) and complete response in paracolic metastatic lesion (Fig. 9.4F, arrows) but no significant change of FDG uptake in lymph nodes involved with sarcoidosis (Fig. 9.4B).

Teaching points

- Pap smear and HPV DNA testing are the two major screening methods for cervical cancer.
- Although the 5-year survival for stage I disease is over 80%, it is only 15% in stage IV.

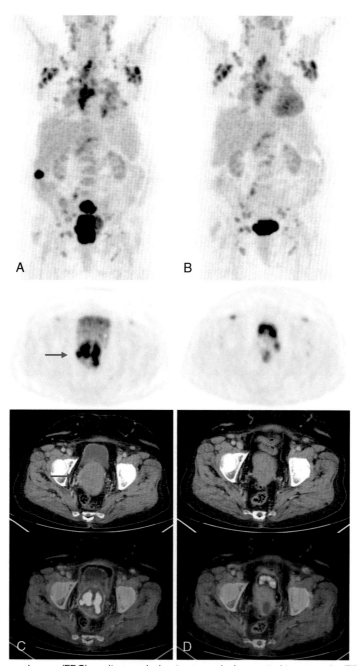

FIG. 9.4 Fludeoxyglucose (FDG) positron emission tomography/computed tomography (FDG PET/CT) showing tracer-avid primary tumor with infiltration to uterus (C, *arrows*). There is an FDG-avid right para-colic soft tissue metastasis (E, *arrows*). Multiple FDG-avid cervical, thoracic, axillary, abdominal, and pelvic lymph nodes are approved to be due to sarcoidosis (A, B). Restaging FDG PET/CT demonstrates major metabolic response in primary tumor (D, *arrows*) and complete response in paracolic metastatic lesion (F, *arrows*) but no significant change of FDG uptake in lymph nodes involved with sarcoidosis (B).

Continued

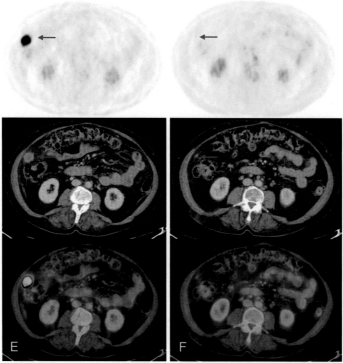

FIG. 9.4, cont'd

- Most cervical cancer recurrences happen within the first 2 years after therapy, with the peak at 9–12 months; therefore a follow-up FDG PET/CT is suggested at least 1 year after therapy of patients with advanced cancer.

Pitfalls
- Sarcoidosis and lymphoma are the common differential diagnoses of multifocal lymphadenopathy when using FDG PET/CT. However, the pattern, localization, and tracer intensity of lymph nodes and a comparison with the tracer intensity of the primary tumor may be helpful for more accurate interpretation.

Case 5: Endometrial Cancer—Recurrence
Findings
A 62-year-old female with recurrent endometrial cancer with a past history of TAH + BSO and lymphadenectomy. FDG PET/CT shows tracer-avid local tumor recurrence in the vagina (Fig. 9.5B, red arrows). There are multiple FDG-avid osseous metastases in pelvic bony structures (Fig. 9.5B, yellow arrows) as well as in bilateral lungs (Fig. 9.5C and D; arrows).

Teaching points
- Endometrial cancer is confined to the uterus in 70%–75% of cases (stage I) at the time of diagnosis.
- TAH + BSO is the cornerstone of treatment.
- FDG PET/CT is superior to conventional imaging modalities for the assessment of local recurrent disease, as well as N and M status.
- Small nodules in the base of the lungs could be missed on FDG PET/CT due to misregistration (Fig. 9.5D, arrows). Applying respiratory gating can be helpful for correct interpretation.

Pitfalls
- Benign lesions like leiomyoma or malignant tumors such as leiomyosarcoma may be intensely FDG-avid and are in the differential diagnosis of endometrial cancer.

Case 6: Recurrent Ovarian Cancer—Atypical Spinal Cord Metastasis
Findings
An 86-year-old female with recurrent serous ovarian cancer, status post TAH + BSO, lymphadenectomy, and chemotherapy. FDG PET/CT shows left

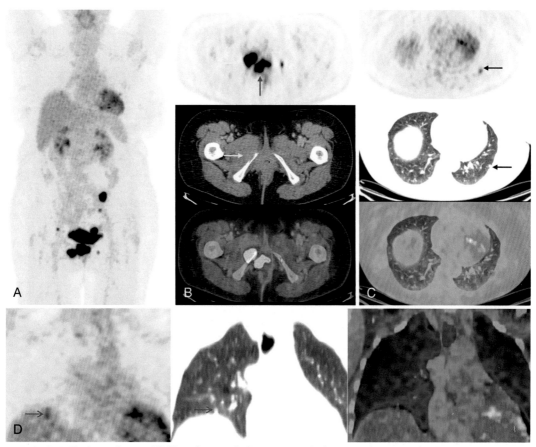

FIG. 9.5 Fludeoxyglucose (FDG) positron emission tomography/computed tomography showing tracer-avid local tumor recurrence in the vagina (B, *red arrows*). There are multiple FDG-avid osseous metastases in pelvic bony structures (B, *yellow arrows*) as well as bilateral lungs (C, D; *arrows*). A, FDG PET MIP image.

paraaortic, left common iliac, and right paracolic lymph node metastases (Fig. 9.6B, arrows). Of incidental note is a focal FDG uptake in the spinal cord, at the level of C1/C2 (Fig. 9.6C, arrows), confirmed in MRI and follow-up images to be metastasis. No bone infiltration on MRI was observed. A mild FDG uptake in the rectum is most likely inflammatory in nature (Fig. 9.6).

Teaching points
- Ovarian cancer presents with advanced stage disease in about 75% of patients.
- Surgery and chemotherapy are the backbone of treatment.
- FDG PET/CT is superior to stand-alone CT or MRI in the assessment of recurrent ovarian cancer, with sensitivity of 91%, 79%, and 75% and specificity of 88%, 84%, and 78%, respectively.

- Stand-alone CT shows limited value in the assessment of small paracolic lymph nodes, whereas FDG PET/CT is able to overcome this limitation.
- FDG PET/CT is promising for the detection of atypical distant metastases (e.g., spinal cord), which may basically be missed on CT alone.

Case 7: Recurrent Ovarian Cancer
Findings
A 66-year-old female with recurrent ovarian cancer. FDG PET/CT shows disseminated tracer-avid peritoneal carcinomatosis. No solid organ or supradiaphragmatic metastatic lesions are noted (Fig. 9.7).

Teaching points
- For the detection of peritoneal carcinomatosis in patients with ovarian cancer, FDG PET/CT has

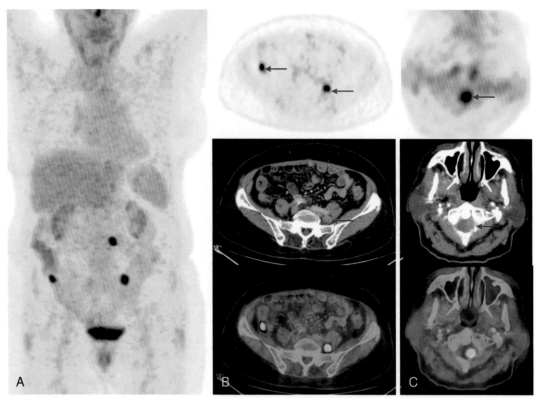

FIG. 9.6 Fludeoxyglucose (FDG) positron emission tomography/computed tomography showing a left paraaortic, left common iliac, and right paracolic lymph node metastases (B, *arrows*). Of incidental note is a focal FDG uptake in the spinal cord, at the level of C1/C2 (C, *arrows*), confirmed in magnetic resonance imaging and follow-up images to be metastasis. A, FDG PET MIP image.

sensitivity, specificity, PPV, NPV, and accuracy of 71%, 100%, 100%, 76%, and 85%, respectively.

- FDG PET/CT may discover the site of recurrence in patients with CA-125 relapse but equivocal or negative conventional imaging.
- It is also superior to stand-alone CT in the assessment of supradiaphragmatic nodal metastases (67% vs 33%).
- It better detects small peritoneal lesions, which are challenging on stand-alone CT.
- FDG PET/CT is cost-effective and redirects the management of patients with recurrent ovarian cancer toward more appropriate therapies.
- Metastatic lesions from the mucinous cystadenocarcinoma subtype are typically calcified.

Pitfalls

- FDG uptake in the rectum is most likely inflammatory in nature and should not be interpreted as metastatic disease.

Case 8: Staging and Restaging Cervical Cancer

Findings

A 68-year-old female with cervical cancer. Staging FDG PET/CT (Fig. 9.8A) shows tracer-avid primary tumor with left iliac, left paraaortic, right retrocrural, and left supraclavicular lymph node metastases (Fig. 9.8A, arrows). Bilateral hydronephrosis is noted. The restaging scan (Fig. 9.8B) demonstrates complete metabolic response after chemotherapy. Bilateral hydronephrosis is also resolved after double-J placement (Fig. 9.8).

Teaching points

- FDG PET/CT is a promising method for the accurate determination of the field of radiation therapy and also treatment monitoring in cervical cancer.
- About 30% of cervical cancers will relapse after treatment. FDG PET/CT discovers recurrent cancer in 11% of patients who are definitively treated and are asymptomatic.

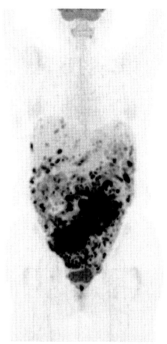

FIG. 9.7 Fludeoxyglucose positron emission tomography MIP image.Showing disseminated tracer-avid peritoneal carcinomatosis.

- FDG PET/CT is more accurate for both staging and restaging of cervical cancer. It is a valuable modality in detecting recurrent disease, with sensitivity, specificity, and accuracy of 95%, 84%, and 88%, respectively.
- FDG PET/CT is an accurate and specifically sensitive modality superior to conventional methods for the detection of distant metastases in patients with advanced cervical cancer.
- The left supraclavicular lymph node (Virchow node) is a common site for distant metastasis from gynecologic cancers.
- In the case of bilateral hydronephrosis, a causative mass lesion in the abdomen or pelvis should be excluded.

Case 9: Recurrent Vulvar Cancer
Findings
A 31-year-old female with recurrent vulvar cancer, status post recent lymphadenectomy. FDG PET/CT shows tracer-avid recurrent cancer with vaginal infiltration (Fig. 9.9A, black arrow). In spite of extended lymphadenectomy, three lymph nodes (two in common and one in external iliac station) are still remaining (Fig. 9.9A and B; red arrows).

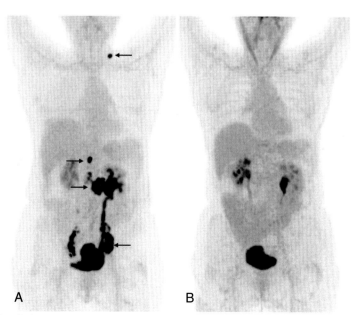

A   B

FIG. 9.8 Staging fludeoxyglucose positron emission tomography/computed tomography (A) showing tracer-avid primary tumor with left iliac, left paraaortic, right retrocrural, and left supraclavicular lymph node metastases (A, *arrows*). Bilateral hydronephrosis is noted. Restaging scan (B) demonstrates complete metabolic response after chemotherapy.

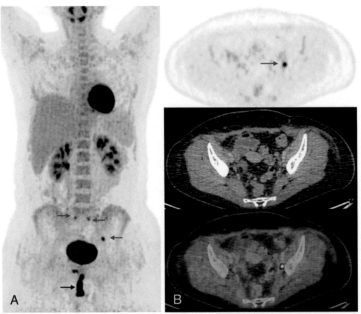

FIG. 9.9 Fludeoxyglucose positron emission tomography/computed tomography tracer-avid recurrent cancer with vaginal infiltration (A, *black arrow*). In spite of extended lymphadenectomy, three lymph nodes (two in common and one in external iliac station) are still remaining (A, B; *red arrows*).

Teaching points
- FDG PET/CT is superior to conventional imaging methods for the assessment of recurrent vulvar cancer.
- It can accurately detect the small lymph nodes (i.e., ≥5 mm) for the assessment of residual disease after lymphadenectomy and accurate determination of the field of radiation therapy.

Pitfalls
- FDG uptake in bilateral tonsils is inflammatory in nature.

Case 10: Staging Cervical Cancer
Findings
A 60-year-old female with basaloid cervical SCC. FDG PET/CT shows tracer-avid primary tumor (arrow). There is disseminated FDG-avid cervical, thoracic, and abdominal lymph node involvement (Fig. 9.10).

Teaching points
- FDG PET/CT is a valuable method in the assessment of pelvic, paraaortic, and distant lymph node metastases in advanced-stage cervical cancers and superior to stand-alone CT and MRI for this purpose.
- FDG PET/CT also showed a significant role in the management of cervix carcinoma and was able to change the treatment approach in up to two-thirds of patients.

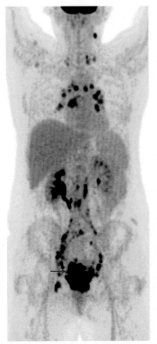

FIG. 9.10 Fludeoxyglucose positron emission tomography/computed tomography showing tracer-avid primary tumor *(arrow)*.

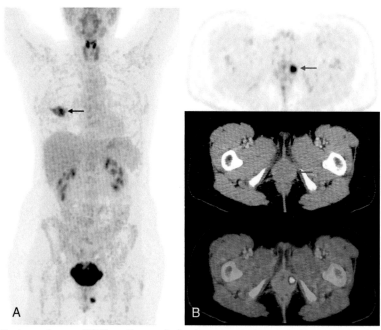

FIG. 9.11 Fludeoxyglucose (FDG) positron emission tomography/computed tomography showing tracer-avid known primary right breast cancer (A, *arrow*). Of incidental note is a focal FDG uptake in the left vaginal/vulvar region (B, *arrows*).

- Novel imaging by FDG PET/MRI showed promising results in staging of cervical cancers.

Pitfalls
- In this patient, the pattern of nodal involvement may resemble sarcoidosis. In such cases, histopathology correlation is imperative for accurate diagnosis. The pathology report confirmed metastatic disease in this patient.

Case 11: Bartholin Cyst Infection
Findings
A 47-year-old female who was initially diagnosed with triple-negative invasive right breast cancer, referred for FDG PET/CT staging. FDG PET/CT shows tracer-avid known primary right breast cancer (Fig. 9.11A, arrow). Of incidental note is a focal FDG uptake in the left vaginal/vulvar region (Fig. 9.11B, arrows).

Teaching points
- A Bartholin cyst or bartholinitis occurs if the gland duct is blocked with resultant inflammation. The infection may lead to an abscess. It most likely happens in females of childbearing age and usually locates at the lower part of the opening of the vagina.
- Although intensive tracer uptake in inflamed Bartholin cyst or abscess is a common pitfall in FDG

PET/CT imaging, its differentiation from malignancy is not possible by this modality. Clinical clarification is strongly recommended.

Pitfalls
- Inflamed lesions can take up FDG and should not be falsely interpreted as malignancy.
- Menstruation, cyst inflammation, and using tampons can cause FDG uptake in the vaginal region.
- Symmetric uptake in vocal cords is physiologic in nature.
- Faint FDG uptake in the thyroid gland could be related with chronic thyroiditis.

Case 12: Endometrial Cancer—Recurrence
Findings
A 69-year-old female with recurrent endometrial cancer. FDG PET/CT shows tracer-avid recurrent malignancy in the vagina (Fig. 9.12A, arrow). There is an FDG-avid left pulmonary nodule, proved in histopathology to be a metastatic lesion (Fig. 9.12B, arrows).

Teaching points
- FDG PET/CT is an accurate method for staging and restaging endometrial cancer.
- It is superior to stand-alone CT for the assessment of vaginal lesions.

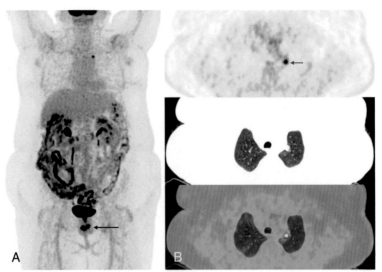

FIG. 9.12 Fludeoxyglucose (FDG) positron emission tomography/computed tomography showing tracer-avid recurrent malignancy in the vagina (A, *arrow*). There is an FDG-avid left pulmonary nodule, proved in histopathology to be a metastatic lesion (B, *arrows*).

- It can successfully differentiate benign lung lesions from metastatic disease with high NPV (>95%).
- For the evaluation of distant metastases, FDG PET/CT showed sensitivity, specificity, NPV, PPV, and accuracy of approximately 93%, 99%, 100%, 81%, and 99%, respectively.
- It was found to be superior to conventional imaging in discovering distant metastases to the abdomen and thorax.
- Preoperative metabolic activity (SUV) of endometrial primary tumor seems to be an independent prognostic factor for malignancy recurrence and mortality, as well as both disease-free and overall survival.

Pitfalls
- A high FDG uptake by bowels may obscure a peritoneal carcinomatosis.

REFERENCES

1. de Abreu AL, Malaguti N, Souza RP, et al. Association of human papillomavirus, *Neisseria gonorrhoeae* and *Chlamydia trachomatis* co-infections on the risk of high-grade squamous intraepithelial cervical lesion. *American Journal of Cancer Research*. 2016;6(6):1371–1383.
2. Saslow D, Solomon D, Lawson HW, et al. American Cancer Society, American Society for Colposcopy and Cervical Pathology, and American Society for Clinical Pathology screening guidelines for the prevention and early detection of cervical cancer. *Journal of Lower Genital Tract Disease*. July 2012;16(3):175–204.
3. Siegel RL, Miller KD, Jemal A. Cancer statistics. *A Cancer Journal for Clinicians*. January–February 2016;66(1):7–30.
4. Hackeng WM, Hruban RH, Offerhaus GJ, Brosens LA. Surgical and molecular pathology of pancreatic neoplasms. *Diagnostic Pathology*. 2016;11(1):47.
5. NCCN Clinical Practice Guidelines in Oncology. *Cervical Cancer*. 2016. Version 1. www.NCCN.org.
6. Alberts S, Goldberg R. Gynecologic cancers. In: Casciato D, ed. *Manual of Clinical Oncology*. 5th ed. Philadelphia, USA: LWW; 2004:254–285.
7. Bilimoria KY, Bentrem DJ, Merkow RP, et al. Application of the pancreatic adenocarcinoma staging system to pancreatic neuroendocrine tumors. *Journal of the American College of Surgeons*. October 2007;205(4):558–563.
8. Imadome K, Iwakawa M, Nakawatari M, et al. Subtypes of cervical adenosquamous carcinomas classified by EpCAM expression related to radiosensitivity. *Cancer Biology & Therapy*. November 15, 2010;10(10):1019–1026.
9. Yao JC, Lombard-Bohas C, Baudin E, et al. Daily oral everolimus activity in patients with metastatic pancreatic neuroendocrine tumors after failure of cytotoxic chemotherapy: a phase II trial. *Journal of Clinical Oncology: Official Journal of the American Society of Clinical Oncology*. January 1, 2010;28(1):69–76.
10. Chaturvedi AK, Kleinerman RA, Hildesheim A, et al. Second cancers after squamous cell carcinoma and adenocarcinoma of the cervix. *Journal of Clinical Oncology: Official Journal of the American Society of Clinical Oncology*. February 20, 2009;27(6):967–973.

11. Uterine cervix. In: Robin P, Hansen JT, eds. *TNM Staging Atlas with Oncoanatomy*. 2nd ed. Philadelphia, USA: Wolters Kluwer|LWW; 2012:520–531.

12. Colombo N, Carinelli S, Colombo A, et al. Cervical cancer: ESMO Clinical Practice Guidelines for diagnosis, treatment and follow-up. *Annals of Oncology: Official Journal of the European Society for Medical Oncology/ ESMO*. October 2012;23(suppl 7):vii27–32.

13. The Royal College of Physicians and the Royal College of Radiologists. *Evidence-based Indications for the Usage of PET-CT in the UK*. London: RCP, RCR; 2016:2016.

14. Fyles A, Walker-Dilks C. *PET Imaging in Cervical Cancer: Evidentiary Base and Consensus Process*. Cancer Care Ontario; 2009.

15. Chu Y, Zheng A, Wang F, et al. Diagnostic value of 18F-FDG-PET or PET-CT in recurrent cervical cancer: a systematic review and meta-analysis. *Nuclear Medicine Communications*. February 2014;35(2):144–150.

16. Ding XP, Feng L, Ma L. Diagnosis of recurrent uterine cervical cancer: PET versus PET/CT: a systematic review and meta-analysis. *Archives of Gynecology and Obstetrics*. October 2014;290(4):741–747.

17. Salem A, Salem AF, Al-Ibraheem A, Lataifeh I, Almousa A, Jaradat I. Evidence for the use PET for radiation therapy planning in patients with cervical cancer: a systematic review. *Hematology/Oncology and Stem Cell Therapy*. 2011;4(4):173–181.

18. Auguste P, Barton P, Meads C, et al. Evaluating PET-CT in routine surveillance and follow-up after treatment for cervical cancer: a cost-effectiveness analysis. *An International Journal of Obstetrics and Gynaecology*. March 2014;121(4):464–476.

19. Arbyn M, Castellsague X, de Sanjose S, et al. Worldwide burden of cervical cancer in 2008. *Annals of Oncology: Official Journal of the European Society for Medical Oncology/ ESMO*. December 2011;22(12):2675–2686.

20. Sankaranarayanan R, Nene BM, Shastri SS, et al. HPV screening for cervical cancer in rural India. *The New England Journal of Medicine*. April 2, 2009;360(14):1385–1394.

21. Pecorelli S. Revised FIGO staging for carcinoma of the vulva, cervix, and endometrium. *International Journal of Gynaecology and Obstetrics: The Official Organ of the International Federation of Gynaecology and Obstetrics*. May 2009;105(2):103–104.

22. Barillot I, Horiot JC, Pigneux J, et al. Carcinoma of the intact uterine cervix treated with radiotherapy alone: a French cooperative study: update and multivariate analysis of prognostics factors. *International Journal of Radiation Oncology, Biology, Physics*. July 15, 1997;38(5):969–978.

23. Perez CA, Grigsby PW, Chao KS, Mutch DG, Lockett MA. Tumor size, irradiation dose, and long-term outcome of carcinoma of uterine cervix. *International Journal of Radiation Oncology, Biology, Physics*. May 1, 1998;41(2):307–317.

24. Peters 3rd WA, Liu PY, Barrett 2nd RJ, et al. Concurrent chemotherapy and pelvic radiation therapy compared with pelvic radiation therapy alone as adjuvant therapy after radical surgery in high-risk early-stage cancer of the cervix. *Journal of Clinical Oncology: Official Journal of the American Society of Clinical Oncology*. April 2000;18(8):1606–1613.

25. Blake MA, Singh A, Setty BN, et al. Pearls and pitfalls in interpretation of abdominal and pelvic PET-CT. *Radiographics: A Review Publication of the Radiological Society of North America, Inc.* September–October 2006;26(5):1335–1353.

26. Gold MA. PET in cervical cancer–implications for 'staging,' treatment planning, assessment of prognosis, and prediction of response. *Journal of the National Comprehensive Cancer Network*. January 2008;6(1):37–45.

27. Son H, Kositwattanarerk A, Hayes MP, et al. PET/CT evaluation of cervical cancer: spectrum of disease. *Radiographics: A Review Publication of the Radiological Society of North America, Inc.* September 2010;30(5):1251–1268.

28. Chou HH, Chang TC, Yen TC, et al. Low value of [18F]-fluoro-2-deoxy-D-glucose positron emission tomography in primary staging of early-stage cervical cancer before radical hysterectomy. *Journal of Clinical Oncology: Official Journal of the American Society of Clinical Oncology*. January 1, 2006;24(1):123–128.

29. Crivellaro C, Guerra L, Dolci C, et al. Preoperative staging of cervical cancer: is FDG PET/CT really effective in patients with Ib1 stage? *Journal of Nuclear Medicine*. 2011;52(suppl 1):144.

30. Driscoll DO, Halpenny D, Johnston C, Sheehy N, Keogan M. 18F-FDG-PET/CT is of limited value in primary staging of early stage cervical cancer. *Abdominal Imaging*. January 2015;40(1):127–133.

31. Tsai CS, Chang TC, Lai CH, et al. Preliminary report of using FDG-PET to detect extrapelvic lesions in cervical cancer patients with enlarged pelvic lymph nodes on MRI/CT. *International Journal of Radiation Oncology, Biology, Physics*. April 1, 2004;58(5):1506–1512.

32. Patel CN, Nazir SA, Khan Z, Gleeson FV, Bradley KM. 18F-FDG PET/CT of cervical carcinoma. *American Journal of Roentgenology*. May 2011;196(5):1225–1233.

33. Rockall AG, Cross S, Flanagan S, Moore E, Avril N. The role of FDG-PET/CT in gynaecological cancers. *Cancer Imaging: The Official Publication of the International Cancer Imaging Society*. 2012;12:49–65.

34. Grigsby PW, Siegel BA, Dehdashti F, Rader J, Zoberi I. Posttherapy [18F] fluorodeoxyglucose positron emission tomography in carcinoma of the cervix: response and outcome. *Journal of Clinical Oncology: Official Journal of the American Society of Clinical Oncology*. June 1, 2004;22(11):2167–2171.

35. Havrilesky LJ, Wong TZ, Secord AA, Berchuck A, Clarke-Pearson DL, Jones EL. The role of PET scanning in the detection of recurrent cervical cancer. *Gynecologic Oncology*. July 2003;90(1):186–190.

36. Belhocine TZ. 18F-FDG PET imaging in posttherapy monitoring of cervical cancers: from diagnosis to prognosis. *Journal of Nuclear Medicine*. October 2004;45(10):1602–1604.

37. Schwarz JK, Grigsby PW, Dehdashti F, Delbeke D. The role of 18F-FDG PET in assessing therapy response in cancer of the cervix and ovaries. *Journal of Nuclear Medicine: Official Publication, Society of Nuclear Medicine.* May 2009;50(suppl 1):64S–73S.

38. Choi J, Kim HJ, Jeong YH, et al. The role of (18) F-FDG PET/CT in assessing therapy response in cervix cancer after concurrent chemoradiation therapy. *Nuclear Medicine and Molecular Imaging.* June 2014;48(2):130–136.

39. Krhili S, Muratet JP, Roche S, et al. Use of metabolic parameters as prognostic factors during concomitant chemoradiotherapy for locally advanced cervical cancer. *American Journal of Clinical Oncology.* March 29, 2016.

40. Xue F, Lin LL, Dehdashti F, Miller TR, Siegel BA, Grigsby PW. F-18 fluorodeoxyglucose uptake in primary cervical cancer as an indicator of prognosis after radiation therapy. *Gynecologic Oncology.* April 2006;101(1):147–151.

41. Kidd EA, Siegel BA, Dehdashti F, Grigsby PW. Pelvic lymph node F-18 fluorodeoxyglucose uptake as a prognostic biomarker in newly diagnosed patients with locally advanced cervical cancer. *Cancer.* March 15, 2010;116(6):1469–1475.

42. Kidd EA, Siegel BA, Dehdashti F, et al. Lymph node staging by positron emission tomography in cervical cancer: relationship to prognosis. *Journal of Clinical Oncology: Official Journal of the American Society of Clinical Oncology.* April 20, 2010;28(12):2108–2113.

43. Waggoner SE. Cervical cancer. *Lancet.* June 28, 2003;361(9376):2217–2225.

44. Yen TC, See LC, Chang TC, et al. Defining the priority of using 18F-FDG PET for recurrent cervical cancer. *Journal of Nuclear Medicine.* October 2004;45(10):1632–1639.

45. Kitajima K, Suenaga Y, Ueno Y, et al. Fusion of PET and MRI for staging of uterine cervical cancer: comparison with contrast-enhanced (18)F-FDG PET/CT and pelvic MRI. *Clinical Imaging.* July–August 2014;38(4):464–469.

46. Kim HJ, Cho A, Yun M, Kim YT, Kang WJ. Comparison of FDG PET/CT and MRI in lymph node staging of endometrial cancer. *Annals of Nuclear Medicine.* February 2016;30(2):104–113.

47. Hwang J, Lyer R, Salo J. *Cancer Management, Esophageal Cancer*; 2015. http://www.cancernetwork.com/cancer-management/esophageal/page/0/3.

48. Brinton LA, Berman ML, Mortel R, et al. Reproductive, menstrual, and medical risk factors for endometrial cancer: results from a case-control study. *American Journal of Obstetrics and Gynecology.* November 1992;167(5):1317–1325.

49. McCluggage WG. My approach to the interpretation of endometrial biopsies and curettings. *Journal of Clinical Pathology.* August 2006;59(8):801–812.

50. McKenney JK, Longacre TA. Low-grade endometrial adenocarcinoma: a diagnostic algorithm for distinguishing atypical endometrial hyperplasia and other benign (and malignant) mimics. *Advances in Anatomic Pathology.* January 2009;16(1):1–22.

51. Hong SJ, Kim TJ, Nam KB, et al. New TNM staging system for esophageal cancer: what chest radiologists need to know. *Radiographics: A Review Publication of the Radiological Society of North America, Inc.* October 2014;34(6):1722–1740.

52. NCCN Clinical Practice Guidelines in Oncology. *Uterine Neoplasms.* 2016. Version 2. www.NCCN.org.

53. *The AJCC Cancer Staging Manual.* 7th ed. Chicago, IL: Springer Science+Business Media, LLC (SBM); 2010.

54. Kurra V, Krajewski KM, Jagannathan J, Giardino A, Berlin S, Ramaiya N. Typical and atypical metastatic sites of recurrent endometrial carcinoma. *Cancer Imaging: The Official Publication of the International Cancer Imaging Society.* 2013;13:113–122.

55. Colombo N, Preti E, Landoni F, et al. Endometrial cancer: ESMO Clinical Practice Guidelines for diagnosis, treatment and follow-up. *Annals of Oncology: Official Journal of the European Society for Medical Oncology/ESMO.* October 2013;24(suppl 6):vi33–38.

56. Group SGOCPECW, Burke WM, Orr J, et al. Endometrial cancer: a review and current management strategies: part II. *Gynecologic Oncology.* August 2014;134(2):393–402.

57. Bollineni VR, Ytre-Hauge S, Bollineni-Balabay O, Salvesen HB, Haldorsen IS. High diagnostic value of 18F-FDG PET/CT in endometrial cancer: systematic review and meta-analysis of the literature. *Journal of Nuclear Medicine: Official Publication, Society of Nuclear Medicine.* June 2016;57(6):879–885.

58. Musto A, Grassetto G, Marzola MC, et al. Role of 18F-FDG PET/CT in the carcinoma of the uterus: a review of literature. *Yonsei Medical Journal.* November 2014;55(6):1467–1472.

59. Kadkhodayan S, Shahriari S, Treglia G, Yousefi Z, Sadeghi R. Accuracy of 18-F-FDG PET imaging in the follow up of endometrial cancer patients: systematic review and meta-analysis of the literature. *Gynecologic Oncology.* February 2013;128(2):397–404.

60. Chang MC, Chen JH, Liang JA, Yang KT, Cheng KY, Kao CH. 18F-FDG PET or PET/CT for detection of metastatic lymph nodes in patients with endometrial cancer: a systematic review and meta-analysis. *European Journal of Radiology.* November 2012;81(11):3511–3517.

61. Verdecchia A, Francisci S, Brenner H, et al. Recent cancer survival in Europe: a 2000-02 period analysis of EUROCARE-4 data. *The Lancet. Oncology.* September 2007;8(9):784–796.

62. Timmermans A, Opmeer BC, Khan KS, et al. Endometrial thickness measurement for detecting endometrial cancer in women with postmenopausal bleeding: a systematic review and meta-analysis. *Obstetrics and Gynecology.* July 2010;116(1):160–167.

63. Kinkel K, Kaji Y, Yu KK, et al. Radiologic staging in patients with endometrial cancer: a meta-analysis. *Radiology.* September 1999;212(3):711–718.

64. Sala E, Rockall A, Kubik-Huch RA. Advances in magnetic resonance imaging of endometrial cancer. *European Radiology.* March 2011;21(3):468–473.

65. Savelli L, Ceccarini M, Ludovisi M, et al. Preoperative local staging of endometrial cancer: transvaginal sonography vs. magnetic resonance imaging. *Ultrasound in Obstetrics & Gynecology: The Official Journal of the International Society of Ultrasound in Obstetrics and Gynecology.* May 2008;31(5):560–566.

66. Hogberg T, Signorelli M, de Oliveira CF, et al. Sequential adjuvant chemotherapy and radiotherapy in endometrial cancer–results from two randomised studies. *European Journal of Cancer.* September 2010;46(13):2422–2431.

67. Lerman H, Metser U, Grisaru D, Fishman A, Lievshitz G, Even-Sapir E. Normal and abnormal 18F-FDG endometrial and ovarian uptake in pre- and postmenopausal patients: assessment by PET/CT. *Journal of Nuclear Medicine: Official Publication, Society of Nuclear Medicine.* February 2004;45(2):266–271.

68. Long NM, Smith CS. Causes and imaging features of false positives and false negatives on F-PET/CT in oncologic imaging. *Insights into Imaging.* December 2011;2(6):679–698.

69. Kitajima K, Suenaga Y, Ueno Y, et al. Value of fusion of PET and MRI for staging of endometrial cancer: comparison with (1)(8)F-FDG contrast-enhanced PET/CT and dynamic contrast-enhanced pelvic MRI. *European Journal of Radiology.* October 2013;82(10):1672–1676.

70. Faria SC, Sagebiel T, Balachandran A, Devine C, Lal C, Bhosale PR. Imaging in endometrial carcinoma. *The Indian Journal of Radiology & Imaging.* April–June 2015;25(2):137–147.

71. Kitajima K, Murakami K, Yamasaki E, et al. Accuracy of 18F-FDG PET/CT in detecting pelvic and paraaortic lymph node metastasis in patients with endometrial cancer. *American Journal of Roentgenology.* June 2008;190(6):1652–1658.

72. Antonsen SL, Jensen LN, Loft A, et al. MRI, PET/CT and ultrasound in the preoperative staging of endometrial cancer - a multicenter prospective comparative study. *Gynecologic Oncology.* February 2013;128(2):300–308.

73. Picchio M, Mangili G, Samanes Gajate AM, et al. High-grade endometrial cancer: value of [(18)F]FDG PET/CT in preoperative staging. *Nuclear Medicine Communications.* June 2010;31(6):506–512.

74. Kitajima K, Murakami K, Yamasaki E, et al. Performance of FDG-PET/CT in the diagnosis of recurrent endometrial cancer. *Annals of Nuclear Medicine.* February 2008;22(2):103–109.

75. Park JY, Kim EN, Kim DY, et al. Clinical impact of positron emission tomography or positron emission tomography/computed tomography in the posttherapy surveillance of endometrial carcinoma: evaluation of 88 patients. *International Journal of Gynecological Cancer: Official Journal of the International Gynecological Cancer Society.* November–December 2008;18(6):1332–1338.

76. Sharma P, Kumar R, Singh H, et al. Carcinoma endometrium: role of 18-FDG PET/CT for detection of suspected recurrence. *Clinical Nuclear Medicine.* July 2012;37(7):649–655.

77. Chung HH, Kang WJ, Kim JW, et al. The clinical impact of [(18)F]FDG PET/CT for the management of recurrent endometrial cancer: correlation with clinical and histological findings. *European Journal of Nuclear Medicine and Molecular Imaging.* June 2008;35(6):1081–1088.

78. Ghooshkhanei H, Treglia G, Sabouri G, Davoodi R, Sadeghi R. Risk stratification and prognosis determination using (18)F-FDG PET imaging in endometrial cancer patients: a systematic review and meta-analysis. *Gynecologic Oncology.* March 2014;132(3):669–676.

79. Nakamura K, Joja I, Fukushima C, et al. The preoperative SUVmax is superior to ADCmin of the primary tumour as a predictor of disease recurrence and survival in patients with endometrial cancer. *European Journal of Nuclear Medicine and Molecular Imaging.* January 2013;40(1):52–60.

80. Ovarian Cancer – Risk Factors and Prevention. http://www.cancer.net/cancer-types/ovarian-cancer/risk-factors-and-prevention.

81. NCCN Clinical Practice Guidelines in Oncology. *Ovarian Cancer Including Fallopian Tube Cancer and Primary Peritoneal Cancer;* 2016. Version 1. www.NCCN.org.

82. Fleming G, Seidman J, Lengyel E. Epithelial ovarian cancer. In: Barakat R, Markman M, Randall M, eds. *Principles and Practice of Gynecologic Oncology.* 6th ed. Philadelphia: Lippincott Williams & Wilkins; 2013:757–847.

83. Ozols R, Rubin S, Thomas G, Robboy S. Epithelial ovarian cancer. In: William J, Carlos A, Robert C, eds. *Principles and Practice of Gynecologic Oncology.* 4th ed. Philadelphia: Lippincott Williams & Wilkins; 2004:841–918.

84. Goff BA, Mandel LS, Drescher CW, et al. Development of an ovarian cancer symptom index: possibilities for earlier detection. *Cancer.* January 15, 2007;109(2):221–227.

85. Agarwal R, Kaye SB. Prognostic factors in ovarian cancer: how close are we to a complete picture? *Annals of Oncology: Official Journal of the European Society for Medical Oncology/ESMO.* January 2005;16(1):4–6.

86. Landrum LM, Java J, Mathews CA, et al. Prognostic factors for stage III epithelial ovarian cancer treated with intraperitoneal chemotherapy: a Gynecologic Oncology Group study. *Gynecologic Oncology.* July 2013;130(1):12–18.

87. Mandic A, Tesic M, Vujkov T, Novta N, Rajovic J. Ovarian cancer stage III/IV: poor prognostic factors. *Archive of Oncology.* 2001;9(1):13–16.

88. Survival Rates for Ovarian Cancer, by Stage. http://www.cancer.org/cancer/ovariancancer/detailedguide/ovarian-cancer-survival-rates.

89. Chen VW, Ruiz B, Killeen JL, Cote TR, Wu XC, Correa CN. Pathology and classification of ovarian tumors. *Cancer.* May 15, 2003;97(10 suppl):2631–2642.

90. Kaku T, Ogawa S, Kawano Y, et al. Histological classification of ovarian cancer. *Medical Electron Microscopy: Official Journal of the Clinical Electron Microscopy Society of Japan.* March 2003;36(1):9–17.

91. Rosen DG, Yang G, Liu G, et al. Ovarian cancer: pathology, biology, and disease models. *Frontiers in Bioscience*. 2009;14:2089–2102.

92. McMahon CJ, Rofsky NM, Pedrosa I. Lymphatic metastases from pelvic tumors: anatomic classification, characterization, and staging. *Radiology*. January 2010;254(1):31–46.

93. Ovary and Fallopian Tube. In: Robin P, Hansen JT, eds. *TNM Staging Atlas with Oncoanatomy*. 2nd ed. Philadelphia, USA: Wolters Kluwer/LWW; 2012:482–495.

94. Prat J, Oncology FCoG. FIGO's staging classification for cancer of the ovary, fallopian tube, and peritoneum: abridged republication. *Journal of Gynecologic Oncology*. April 2015;26(2):87–89.

95. Colombo N, Peiretti M, Garbi A, et al. Non-epithelial ovarian cancer: ESMO Clinical Practice Guidelines for diagnosis, treatment and follow-up. *Annals of Oncology: Official Journal of the European Society for Medical Oncology/ESMO*. October 2012;23(suppl 7):vii20–26.

96. Ledermann JA, Raja FA, Fotopoulou C, et al. Newly diagnosed and relapsed epithelial ovarian carcinoma: ESMO Clinical Practice Guidelines for diagnosis, treatment and follow-up. *Annals of Oncology: Official Journal of the European Society for Medical Oncology/ESMO*. October 2013;24(suppl 6):vi24–vi32.

97. Wright AA, Bohlke K, Armstrong DK, et al. Neoadjuvant chemotherapy for newly diagnosed, advanced ovarian cancer: Society of Gynecologic Oncology and American Society of Clinical Oncology clinical practice guideline. *Journal of Clinical Oncology: Official Journal of the American Society of Clinical Oncology*. October 2016;1; 34(28):3460–3473.

98. Schmidt S, Meuli RA, Achtari C, Prior JO. Peritoneal carcinomatosis in primary ovarian cancer staging: comparison between MDCT, MRI, and 18F-FDG PET/CT. *Clinical Nuclear Medicine*. May 2015;40(5):371–377.

99. Gu P, Pan LL, Wu SQ, Sun L, Huang GCA. 125, PET alone, PET-CT, CT and MRI in diagnosing recurrent ovarian carcinoma: a systematic review and meta-analysis. *European Journal of Radiology*. July 2009;71(1):164–174.

100. Limei Z, Yong C, Yan X, Shuai T, Jiangyan X, Zhiqing L. Accuracy of positron emission tomography/computed tomography in the diagnosis and restaging for recurrent ovarian cancer: a meta-analysis. *International Journal of Gynecological Cancer: Official Journal of the International Gynecological Cancer Society*. May 2013;23(4):598–607.

101. Ruiz-Hernandez G, Delgado-Bolton RC, Fernandez-Perez C, Lapena-Gutierrez L, Carreras-Delgado JL. Meta-analysis of the diagnostic efficacy of FDG-PET in patients with suspected ovarian cancer recurrence. *Revista espanola de medicina nuclear*. May–June 2005;24(3):161–173.

102. Mansueto M, Grimaldi A, Mangili G, et al. Positron emission tomography/computed tomography introduction in the clinical management of patients with suspected recurrence of ovarian cancer: a cost-effectiveness analysis. *European Journal of Cancer Care*. November 2009;18(6):612–619.

103. Kim S, Chung JK, Kang SB, et al. [18F]FDG PET as a substitute for second-look laparotomy in patients with advanced ovarian carcinoma. *European Journal of Nuclear Medicine and Molecular Imaging*. February 2004;31(2):196–201.

104. Smith GT, Hubner KF, McDonald T, Thie JA. Cost Analysis of FDG PET for managing patients with ovarian cancer. *Clinical Positron Imaging: Official Journal of the Institute for Clinical P.E.T.* March 1999;2(2):63–70.

105. Lerner JP, Timor-Tritsch IE, Federman A, Abramovich G. Transvaginal ultrasonographic characterization of ovarian masses with an improved, weighted scoring system. *American Journal of Obstetrics and Gynecology*. January 1994;170(1 Pt 1):81–85.

106. du Bois A, Reuss A, Pujade-Lauraine E, Harter P, Ray-Coquard I, Pfisterer J. Role of surgical outcome as prognostic factor in advanced epithelial ovarian cancer: a combined exploratory analysis of 3 prospectively randomized phase 3 multicenter trials: by the Arbeitsgemeinschaft Gynaekologische Onkologie Studiengruppe Ovarialkarzinom (AGO-OVAR) and the Groupe d'Investigateurs Nationaux Pour les Etudes des Cancers de l'Ovaire (GINECO). *Cancer*. March 15, 2009;115(6):1234–1244.

107. Swart A. Long-term follow-up of women enrolled in a randomized trial of adjuvant chemotherapy for early stage ovarian cancer (ICON1). *Journal of Clinical Oncology: Official Journal of the American Society of Clinical Oncology*. 2007;25(18S):5509.

108. Perren TJ, Swart AM, Pfisterer J, et al. A phase 3 trial of bevacizumab in ovarian cancer. *The New England Journal of Medicine*. December 29, 2011;365(26):2484–2496.

109. Aghajanian C, Blank SV, Goff BA, et al. OCEANS: a randomized, double-blind, placebo-controlled phase III trial of chemotherapy with or without bevacizumab in patients with platinum-sensitive recurrent epithelial ovarian, primary peritoneal, or fallopian tube cancer. *Journal of Clinical Oncology: Official Journal of the American Society of Clinical Oncology*. June 10, 2012;30(17):2039–2045.

110. Pujade-Lauraine E, Hilpert F, Weber B, Reuss A. AURELIA: a randomized phase III trial evaluating bevacizumab (BEV) plus chemotherapy (CT) for platinum (PT)-resistant recurrent ovarian cancer (OC). *Journal of Clinical Oncology: Official Journal of the American Society of Clinical Oncology*. 2012;30S:LBA5002.

111. Rustin G, van der Burg M. A randomized trial in ovarian cancer (OC) of early treatment of relapse based on CA125 level alone versus delayed treatment based on conventional clinical indicators (MRC OV05/EORTC 55955 trials). *Journal of Clinical Oncology: Official Journal of the American Society of Clinical Oncology*. 2009;27(18S):1.

112. Carter K, Kotlyarov E. Common causes of false positive F18 FDG PET/CT scans in oncology. *Brazilian Archives of Biology and Technology*. 2007;50:29–35.

113. De Iaco P, Musto A, Orazi L, et al. FDG-PET/CT in advanced ovarian cancer staging: value and pitfalls in detecting lesions in different abdominal and pelvic quadrants compared with laparoscopy. *European Journal of Radiology*. November 2011;80(2):e98–e103.

114. Fenchel S, Grab D, Nuessle K, et al. Asymptomatic adnexal masses: correlation of FDG PET and histopathologic findings. *Radiology*. June 2002;223(3):780–788.

115. Nishizawa S, Inubushi M, Okada H. Physiological 18F-FDG uptake in the ovaries and uterus of healthy female volunteers. *European Journal of Nuclear Medicine and Molecular Imaging*. May 2005;32(5):549–556.

116. Prakash P, Cronin CG, Blake MA. Role of PET/CT in ovarian cancer. *American Journal of Roentgenology*. June 2010;194(6):W464–W470.

117. Woodward PJ, Hosseinzadeh K, Saenger JS. From the archives of the AFIP: radiologic staging of ovarian carcinoma with pathologic correlation. *Radiographics: A Review Publication of the Radiological Society of North America, Inc*. January–February 2004;24(1):225–246.

118. Rieber A, Nussle K, Stohr I, et al. Preoperative diagnosis of ovarian tumors with MR imaging: comparison with transvaginal sonography, positron emission tomography, and histologic findings. *American Journal of Roentgenology*. July 2001;177(1):123–129.

119. Castellucci P, Perrone AM, Picchio M, et al. Diagnostic accuracy of 18F-FDG PET/CT in characterizing ovarian lesions and staging ovarian cancer: correlation with transvaginal ultrasonography, computed tomography, and histology. *Nuclear Medicine Communications*. August 2007;28(8):589–595.

120. Kitajima K, Murakami K, Yamasaki E, et al. Diagnostic accuracy of integrated FDG-PET/contrast-enhanced CT in staging ovarian cancer: comparison with enhanced CT. *European Journal of Nuclear Medicine and Molecular Imaging*. October 2008;35(10):1912–1920.

121. Yoshida Y, Kurokawa T, Tsujikawa T, Okazawa H, Kotsuji F. Positron emission tomography in ovarian cancer: 18F-deoxy-glucose and 16alpha-18F-fluoro-17beta-estradiol PET. *Journal of Ovarian Research*. 2009;2(1):7.

122. Signorelli M, Guerra L, Pirovano C, et al. Detection of nodal metastases by 18F-FDG PET/CT in apparent early stage ovarian cancer: a prospective study. *Gynecologic Oncology*. November 2013;131(2):395–399.

123. Hynninen J, Auranen A, Carpen O, et al. FDG PET/CT in staging of advanced epithelial ovarian cancer: frequency of supradiaphragmatic lymph node metastasis challenges the traditional pattern of disease spread. *Gynecologic Oncology*. July 2012;126(1):64–68.

124. Iagaru AH, Mittra ES, McDougall IR, Quon A, Gambhir SS. 18F-FDG PET/CT evaluation of patients with ovarian carcinoma. *Nuclear Medicine Communications*. December 2008;29(12):1046–1051.

125. Yoshida Y, Kurokawa T, Kawahara K, et al. Incremental benefits of FDG positron emission tomography over CT alone for the preoperative staging of ovarian cancer. *American Journal of Roentgenology*. January 2004;182(1):227–233.

126. Lee SI, Catalano OA, Dehdashti F. Evaluation of gynecologic cancer with MR imaging, 18F-FDG PET/CT, and PET/MR imaging. *Journal of Nuclear Medicine: Official Publication, Society of Nuclear Medicine*. March 2015;56(3):436–443.

127. Fularz M, Adamiak P, Czepczynski R, et al. Utility of PET/CT in the diagnosis of recurrent ovarian cancer depending on CA 125 serum level. *Nuklearmedizin. Nuclear Medicine*. 2015;54(4):158–162.

128. Hauth EA, Antoch G, Stattaus J, et al. Evaluation of integrated whole-body PET/CT in the detection of recurrent ovarian cancer. *European Journal of Radiology*. November 2005;56(2):263–268.

129. Sebastian S, Lee SI, Horowitz NS, et al. PET-CT vs. CT alone in ovarian cancer recurrence. *Abdominal Imaging*. January–February 2008;33(1):112–118.

130. You JJ, Cline KJ, Gu CS, et al. (18)F-fluorodeoxyglucose positron-emission tomography-computed tomography to diagnose recurrent cancer. *British Journal of Cancer*. May 26, 2015;112(11):1737–1743.

131. Thrall MM, DeLoia JA, Gallion H, Avril N. Clinical use of combined positron emission tomography and computed tomography (FDG-PET/CT) in recurrent ovarian cancer. *Gynecologic Oncology*. April 2007;105(1):17–22.

132. De Gaetano AM, Calcagni ML, Rufini V, et al. Imaging of gynecologic malignancies with FDG PET-CT: case examples, physiologic activity, and pitfalls. *Abdominal Imaging*. November 2009;34(6):696–711.

133. Avril N, Sassen S, Schmalfeldt B, et al. Prediction of response to neoadjuvant chemotherapy by sequential F-18-fluorodeoxyglucose positron emission tomography in patients with advanced-stage ovarian cancer. *Journal of Clinical Oncology: Official Journal of the American Society of Clinical Oncology*. October 20, 2005;23(30):7445–7453.

134. Kumar Dhingra V, Kand P, Basu S. Impact of FDG-PET and -PET/CT imaging in the clinical decision-making of ovarian carcinoma: an evidence-based approach. *Women's Health*. March 2012;8(2):191–203.

135. Martoni AA, Fanti S, Zamagni C, et al. [18F]FDG-PET/CT monitoring early identifies advanced ovarian cancer patients who will benefit from prolonged neo-adjuvant chemotherapy. *The Quarterly Journal of Nuclear Medicine and Molecular Imaging: Official Publication of the Italian Association of Nuclear Medicine*. February 2011;55(1):81–90.

136. Brunetti JC. Fludeoxyglucose F 18 PET-computed tomography: management changes effecting patient outcomes in gynecologic malignancies. *PET Clinics*. July 2015;10(3):395–409.

137. Nishiyama Y, Yamamoto Y, Kanenishi K, et al. Monitoring the neoadjuvant therapy response in gynecological cancer patients using FDG PET. *European Journal of Nuclear Medicine and Molecular Imaging*. February 2008;35(2):287–295.

138. Caobelli F, Alongi P, Evangelista L, et al. Predictive value of (18)F-FDG PET/CT in restaging patients affected by ovarian carcinoma: a multicentre study. *European Journal of Nuclear Medicine and Molecular Imaging*. March 2016;43(3):404–413.

139. Lee M, Lee H, Cheon GJ, et al. Prognostic value of preoperative intratumoral FDG uptake heterogeneity in patients with epithelial ovarian cancer. *European Radiology*. January 2017;27(1):16–23.

140. Kim CY, Jeong SY, Chong GO, et al. Quantitative metabolic parameters measured on F-18 FDG PET/CT predict survival after relapse in patients with relapsed epithelial ovarian cancer. *Gynecologic Oncology*. March 2015;136(3):498–504.

141. Chung HH, Kwon HW, Kang KW, et al. Preoperative [F] FDG PET/CT predicts recurrence in patients with epithelial ovarian cancer. *Journal of Gynecologic Oncology*. January 2012;23(1):28–34.

142. Evangelista L, Palma MD, Gregianin M, et al. Diagnostic and prognostic evaluation of fluorodeoxyglucose positron emission tomography/computed tomography and its correlation with serum cancer antigen-125 (CA125) in a large cohort of ovarian cancer patients. *Journal of the Turkish German Gynecological Association*. 2015;16(3):137–144.

143. Mangili G, Picchio M, Sironi S, et al. Integrated PET/ CT as a first-line re-staging modality in patients with suspected recurrence of ovarian cancer. *European Journal of Nuclear Medicine and Molecular Imaging*. May 2007;34(5):658–666.

144. Simcock B, Neesham D, Quinn M, Drummond E, Milner A, Hicks RJ. The impact of PET/CT in the management of recurrent ovarian cancer. *Gynecologic Oncology*. October 2006;103(1):271–276.

145. Takeuchi S, Lucchini M, Schmeler KM, et al. Utility of 18F-FDG PET/CT in follow-up of patients with low-grade serous carcinoma of the ovary. *Gynecologic Oncology*. April 2014;133(1):100–104.

CHAPTER 10

Prostate Cancer

MOHSEN BEHESHTI • HEIKO SCHÖDER • JOCHEN WALZ •
ALIREZA REZAEE • WERNER LANGSTEGER

BACKGROUND

General[1-3]

- Prostate cancer is the second most common malignancy among men.
- Prostate cancer is the sixth leading cause of cancer-related death worldwide.
- It is diagnosed in 30%–70% of autopsies in patients older than 60 years who died because of other causes.
- Metastatic disease as the initial presentation of prostate cancer declined from >70% to <30% after the global prostate-specific antigen (PSA) screening was started because of early detection of primary disease in the prostate gland.

Early Clinical Symptoms[4]

- There are no signs or symptoms in the early stages.
- In the advanced stages, symptoms include pelvic discomfort/pain, dysuria, nocturia, hematuria, and renal insufficiency caused by upper tract obstruction.
- Bone pain and skeletal-related events are seen in metastatic disease.

Primary Diagnostic Procedure[3]

- PSA testing
- Digital rectal examination
- Sonography
- Transrectal biopsy

Standard Treatment[5]

The standard treatment is usually considered for patients with life expectancy >10 years.

- Low-risk prostate cancer: active surveillance/watchful waiting, radical prostatectomy, radiation therapy, brachytherapy, focal therapy, clinical trials
- Intermediate-risk prostate cancer: radical prostatectomy, radiation therapy + short-term androgen deprivation therapy, brachytherapy, clinical trials
- High-risk prostate cancer: radical prostatectomy, radiation therapy + long-term androgen deprivation therapy, brachytherapy, clinical trials
- Metastatic disease: androgen deprivation therapy + chemotherapy, androgen deprivation therapy alone, management of metastasis, clinical trials

Prognostic Factors[6]

- Gleason score
- PSA
- Clinical and pathologic stage
- Surgical margins
- Tumor volume
- Gene profiles

Five-Year Survival[7]

- Local disease (cancer confined to prostate gland) ~100%
- Regional disease (cancer with local invasion/pelvic lymph node metastases) ~100%
- Distant disease (distant lymph node and organ involvement) ~28%

TUMOR CHARACTERISTICS AND TYPICAL BEHAVIOR

Histopathology[8,9]

- Adenocarcinoma >95%
- Others (mucinous/signet ring cell and adenoid cystic carcinomas, neuroendocrine tumors, large prostatic duct carcinoma, small-cell undifferentiated cancers) <5%

Cancer Distribution[10,11]

- Peripheral zone: 75%–85%
- Transitional zone: ≤25%
- Central zone: 1%

COMMON PATTERN OF SPREAD[10,11]

Lymph Nodes

- Regional pelvic lymph nodes
- Distant extrapelvic lymph nodes

Distant Metastasis

- Most common sites:
  - Bone (90%)
  - Lung (46%)
  - Liver (25%)
  - Pleura (21%)
  - Adrenal glands (13%)

TNM AND EAU TNM CLASSIFICATION[12,13]

TNM and European Association of Urology (EAU) TNM classifications are given in Tables 10.1 and 10.2.

TABLE 10.1 Prostate Cancer TNM Classification				
TNM	**T1**	**T2**	**T3**	**T4**
N0	I	II	III	IV
N1	IV	IV	IV	IV
M1	IV	IV	IV	IV

CLINICAL GUIDELINES FOR USING PET/CT[13–15]

Primary Staging

- PET/CT is not recommended by the EAU, European Society for Medical Oncology, and National Comprehensive Cancer Network (NCCN).

Recurrent Disease

- **EAU**: Choline PET/CT is not recommended in patients with biochemical recurrence and a PSA level <1 ng/mL (Table 10.3).
- **NCCN**: Choline PET/CT is indicated in the evaluation of patients with biochemical recurrence after radical prostatectomy or radiation therapy, as well as in the evaluation of distant metastases and workup of patients scheduled for local treatment.

EVIDENCE-BASED VIEWPOINTS

- To date, there is no role defined for PET/CT imaging for the primary diagnosis of prostate cancer.

TABLE 10.2 European Association of Urology Prostate Cancer TNM Classification		
CLINICAL STAGE		
Primary Tumor (T)	**Lymph Nodes (N)**	**Distant Metastasis (M)**
T1: Clinically inapparent tumor not palpable or visible by imaging, diagnosed by prostate-specific antigen or surgery for benign prostatic hyperplasia T2: Palpable tumor confined within prostate; tumors found in one (T2a-b) or both lobes (T2c) T3: Palpable tumor extends beyond the prostatic capsule (T3a) or into the seminal vesicles (T3b) T4: Palpable tumor fixed or invades adjacent structures other than seminal vesicles (e.g., bladder, rectum, levator muscles, and/or pelvic wall)	N0: No regional lymph node metastasis N1: Metastasis in regional lymph node(s)	M0: No distant metastasis M1: Distant metastasis
PATHOLOGIC STAGE		
Primary Tumor (T)	**Lymph Nodes (N)**	**Distant Metastasis (M)**
pT1: Diagnosed by surgery for benign prostatic hyperplasia <5% (pT1a) or >5% (pT1b) of tissue pT2: Tumor confined within prostate; tumors found in one (pT2a-b) or both lobes (pT2c) pT3: Tumor with extraprostatic extension (pT3a) or infiltration of the seminal vesicles (pT3b) pT4: Tumor extends into adjacent organs other than seminal vesicles (e.g., bladder, rectum, levator muscles, and/or pelvic wall)	pN0: No regional lymph node metastasis pN1: Metastasis in regional lymph node(s)	M0: No distant metastasis M1: Distant metastasis

TABLE 10.3
EAU Risk Groups for Biochemical Recurrence of Localised and Locally Advanced Prostate Cancer

	Low-risk	Intermediate-risk	High-risk	
Definition	PSA < 10 ng/mL and GS < 7 and cT1–2a	PSA 10–20 ng/mL or GS 7 or cT2b	PSA > 20 ng/mL or GS > 7 or cT2c	any PSA any GS cT3–4 or cN+
		Localised		Locally advanced

GS, Gleason score; PSA, prostate-specific antigen.
From Mottet N, Bellmunt J, Bolla M, et al. EAU-ESTRO-SIOG Guidelines on Prostate Cancer. *Eur Urol* 2017;71(4):618–629.

- Fludeoxyglucose (FDG) PET/CT is not useful in the evaluation of initial or early recurrent prostate cancer. However, FDG PET/CT provides prognostic value and may be beneficial for therapy monitoring in castrate-resistant metastatic disease with poorly differentiated tumor.[16–18]
- Radiopharmaceuticals such as [11]C- and ^{18}F-choline, as well as ^{11}C-acetate, seem to be promising in staging of high-risk prostate cancer.[19,20] PET/CT using [11]C- or ^{18}F-choline is an accurate modality for detecting lymph node and/or distant metastatic lesions in patients with biochemical relapse and PSA value >1 ng/mL.[21,22]
- [11]C- or ^{18}F-choline PET/CT showed a good performance in the therapy monitoring of patients with metastatic prostate cancer. Nevertheless, its value in the assessment of densely sclerotic lesions is under debate.
- ^{68}Ga-prostate-specific membrane antigen (PSMA) PET/CT is more sensitive than CT or MRI for the detection of metastatic disease in patients with intermediate- to high-risk prostate cancer, even at low serum PSA values. Thus, although current knowledge is still limited and derived mostly from retrospective series, ^{68}Ga-PSMA-based imaging holds great promise to improve prostate cancer management.[23]
- ^{18}F-NaF PET/CT is superior to conventional bone scintigraphy and provides excellent performance in the assessment of bone metastasis.

CLINICAL POINT OF VIEW

The following statements are of clinical relevance to define imaging of choice in the assessment of patients with prostate cancer:
- Critical assessment of available studies, their quality, the used reference test for validation of the results, and clinical meaning
- Detection of intraprostatic prostate cancer lesions for initial diagnosis

- Initial staging after the diagnosis to rule in or out lymph node or distant metastasis before treatment with curative intent
- Staging at the time point of biochemical recurrence to rule in or out local recurrence, regional recurrence to lymph nodes, or distant recurrence
- Detection of intraprostatic prostate cancer lesions when suspecting local recurrence after radiotherapy or ablative treatments
- Monitoring of treatment response in patients treated for metastatic prostate cancer
- Information about cancer size/volume
- Number of metastatic lesions
- Location/organ of metastatic lesion
- Quantification of tracer intensity
- Use of test in the correct clinical setting and when result will change treatment strategies
- Information about incidental findings and possible clinical meaning
- Comparison between tracers and critical assessment of differences
- Availability of tracers and their individual limitation

PITFALLS[24,25]
False Positive
- Inflammation and infections, such as prostatitis
- Benign conditions, such as prostatic hyperplasia (BPH)
- Reactive lymph nodes

False Negative
- Neuroendocrine neoplasia in the prostate (except for neuroendocrine tumor-specific tracers)
- Low metabolic cancer tissue
- Poorly differentiated cancer on non-FDG tracers
- Micrometastases in the locoregional lymph node
- Common false negative in all cancers: early-stage malignancy, small lesions (<8 mm)

DISCUSSION
Fludeoxyglucose PET/CT

As previously reviewed, the major guidelines do not support utilization of FDG PET/CT for the evaluation of prostate cancer. Although the vast majority of these tumors are adenocarcinomas, they usually exhibit a low level of glucose metabolism, which causes false-negative FDG PET. On the other hand, the kidneys excrete radioactive urine into the urinary bladder at the vicinity of the prostate gland, which may obscure potential FDG-avid primary or regional metastatic lesions. Another reason is false-positive images caused by inflammatory changes in the prostate gland, as well as a high uptake in benign prostatic hyperplasia (BPH).

Nonetheless, the poorly differentiated advanced cancers with high Gleason scores (≥ 8) could be FDG avid. Thus a high FDG uptake might be a prognostic factor in prostate cancer imaging.

Although FDG PET/CT is not recommended to be routinely used for the evaluation of prostate cancer, it may have a complementary role for the detection of nodal and soft tissue metastatic disease.[25] Also, it is revealed that the FDG uptake of malignant tumor diminishes with effective therapy corresponding to clinical parameters (e.g., serum PSA levels).[16]

[11]C-Acetate PET/CT

[11]C-acetate is one of the positron-emitting tracers that have been used for the evaluation of prostate cancer. Acetate is a precursor for lipid synthesis, a process that enhances within the cytoplasm of cancerous cells. However, because of overactivation of the β-oxidation pathway in prostate cancer cells, in contrast to most other malignancies, fatty acid metabolism is the dominant source of energy instead of glycolysis. The upregulation of the key enzyme "fatty acid synthase" results in the accumulation of this radiotracer in prostate malignant tissue.[25] ^{11}C-acetate is not excreted from the urinary tract, which allows better imaging of the pelvis compared with ^{18}F-labeled radiotracers. However, because of the short half-life (20 min), its production for routine clinical use needs an on-site cyclotron, which limits its commercial use.

In the detection of primary prostate cancer using ^{11}C-acetate PET/CT, a systematic review and meta-analysis from 23 studies showed a pooled sensitivity and specificity of 75.1% and 75.8%, respectively.[26] However, this agent may have a low sensitivity of only 38% in detecting pelvic lymph node metastases.[26] On the other hand, ^{11}C-acetate PET/CT seems to be promising in the early detection of bone metastases in prostate cancer with a sensitivity, specificity,

PPV, and NPV of 89.7%, 96.1%, 94.6%, and 92.2%, respectively.[27]

Furthermore, ^{11}C-acetate PET/CT showed promise in the detection and localization of prostate cancer recurrence, with a sensitivity and specificity of 86.6% and 65.8%, respectively, when a PSA level of greater than 1.24 ng/mL was used as the threshold for scanning.[28]

[18]F-Fluoromethylcholine and ^{11}C-Choline PET/CT

Choline is a chemical component of phosphatidylcholine, which is a phospholipid that is integrated in the cell membrane. Therefore, radiolabeled choline uptake may reflect accelerated cell membrane proliferation in cancer cells. One of the positron emitter radiopharmaceuticals is ^{18}F-fluoromethylcholine (FCH), which is physiologically excreted by the kidneys. Another member of this group is ^{11}C-choline, which is favorably less excreted in urine; however, the short half-life of ^{11}C limits its clinical use.[25]

FCH PET/CT is successfully used to guide prostate cancer biopsy and evaluate primary prostate cancer. The reported sensitivity and specificity for the detection of primary prostate cancer are diverse in the medical literature, ranging from 65% to 100% and from 45% to 90%, respectively.[20,25,29] Considering false-positive results with prostatitis, high-grade prostatic intraepithelial neoplasia, and BPH, the modality is not recommended by some investigators as the first-line diagnostic imaging of primary prostate cancer.[30]

A systematic review and meta-analysis assessed the role of radiolabeled choline PET/CT in prostate cancer. In staging cases, the authors reported a pooled sensitivity and specificity of 84% and 79% on a per-patient basis and 66% and 92% on a per-lesion basis, respectively. They also found a pooled sensitivity and specificity of 85% and 88%, respectively, in patients with biochemical recurrence after local treatment with curative intent.[31] The value of FCH PET/CT in recurrent disease was confirmed in a systematic review and meta-analysis of 29 studies with 2686 patients, with a pooled sensitivity and specificity of about 89%.[21] However, FCH PET/CT has its best performance (91% detection rate) in patients with both PSA level >2 ng/mL and Gleason score (GS) > 7, which may suggest a prognostic role for FCH PET/CT in this group of patients.[32] A limitation of choline PET in the setting of biochemical recurrence is the problem of low detection rates at the clinically relevant low PSA ranges (0.2 ng/mL) at the time of early recurrence. This is the time point when local or regional salvage treatments are most effective, but the choline PET is informative only in few of these patients.

In the evaluation of metastatic involvement of lymph nodes ≥ 0.5 cm in size, sensitivity, specificity,

NPV, and PPV were calculated as 66%, 96%, 92%, and 82% for FCH PET/CT, respectively. However, disregarding the lymph nodes' size, the sensitivity dropped to only 45%. This indicates that for the evaluation of small lymph nodes, FCH PET/CT is not sensitive enough and cannot replace lymph node dissection.[20]

The role of choline PET/CT in the evaluation of osseous metastatic disease from prostate cancer is well investigated in the medical literature. Choline PET/CT was found to be superior to both single-photon emission CT and conventional whole-body bone scintigraphy on a per-lesion basis in a comprehensive meta-analysis of 27 studies. However, MRI was the most sensitive modality (97%) on a per-patient basis.[33] In addition, FCH PET/CT was able to change management in 20% of high-risk patients.[20]

Choline PET/CT is also an effective technique in prostate cancer radiation therapy planning. It has the potential to accurately define the field of radiotherapy and guide external beam radiation to the FCH PET-positive lesions.[30,34-37]

In the last few years, clinical guidelines have tried to provide a statement regarding the role of choline PET/CT in the assessment of patients with prostate cancer.[13,15]

According to NCCN guidelines, choline PET is indicated in the evaluation of patients with biochemical recurrence after radical prostatectomy or radiation therapy, as well as in the evaluation of distant metastases and workup of patients scheduled for local treatment.

However, EAU guidelines do not recommend choline PET/CT for the initial staging of patients with prostate cancer independent of the risk for extraglandular metastases. Also, this test is not recommended for restaging of patients with biochemical recurrence after radical prostatectomy if PSA is <1 ng/mL or after radiation therapy.

68Ga-Prostate-Specific Membrane Antigen PET/CT

PSMA is a cell membrane protein with enzymatic activity that is highly expressed in prostate cancer cells but not on normal prostate tissue or benign lesions.[38] Accordingly, the 68Ga-PSMA probe has been developed, which proved to be promising in the assessment of patients with prostate cancer in preliminary investigations.

It is noteworthy that the detection rate of 68Ga-PSMA PET/CT may reach 100% even in patients with serum PSA levels >2.2 ng/mL. This rate is approximately 60% at PSA levels of <2.2 ng/mL.[39] In a study on 112 prostate segments with this modality to detect cancer, a sensitivity and specificity of 92%, and a PPV and NPV of 96% and 85%, were calculated, respectively.[40]

In spite of the high accuracy of 68Ga-PSMA PET/CT in detecting primary prostate tumor, controversial results have been reported concerning its value in detecting lymph node metastases. A retrospective study compared the results of 68Ga-PSMA PET/CT with postsurgical nodal pathology in patients with prostate cancer and calculated a sensitivity, specificity, NPV, and PPV of 33%, 100%, 69%, and 100%, respectively. The low sensitivity for nodal detection was most likely because of the small size of the included lymph nodes.[41] In contrast, an approximate sensitivity, specificity, NPV, and PPV of 94%, 99%, 100%, and 89%, respectively, have been reported for malignant pelvic lymph node detection in another study.[42] This difference may be related to the size of the metastatic lymph nodes in various studies. Given the fact that the tumor to background ratio increases over time in malignant lesions, a biphasic PET scan may help to more efficiently specify the pathologic lesions.[43]

In addition, 68Ga-PSMA PET/CT has been regarded by many investigators as a significant step forward for nodal and metastasis staging of patients with recurrent prostate cancer.[44]

Studies have reported that this modality is able to detect cancer lesions even in patients with serum PSA levels of as low as 0.5 ng/mL.[45-47]

In a large-cohort study of 319 patients with recurrent prostate cancer, PSMA PET/CT revealed a sensitivity, specificity, PPV, and NPV of approximately 77%, 100%, 100%, and 91%, respectively, on a lesion-based analysis. However, in patient-based analysis, the sensitivity reached 88%.[48]

Moreover, some studies addressed the substantial influence of 68Ga-PSMA PET/CT on patients' management, changing therapy in about 29%–54% of cases.[46-50]

Considering the high level of PSMA on metastatic lesions from prostate cancer, investigators tried to use radiolabeled PSMA for endoradiotherapeutic purposes. The efforts resulted in the production of 177Lu-PSMA for the treatment of patients with metastatic and castration-resistant prostate cancer. The first proof-of-concept human study introduced the pharmaceutical as an appropriate endoradiotherapeutic agent.[51]

Anti1-Amino-3-18F-Fluorocyclobutane-1-Carboxylic Acid PET/CT

18F-FACBC (anti1-amino-3-18F-fluorocyclobutane-1-carboxylic acid) is a novel synthetic amino acid analogue positron emitter with a relatively minimal urinary excretion, which was tested for the evaluation of recurrent prostate cancer. When compared with conventional CT, it is superior in diagnostic performance and differentiation of intraprostatic from extraprostatic relapse. This modality provided a sensitivity, specificity, NPV, PPV, and accuracy of approximately 89%, 56%, 69%, 82%, and 78%, respectively. The values for extra-prostatic recurrence were calculated as 46%, 100%, 52%, 100%, and 66%, respectively. Both sets of values are significantly higher than those of CT.[52] It is also superior to ^{11}C-choline PET/CT in patients with bio-chemical prostate cancer relapse after radical prostatec-tomy with better sensitivity (37% vs. 32%), specificity (67% vs. 40%), PPV (97% vs. 90%), and accuracy (38% vs. 32%).[53] However, more investigations are warranted to clarify its role in the evaluation of prostate cancer.

[18]F-Sodium Fluoride PET/CT

[99m]Tc-methylene diphosphonate (MDP) whole-body bone scan is a widely available and relatively inexpensive imaging method with reasonable sensitivity for detect-ing prostate cancer bone metastases. However, this test suffers from a relatively low specificity. ^{18}F-NaF as an old bone-seeking positron emitter has been reintroduced to PET clinics mainly because of its excellent performance and more availability of PET/CT scanners. The mecha-nism of action is not quite clear but is most likely by chemisorption to hydroxyapatite at the bone turnover site. Overall, it is indicated in the detection of primary and secondary bone cancers, therapy monitoring, and clarification of equivocal findings of other imaging tools, such as plain radiography or CT.[54] Review of correlated sensitivity and specificity of ^{18}F-NaF PET/CT in the medi-cal literature shows different results. Even-Sapir and col-leagues calculated a sensitivity and specificity of 100%,[55] whereas Poulsen and colleagues reported a high sensitiv-ity of 93% but surprisingly low specificity of only 54%, most likely because of a large number of false-positive lesions associated with degenerative or inflammatory changes in older patients.[56]

As mentioned earlier, ^{18}F-NaF PET/CT is capable of evaluating the response of osseous metastatic disease to therapy. However, nuclear physicians should be aware of the "flare phenomenon," which may resemble progressive disease with increasing intensity of lesions (and even appearance of new lesions), but is indeed a sign of favorable response, shortly after commence-ment of therapy.[57] For this reason, the prostate cancer working group recommends calling progression only after an increasing number of lesions is detected in at least two consecutive studies.[58]

[18]F-NaF PET/CT shows comparable accuracy with the aforementioned prostate-specific PET radiotracers; however, the latter may depict marrow-based metasta-ses earlier.[59]

TEACHING CASES
Case 1: FDG PET/CT—Staging
Findings

A 75-year-old male with high-risk prostate cancer, PSA = 8 ng/mL and GS = 10. FDG PET/CT shows tracer-avid cervical, mediastinal, and retroperitoneal lymph node metastases (Fig. 10.1).

Teaching points
- FDG PET/CT has limited sensitivity for the assess-ment of prostate cancer. However, it could be posi-tive in high-grade prostatic cancers. These patients have poorer prognosis compared with patients with FDG-negative malignancies.
- In patients with disseminated lymph node involve-ment, further evaluation should be performed to exclude lymphoma or sarcoidosis.

Case 2: ^{18}F-Choline PET/CT—Staging
Findings

A 78-year-old male with intermediate-risk prostate cancer, PSA = 3.9 ng/mL and GS = 7. ^{18}F-choline PET/CT shows tracer-avid primary tumor in the pros-tate gland with pelvic lymph node involvement (A–C, white arrow), as well as metastatic lesions in the left rib and left ischium (A–C, yellow arrow). Focal FDG uptake within the right pelvis (C, blue arrow) represents radioactive urine in the ureter (Fig. 10.2).

Teaching points
- ^{18}F-choline PET/CT may provide useful information in patients with intermediate- and high-risk prostate cancer.
- It can change the staging in 20% of high-risk patients, which causes alteration of management as well.
- The modality has limited sensitivity for the detec-tion of small lymph nodes (i.e., <5 mm in size).
- ^{18}F-choline PET/CT has limited value in differentiat-ing benign from malignant prostate lesions.

Pitfalls
- Correlation with CT and review of early dynamic scan may help in differentiating small lymph node from nonspecific tracer retention in the ureter.
- A heterogeneous uptake of tracer in bone marrow is physiologic and should not be interpreted as metastasis.
- Although chronic degenerative changes are nega-tive on ^{18}F-choline PET/CT, recent traumatic lesions could be positive and should not be interpreted as metastasis.

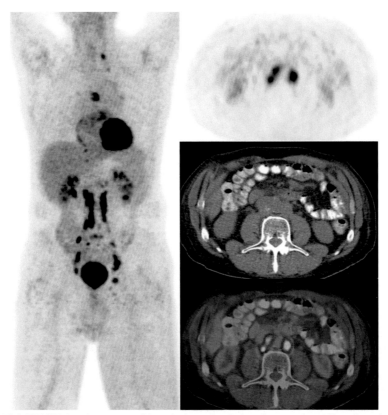

FIG. 10.1 FDG PET/CT showing tracer-avid cervical, mediastinal, and retroperitoneal lymph node metastases.

Case 3: ^{68}Ga-PSMA PET/CT—Staging

Findings

An 80-year-old male with high-risk prostate cancer, PSA = 55 ng/mL and GS = 9. ^{68}Ga-PSMA PET/CT shows tracer-avid primary prostate cancer (B, arrow) and multiple pelvic lymph nodes (C, white arrow), as well as a focal uptake in the left iliac bone (C, yellow arrow) and left supraclavicular lymph node (E, arrow). Of incidental note is a focal uptake in the right rib (D, arrow) (Fig. 10.3).

Teaching points

- Prostate malignancy could be differentiated on ^{68}Ga-PSMA PET/CT from benign prostatic hyperplasia or prostatitis because of PSMA overexpression on the malignant cells.
- ^{68}Ga-PSMA PET/CT could be used for guiding prostate biopsy.
- It is a highly sensitive modality with high resolution for the evaluation of small lymph nodes.
- Atypical lymph node metastasis (e.g., mediastinal and/or supraclavicular) without involvement of retroperitoneal lymph nodes could also happen.

Pitfalls

- Faint ^{68}Ga-PSMA uptake in the bone with no corresponding morphologic lesion on CT should be cautiously interpreted as metastatic disease. Correlation with other imaging modalities, particularly for solitary bone lesions, is strongly recommended.
- Recent rib fracture can take up ^{68}Ga-PSMA and should not be reported as metastatic disease.

Case 4: ^{18}F-Choline PET/CT—Biochemical Recurrence

Findings

A 78-year-old male with biochemical recurrence of intermediate-risk prostate cancer, initial PSA = 3.9 ng/mL and GS = 7, PSA at the time of recurrence = 4.7 ng/mL. ^{18}F-choline PET/CT shows a tracer-avid right pararectal lymph node (B, arrow) (Fig. 10.4).

Teaching points

- ^{18}F-choline PET/CT is approved as an accurate imaging method in the detection and localization of recurrent prostate cancer.

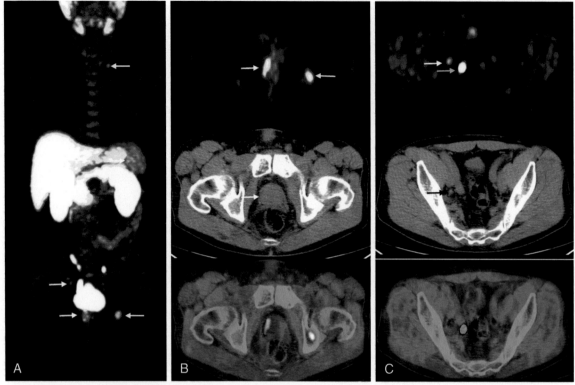

FIG. 10.2 ¹⁸F-choline PET/CT showing tracer-avid primary tumor in the prostate gland with pelvic lymph node involvement (A–C, *white arrows*) and metastatic lesions in the left rib and left ischium (A and B, *yellow arrow*). Focal FDG uptake within the right pelvis (C, *blue arrow*) represents radioactive urine in the ureter.

- There is significant correlation between the PSA value and ¹¹C- or ¹⁸F-choline PET positivity in biochemical recurrence.
- This modality is recommended for the evaluation of patients with recurrent prostate cancer and PSA level >1 ng/mL.
- Differentiation of local recurrence from distant metastases is of crucial clinical relevance for the defining of treatment approach.

Pitfalls
- Urinary excretion of radiotracer and intensive bowel activity may affect interpretation by obscuring small malignant lesions.

Case 5: ⁶⁸Ga-PSMA PET/CT — Biochemical Recurrence
Findings
A 63-year-old male with biochemical recurrence of high-risk prostate cancer, initial PSA = 10,2 ng/mL and

GS = 8, PSA at the time of recurrence = 0.33 ng/mL. ⁶⁸Ga-PSMA PET/CT shows focal uptake in the right prostate bed (B, arrow), suggestive of malignancy recurrence (Fig. 10.5).

Teaching points
- ⁶⁸Ga-PSMA PET/CT is a promising modality for the assessment of recurrent prostate cancer with excellent sensitivity and high tumor to background ratio.
- It provides useful information even at low PSA levels (i.e., <1 ng/mL).

Pitfalls
- Radioactive urine accumulation in the bladder may obscure small local recurrence. Thus, complementary delayed scans (i.e., after 90 to 120 min) may overcome this limitation.
- A faint tracer uptake may be seen in celiac and stellate ganglia, which should be considered as a nonspecific finding and not metastatic disease.

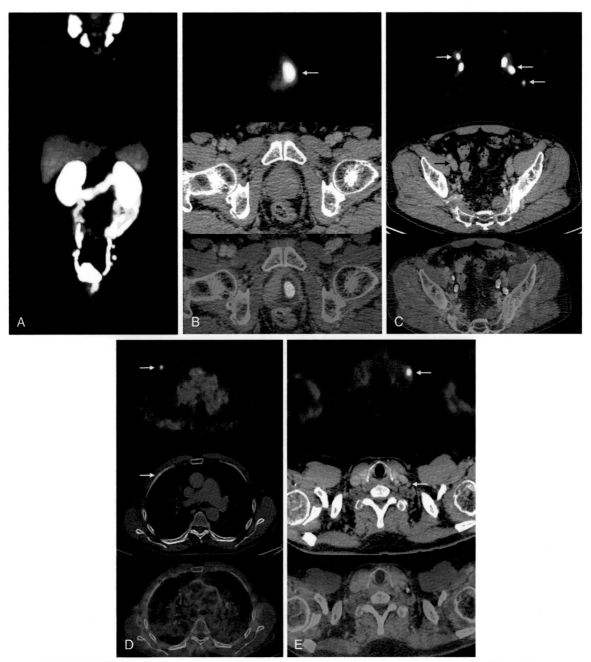

FIG. 10.3 ⁶⁸Ga-PSMA PET/CT showing tracer-avid primary prostate cancer (B, *arrow*) and multiple pelvic lymph nodes (C, *white arrows*), as well as a focal uptake in the left iliac bone (C, *yellow arrow*) and left supraclavicular lymph node (E, *arrows*). Of incidental note is a focal uptake in the right rib (D, *arrows*). A, ⁶⁸Ga-PSMA PET MIP image.

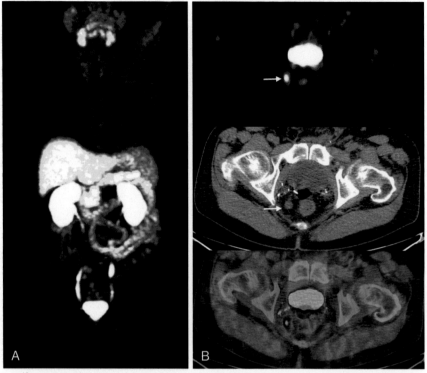

FIG. 10.4 ^{18}F-choline PET/CT showing a tracer-avid right pararectal lymph node (B, *arrows*). A, ^{18}F-choline PET MIP image.

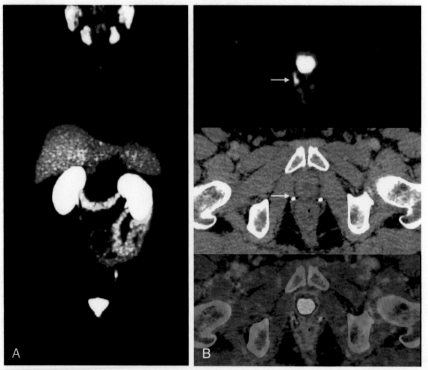

FIG. 10.5 ^{68}Ga-PSMA PET/CT showing focal uptake in the right prostate bed (B, *arrows*), suggestive of malignancy recurrence. A, ^{68}Ga-PSMA PET MIP image.

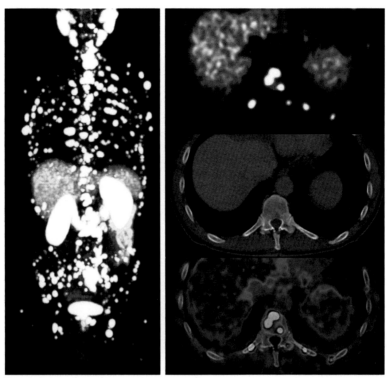

FIG. 10.6 ^{68}Ga-PSMA PET/CT showing generalized bone marrow metastases without significant CT correlation.

Case 6: ^{68}Ga-PSMA PET/CT, Extensive Recurrent Metastatic Disease

Findings

A 68-year-old male with biochemical recurrence of primary intermediate-risk prostate cancer, initial PSA = 10.6 ng/mL and GS = 7. ^{68}Ga-PSMA PET/CT shows generalized bone marrow metastases without significant CT correlation (Fig. 10.6).

Teaching points

- Functional imaging modalities, such as ^{68}Ga-PSMA and ^{18}F-choline PET/CT, are able to detect early bone marrow metastases before morphologic changes are evident.
- PET/CT is a feasible modality for examining the whole body in one acquisition.
- Specific targets, such as PSMA, can be used for both diagnostic and therapeutic (transonic) purposes.

Case 7: ^{18}F-Choline PET/CT—Therapy Monitoring

Findings

A 58-year-old male with high-risk prostate cancer, initial PSA = 18.2 ng/mL and GS = 9. ^{18}F-choline PET/CT shows tracer-avid bone metastases and cervical, mediastinal, and retroperitoneal lymph node involvement (A). A follow-up scan shows an excellent metabolic response to therapy (B) (Fig. 10.7).

Teaching points

- ^{18}F-choline PET/CT is a useful modality in the evaluation of therapy monitoring in patients with prostate cancer.
- It may have limited value in the assessment of therapy response in densely sclerotic bone metastases.
- If the uptake of ^{18}F-choline is negative in densely sclerotic lesions (i.e., Hounsfield unit >800), additional evaluation with a bone-seeking agent imaging (e.g., ^{18}F-NaF PET/CT) is recommended.

Pitfalls

- A focal increased tracer uptake in the colon should be further evaluated to exclude secondary malignancy.
- A mild to moderate increased ^{18}F-choline uptake is frequently seen in the hilar, axillary, and inguinal lymph nodes, which is most likely reactive in nature.

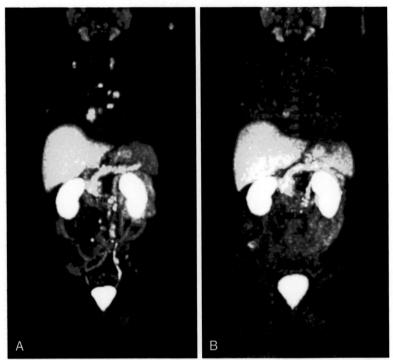

FIG. 10.7 ^18F-choline PET/CT showing tracer-avid bone metastases and cervical, mediastinal, and retro-peritoneal lymph node involvement (A). A follow-up scan shows an excellent metabolic response to therapy (B).

Case 8: Bone Metastases—Functional Versus Anatomic Imaging

Findings

An 85-year-old male with prostate cancer, PSA = 12.8 ng/mL, referred for imaging after therapy. Follow-up PET/CT imaging shows sclerotic lesions on CT, which are negative on ^18F-choline (A, arrow), positive on initial ^18F-NaF (B, arrow), and negative on posttherapy ^18F-NaF PET/CT (C, arrow) (Fig. 10.8).

Teaching points

- A small tumor volume and low perfusion may limit the accuracy of ^11C- and/or ^18F-choline PET/CT in the assessment of densely sclerotic lesions.
- Although CT shows stability or progression of disease, functional imaging proved nonviable sclerotic lesions (e.g., complete metabolic remission). It shows the superiority of functional over anatomic imaging in the assessment of prostate cancer.
- In the case of ^18F-choline-negative sclerotic lesions, further evaluation with a bone-seeking agent imaging (e.g., ^18F-NaF PET/CT) is recommended.

Case 9: ^18F-Choline PET/CT—Treatment Monitoring, Flip-Flop Phenomenon

Findings

An 81-year-old male with intermediate-risk prostate cancer, initial PSA = 11.7 ng/mL and GS = 7. Follow-up ^18F-choline PET/CT shows progressive disease (B). CT demonstrates progression of sclerotic lesion in the thoracic vertebral body (C,D; arrow); however, correlated ^18F-choline PET shows complete resolution of ^18F-choline uptake, representing an excellent metabolic response to therapy. There is a new tracer-avid lesion at the vicinity of old metastasis (D, arrow), with no corresponding morphologic changes on CT, which represents a progressive disease most likely because of new bone marrow involvement (Fig. 10.9).

Teaching points

- Functional imaging is superior to morphologic imaging for the evaluation of response to therapy and early detection of bone marrow involvement.

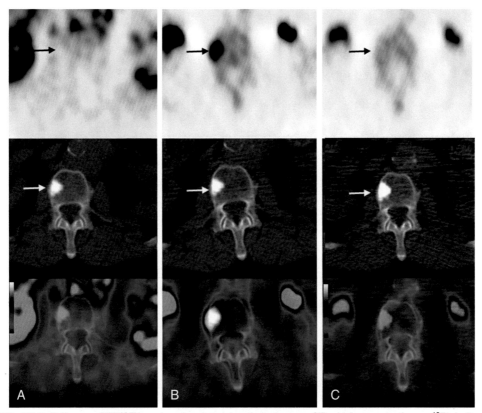

FIG. 10.8 Follow-up PET/CT imaging showing sclerotic lesions on CT, which are negative on ^{18}F-choline (A, *arrows*), positive on initial ^{18}F-NaF (B, *arrows*), and negative on posttherapy ^{18}F-NaF PET/CT (C, *arrows*).

Pitfalls
- Tracer uptake in the vein of injection is a benign finding (B).
- A mild diffuse faint uptake of ^{18}F-choline in the thyroid gland could be suggestive of thyropathy. However, the focal uptakes should be further clarified.
- An intense uptake of ^{18}F-choline in the salivary glands is physiologic.

Case 10: ^{68}Ga-PSMA PET/CT—Metastatic Bone Disease
Findings
A 70-year-old male with primary low-risk prostate cancer, initial PSA = 9.2 ng/mL and GS = 5. ^{68}Ga-PSMA PET/CT shows disseminated tracer-avid bone metastases (A) with an excellent response to therapy (B) (Fig. 10.10).

Teaching points
- In spite of a constant or progressive pattern of bone metastases on CT, complete remission is evident by metabolic imaging using ^{68}Ga-PSMA, which

emphasizes again on the value of functional imaging for the evaluation of response to therapy.

Pitfalls
- A focal uptake from radioactive urine in the ureter should not be interpreted as metastatic disease (A,B; arrow).

Case 11: ^{18}F-Choline Versus ^{68}Ga-PSMA PET/CT—Therapy Monitoring
Findings
A 59-year-old male with biochemical recurrence of high-risk prostate cancer, initial PSA = 43 ng/mL, GS = 9; PSA level at the time of recurrence = 38 ng/mL, 4 months after androgen deprivation therapy. ^{18}F-choline PET/CT shows an excellent response of thoracic and lumbar sclerotic metastatic bone disease to therapy (A,B). The finding is concordant with markedly diminished serum PSA levels. ^{68}Ga-PSMA PET/CT shows tracer uptake in the sclerotic metastatic lesion within the lumbar vertebral body,

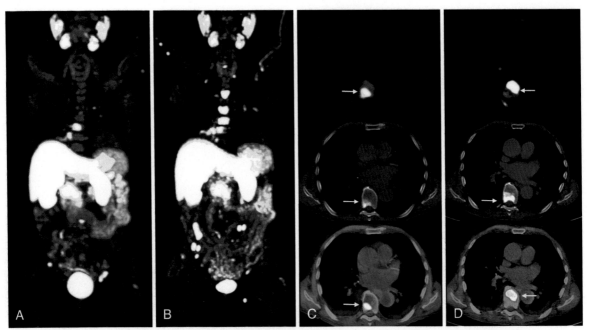

FIG. 10.9 Follow-up ¹⁸F-choline PET/CT showing progressive disease (B). CT demonstrates progression of sclerotic lesion in the thoracic vertebral body (C,D; *arrow*); however, correlated ¹⁸F-choline PET shows complete resolution of ¹⁸F-choline uptake, representing an excellent metabolic response to therapy. There is a new tracer-avid lesion at the vicinity of old metastasis (D, *arrow*) with no corresponding morphologic changes on CT, which represents a progressive disease most likely caused by new bone marrow involvement. A, ¹⁸F-choline PET MIP image.

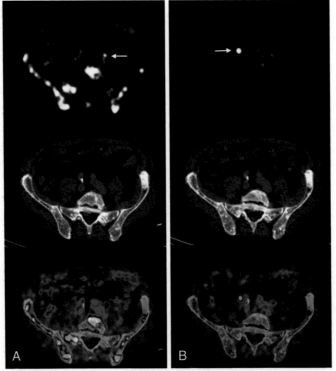

FIG. 10.10 ⁶⁸Ga-PSMA PET/CT showing disseminated tracer-avid bone metastases (A) with an excellent response to therapy (B). Focal uptake from radioactive urine in the ureter should not be interpreted as metastatic disease (A and B, *arrow*).

but no uptake in thoracic spine osseous metastasis. Although the rib lesion (D, yellow arrow) is resolved on follow-up ^{18}F-choline PET/CT (E, yellow arrow), it is still tracer avid on ^{68}Ga-PSMA PET/CT (F, yellow arrow). Increased sclerosis in the thoracic vertebral lesion (D–F, white arrow) is consistent with favorable response to therapy (Fig. 10.11).

Teaching points

- ^{68}Ga-PSMA seems to be superior to ^{18}F-choline PET/CT for the evaluation of metastatic prostate cancer to skeleton and lymph nodes.
- Metastases can have characteristics different from those of the primary tumor, with a different pattern of response to therapy.
- PET/CT using different specific tracers may provide the most accurate statement regarding response to therapy.

Pitfalls

- ^{68}Ga-PSMA uptake in cervicothoracic ganglia is a nonspecific finding.

Case 12: ^{18}F-Choline Versus ^{68}Ga-PSMA PET/CT—Staging
Findings

A 69-year-old male with high-risk prostate cancer, PSA = 25 ng/mL and GS = 8. Although ^{18}F-choline PET/CT shows a faint uptake by the primary tumor and multiple abdominal lymph nodes, they are intensely ^{68}Ga-PSMA avid (Fig. 10.12).

Teaching points

- ^{68}Ga-PSMA provides excellent tumor to background resolution and is superior to ^{18}F-choline PET/CT for N-staging of prostate cancer.
- The detection rate of ^{68}Ga-PSMA PET/CT may reach 100% even in patients with serum PSA levels <2.2 ng/mL.

Case 13: ^{68}Ga-PSMA Versus ^{18}F-Choline PET/CT—Restaging
Findings

A 61-year-old male with biochemical recurrence of primary high-risk prostate cancer, initial PSA = 11.8 ng/mL and GS = 9. Multiple tracer-avid pelvic lymph node metastases are evident on both imaging modalities (A,B; arrows); however, ^{68}Ga-PSMA PET/CT is more sensitive particularly in the detection of small lymph node metastases. CT shows a small sclerotic lesion within the T6 vertebral body, which is positive on ^{18}F-choline (C, arrow) but negative on ^{68}Ga-PSMA PET (D, arrow) (Fig. 10.13).

Teaching points

- ^{68}Ga-PSMA is more sensitive than ^{18}F-choline for the detection of small lymph node metastases.
- The value of ^{68}Ga-PSMA in the detection of bone metastasis should be further evaluated because osseous metastatic lesions may show different characteristics.

Pitfalls

- In obese patients, ^{68}Ga-PSMA PET images may be heterogeneous, which could cause false-positive reports.

Case 14: ^{18}F-Choline Versus ^{18}F-NaF PET/CT—Bone Metastases
Findings

A 58-year-old male with metastatic high-risk prostate cancer to skeleton, initial PSA = 3.8 ng/mL and GS = 8. A focal bone marrow involvement is positive in T12 on ^{18}F-choline (D, red arrow) but negative on ^{18}F-NaF PET/CT (C, red arrow). Bone metastases in L2 and sacrum are positive on both ^{18}F-NaF and ^{18}F-choline PET/CT (A,B; black arrow). Degenerative lesion is positive on ^{18}F-NaF (A, blue arrow) but negative on ^{18}F-choline PET/CT (B) (Fig. 10.14).

Teaching points

- Chronic degenerative changes in the skeleton do not take up ^{18}F-choline.
- ^{18}F-choline PET/CT shows a comparable sensitivity but significantly higher specificity in the detection of bone metastases compared with ^{18}F-NaF PET/CT.
- ^{18}F-choline PET/CT was found to be superior in the early detection of osseous metastases to PET/CT studies with bone-seeking agents.

Pitfalls

- Degenerative changes are an important source of false-positive reports for ^{18}F-NaF PET/CT. Correlation with morphologic changes on CT improves the specificity of this modality.
- An asymmetric pattern of choline uptake in the submandibular salivary glands is most likely functional in origin (e.g., unilateral hypogenesis or agenesis).

Case 15: ^{18}F-NaF PET/CT Versus ^{68}Ga-PSMA—Bone Metastases
Findings

An 81-year-old male with primary intermediate-risk prostate cancer, initial PSA = 12 ng/mL and GS = 7. ^{68}Ga-PSMA detects more lesions (B) than ^{18}F-NaF PET/CT (A), which is most likely because of prominent marrow compared with cortical involvement (Fig. 10.15).

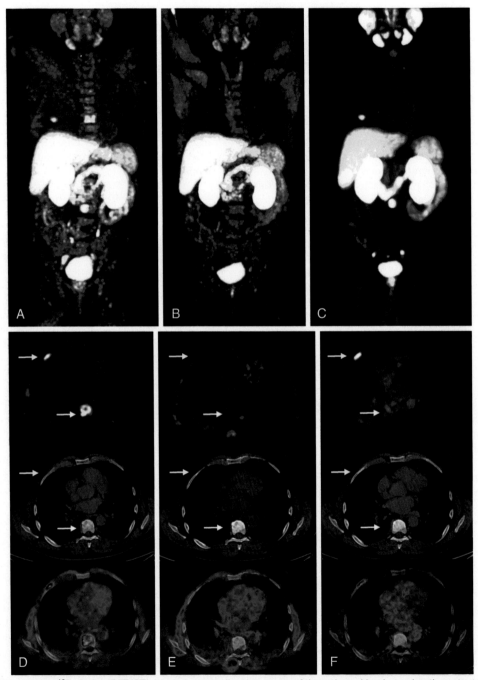

FIG. 10.11 ^{18}F-choline PET/CT showing an excellent response of thoracic and lumbar sclerotic metastatic bone disease to therapy (A,B). ^{68}Ga-PSMA PET/CT shows tracer uptake in the sclerotic metastatic lesion within the lumbar vertebral body but no uptake in thoracic spine osseous metastasis (C). Although the rib lesion (D, *yellow arrows*) is resolved on follow-up ^{18}F-choline PET/CT (E, *yellow arrows*), it is still tracer avid on ^{68}Ga-PSMA PET/CT (F, *yellow arrows*). Increased sclerosis in the thoracic vertebral lesion (D–F, *white arrows*) is consistent with a favorable response to therapy.

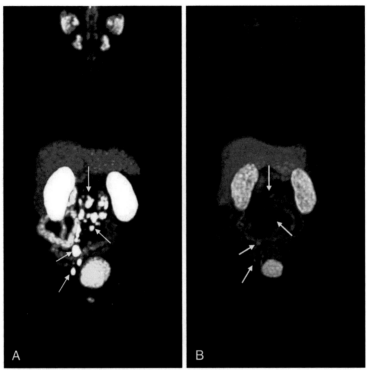

FIG. 10.12 Although 18F-choline PET/CT shows a faint uptake by the primary tumor and multiple abdominal lymph nodes (B, *arrows*), they are intensely 68Ga-PSMA avid (A, *arrows*).

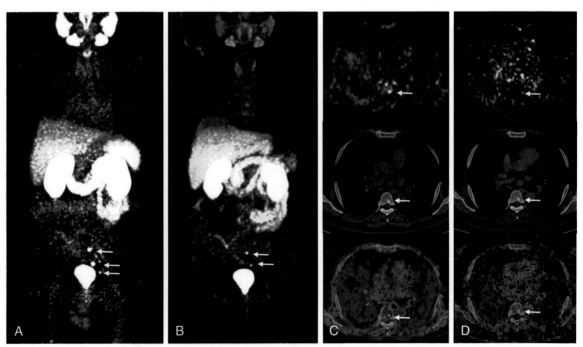

FIG. 10.13 Multiple tracer-avid pelvic lymph node metastases are evident on both imaging modalities (A,B; *arrows*); however, 68Ga-PSMA PET/CT is more sensitive particularly in the detection of small lymph node metastases. CT shows a small sclerotic lesion within the T6 vertebral body, which is positive on 18F-choline (C, *arrows*) but negative on 68Ga-PSMA PET (D, *arrows*).

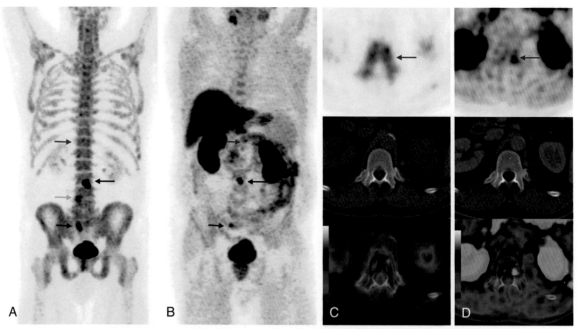

FIG. 10.14 A focal bone marrow involvement is positive in T12 on ¹⁸F-choline (D, *red arrows*) but negative on ¹⁸F-NaF PET/CT (C, *red arrows*). Bone metastases in L2 and sacrum are positive on both ¹⁸F-NaF
and ¹⁸F-choline PET/CT (A,B; *black arrows*). Degenerative lesion is positive on ¹⁸F-NaF (A, *blue arrow*) but
negative on ¹⁸F-choline PET/CT (B).

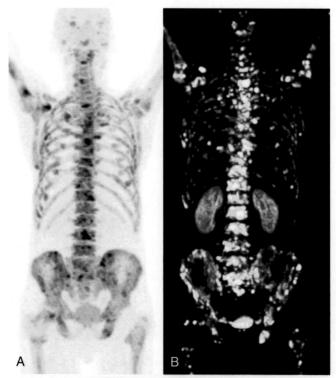

FIG. 10.15 ⁶⁸Ga-PSMA detects more lesions (B) than ¹⁸F-NaF PET/CT (A), which is most likely because
of prominent marrow compared with cortical involvement.

Teaching points
- ^{68}Ga-PSMA PET/CT seems to be superior to ^{18}F-NaF PET/CT, with a higher sensitivity for the early detection of bone marrow–based metastatic lesions.

Pitfalls
- Early bone marrow involvement could be missed on ^{18}F-NaF PET/CT as a false-negative lesion.

REFERENCES

1. Center MM, Jemal A, Lortet-Tieulent J, et al. International variation in prostate cancer incidence and mortality rates. *European Urology.* 2012;61(6):1079–1092.
2. Ferlay J, Shin HR, Bray F, Forman D, Mathers C, Parkin DM. Estimates of worldwide burden of cancer in 2008: GLOBOCAN 2008. *International Journal of Cancer.* 2010;127(12):2893–2917.
3. Welch HG, Gorski DH, Albertsen PC. Trends in metastatic breast and prostate cancer–lessons in cancer dynamics. *The New England Journal of Medicine.* 2015;373(18): 1685–1687.
4. Collin SM, Metcalfe C, Donovan JL, et al. Associations of sexual dysfunction symptoms with PSA-detected localised and advanced prostate cancer: a case-control study nested within the UK population-based ProtecT (prostate testing for cancer and treatment) study. *European Journal of Cancer.* 2009;45(18):3254–3261.
5. American Cancer Society. Initial Treatment of Prostate Cancer, by Stage. http://www.cancer.org/cancer/prostate-cancer/detailedguide/prostate-cancer-treating-by-stage.
6. Buhmeida A, Pyrhonen S, Laato M, Collan Y. Prognostic factors in prostate cancer. *Diagnostic Pathology.* 2006;1:4.
7. American Cancer Society. Survival Rates for Prostate Cancer. http://www.cancer.org/cancer/prostatecancer/detailed guide/prostate-cancer-survival-rates.
8. Bostwick DG. The pathology of early prostate cancer. *CA: A Cancer Journal for Clinicians.* 1989;39(6):376–393.
9. McWilliam LJ, Manson C, George NJ. Neuroendocrine differentiation and prognosis in prostatic adenocarcinoma. *British Journal of Urology.* 1997;80(2):287–290.
10. Akin O, Sala E, Moskowitz CS, et al. Transition zone prostate cancers: features, detection, localization, and staging at endorectal MR imaging. *Radiology.* 2006;239(3):784–792.
11. Bubendorf L, Schopfer A, Wagner U, et al. Metastatic patterns of prostate cancer: an autopsy study of 1,589 patients. *Human Pathology.* 2000;31(5):578–583.
12. AJCC Prostate Cancer TNM Staging. 7th ed. American Cancer Society; 2009.
13. Mottet N, Bellmunt J, Briers E, et al. EAU guidelines on prostate cancer. *European Association of Urology.* 2015.
14. Parker C, Gillessen S, Heidenreich A, Horwich A, Committee EG. Cancer of the prostate: ESMO clinical practice guidelines for diagnosis, treatment and follow-up. *Annals of Oncology: Official Journal of the European Society for Medical Oncology.* 2015;26(suppl 5):v69–77.
15. Feinstein AR, Arevalo AC. Manifestations and treatment of congestive heart failure in young patients with rheumatic heart disease. *Pediatrics.* 1964;33:661–671.
16. Jadvar H. FDG PET in prostate cancer. *PET Clinics.* 2009;4(2):155–161.
17. Morris MJ, Akhurst T, Larson SM, et al. Fluorodeoxyglucose positron emission tomography as an outcome measure for castrate metastatic prostate cancer treated with antimicrotubule chemotherapy. *Clinical Cancer Research.* 2005;11(9):3210–3216.
18. Meirelles GS, Schoder H, Ravizzini GC, et al. Prognostic value of baseline [18F] fluorodeoxyglucose positron emission tomography and 99mTc-MDP bone scan in progressing metastatic prostate cancer. *Clinical Cancer Research.* 2010;16(24):6093–6099.
19. Kelloff GJ, Choyke P, Coffey DS. Prostate Cancer Imaging Working Group. Challenges in clinical prostate cancer: role of imaging. *American Journal of Roentgenology.* 2009;192(6):1455–1470.
20. Beheshti M, Imamovic L, Broinger G, et al. 18F choline PET/CT in the preoperative staging of prostate cancer in patients with intermediate or high risk of extracapsular disease: a prospective study of 130 patients. *Radiology.* 2010;254(3):925–933.
21. Fanti S, Minozzi S, Castellucci P, et al. PET/CT with (11) C-choline for evaluation of prostate cancer patients with biochemical recurrence: meta-analysis and critical review of available data. *European Journal of Nuclear Medicine and Molecular Imaging.* 2016;43(1):55–69.
22. Beheshti M, Haim S, Zakavi R, et al. Impact of 18F-choline PET/CT in prostate cancer patients with biochemical recurrence: influence of androgen deprivation therapy and correlation with PSA kinetics. *Journal of Nuclear Medicine: Official Publication, Society of Nuclear Medicine.* 2013;54(6):833–840.
23. Maurer T, Eiber M, Schwaiger M, Gschwend JE. Current use of PSMA-PET in prostate cancer management. *Nature Reviews Urology.* 2016;13(4):226–235.
24. Haroon A, Zanoni L, Celli M, et al. Multicenter study evaluating extraprostatic uptake of 11C-choline, 18F-methylcholine, and 18F-ethylcholine in male patients: physiological distribution, statistical differences, imaging pearls, and normal variants. *Nuclear Medicine Communications.* 2015;36(11):1065–1075.
25. Jadvar H. Prostate cancer: PET with 18F-FDG, 18F- or 11C-acetate, and 18F- or 11C-choline. *Journal of Nuclear Medicine: Official Publication, Society of Nuclear Medicine.* 2011;52(1):81–89.
26. Mohsen B, Giorgio T, Rasoul ZS, et al. Application of C-11-acetate positron-emission tomography (PET) imaging in prostate cancer: systematic review and meta-analysis of the literature. *BJU International.* 2013;112(8): 1062–1072.
27. Spick C, Polanec SH, Mitterhauser M, et al. Detection of bone metastases using 11C-Acetate PET in patients with prostate cancer with biochemical recurrence. *Anticancer Research.* 2015;35(12):6787–6791.

28. Dusing RW, Peng W, Lai SM, et al. Prostate-specific antigen and prostate-specific antigen velocity as threshold indicators in 11C-acetate PET/CTAC scanning for prostate cancer recurrence. *Clinical Nuclear Medicine.* 2014;39(9): 777–783.

29. Vali R, Loidl W, Pirich C, Langesteger W, Beheshti M. Imaging of prostate cancer with PET/CT using (18)F-fluorocholine. *American Journal of Nuclear Medicine and Molecular Imaging.* 2015;5(2):96–108.

30. Schwarzenbock SM, Kurth J, Gocke C, Kuhnt T, Hildebrandt G, Krause BJ. Role of choline PET/CT in guiding target volume delineation for irradiation of prostate cancer. *European Journal of Nuclear Medicine and Molecular Imaging.* 2013;40(suppl 1):S28–S35.

31. Umbehr MH, Muntener M, Hany T, Sulser T, Bachmann LM. The role of 11C-choline and 18F-fluorocholine positron emission tomography (PET) and PET/CT in prostate cancer: a systematic review and meta-analysis. *European Urology.* 2013;64(1):106–117.

32. Cimitan M, Evangelista L, Hodolic M, et al. Gleason score at diagnosis predicts the rate of detection of 18F-choline PET/CT performed when biochemical evidence indicates recurrence of prostate cancer: experience with 1,000 patients. *Journal of Nuclear Medicine: Official publication, Society of Nuclear Medicine.* 2015;56(2):209–215.

33. Shen G, Deng H, Hu S, Jia Z. Comparison of choline-PET/CT, MRI, SPECT, and bone scintigraphy in the diagnosis of bone metastases in patients with prostate cancer: a meta-analysis. *Skeletal Radiology.* 2014;43(11):1503–1513.

34. Garcia JR, Cozar M, Soler M, Bassa P, Riera E, Ferrer J. Salvage radiotherapy in prostate cancer patients. Planning, treatment response and prognosis using C-choline PET/CT. *Revista espanola de medicina nuclear e imagen molecular.* 2016;35(4):238–245.

35. Alongi F, Fersino S, Giaj Levra N, et al. Impact of 18F-choline PET/CT in the decision-making strategy of treatment volumes in definitive prostate cancer volumetric modulated radiation therapy. *Clinical Nuclear Medicine.* 2015;40(11):e496–500.

36. Lopez E, Lazo A, Gutierrez A, Arregui G, Nunez I, Sacchetti A. Influence of (11)C-choline PET/CT on radiotherapy planning in prostate cancer. *Reports of Practical Oncology and Radiotherapy: Journal of Greatpoland Cancer Center in Poznan and Polish Society of Radiation Oncology.* 2015;20(2): 104–112.

37. Wurschmidt F, Petersen C, Wahl A, Dahle J, Kretschmer M. [18F]fluoroethylcholine-PET/CT imaging for radiation treatment planning of recurrent and primary prostate cancer with dose escalation to PET/CT-positive lymph nodes. *Radiation Oncology.* 2011;6:44.

38. Chang SS. Overview of prostate-specific membrane antigen. *Reviews in Urology.* 2004;6(suppl 10):S13–S18.

39. Afshar-Oromieh A, Malcher A, Eder M, et al. PET imaging with a [68Ga]gallium-labelled PSMA ligand for the diagnosis of prostate cancer: biodistribution in humans and first evaluation of tumour lesions. *European Journal of Nuclear Medicine and Molecular Imaging.* 2013;40(4):486–495.

40. Rahbar K, Weckesser M, Huss S, et al. Correlation of intraprostatic tumor extent with 68Ga-PSMA distribution in patients with prostate cancer. *Journal of Nuclear Medicine: Official Publication, Society of Nuclear Medicine.* 2016;57(4):563–567.

41. Budaus L, Leyh-Bannurah SR, Salomon G, et al. Initial experience of (68)Ga-PSMA PET/CT imaging in high-risk prostate cancer patients prior to radical prostatectomy. *European Urology.* 2016;69(3):393–396.

42. Hijazi S, Meller B, Leitsmann C, et al. Pelvic lymph node dissection for nodal oligometastatic prostate cancer detected by 68Ga-PSMA-positron emission tomography/computerized tomography. *The Prostate.* 2015;75(16): 1934–1940.

43. Sahlmann CO, Meller B, Bouter C, et al. Biphasic (68) Ga-PSMA-HBED-CC-PET/CT in patients with recurrent and high-risk prostate carcinoma. *European Journal of Nuclear Medicine and Molecular Imaging.* 2016;43(5): 898–905.

44. Ceci F, Uprimny C, Nilica B, et al. (68)Ga-PSMA PET/CT for restaging recurrent prostate cancer: which factors are associated with PET/CT detection rate? *European Journal of Nuclear Medicine and Molecular Imaging.* 2015;42(8):1284–1294.

45. Verburg FA, Pfister D, Heidenreich A, et al. Extent of disease in recurrent prostate cancer determined by [(68)Ga] PSMA-HBED-CC PET/CT in relation to PSA levels, PSA doubling time and Gleason score. *European Journal of Nuclear Medicine and Molecular Imaging.* 2016;43(3):397–403.

46. van Leeuwen PJ, Stricker P, Hruby G, et al. (68) Ga-PSMA has a high detection rate of prostate cancer recurrence outside the prostatic fossa in patients being considered for salvage radiation treatment. *BJU International.* 2016;117(5):732–739.

47. Eiber M, Maurer T, Souvatzoglou M, et al. Evaluation of Hybrid (6)(8)Ga-PSMA ligand PET/CT in 248 patients with biochemical recurrence after radical prostatectomy. *Journal of Nuclear Medicine: Official Publication, Society of Nuclear Medicine.* 2015;56(5):668–674.

48. Afshar-Oromieh A, Avtzi E, Giesel FL, et al. The diagnostic value of PET/CT imaging with the (68)Ga-labelled PSMA ligand HBED-CC in the diagnosis of recurrent prostate cancer. *European Journal of Nuclear Medicine and Molecular Imaging.* 2015;42(2):197–209.

49. Sterzing F, Kratochwil C, Fiedler H, et al. (68)Ga-PSMA-11 PET/CT: a new technique with high potential for the radiotherapeutic management of prostate cancer patients. *European Journal of Nuclear Medicine and Molecular Imaging.* 2016;43(1):34–41.

50. Morigi JJ, Stricker PD, van Leeuwen PJ, et al. Prospective comparison of 18F-fluoromethylcholine versus 68Ga-PSMA PET/CT in prostate cancer patients who have rising PSA after curative treatment and are being considered for targeted therapy. *Journal of Nuclear Medicine: Official Publication, Society of Nuclear Medicine.* 2015;56(8):1185–1190.

51. Weineisen M, Schottelius M, Simecek J, et al. 68Ga- and 177Lu-Labeled PSMA I&T: optimization of a PSMA-targeted theranostic concept and first proof-of-concept human studies. *Journal of Nuclear Medicine: Official Publication, Society of Nuclear Medicine.* 2015;56(8):1169–1176.

52. Odewole OA, Tade FI, Nieh PT, et al. Recurrent prostate cancer detection with anti-3-[F]FACBC PET/CT: comparison with CT. *European Journal of Nuclear Medicine and Molecular Imaging.* 2016;43(10):1173–1783.

53. Nanni C, Zanoni L, Pultrone C, et al. F-FACBC (anti1-amino-3-F-fluorocyclobutane-1-carboxylic acid) versus C-choline PET/CT in prostate cancer relapse: results of a prospective trial. *European Journal of Nuclear Medicine and Molecular Imaging.* 2016;43(9):1601–1610.

54. Bastawrous S, Bhargava P, Behnia F, Djang DS, Haseley DR. Newer PET application with an old tracer: role of 18F-NaF skeletal PET/CT in oncologic practice. *Radiographics: A Review Publication of the Radiological Society of North America, Inc.* 2014;34(5):1295–1316.

55. Even-Sapir E, Metser U, Mishani E, Lievshitz G, Lerman H, Leibovitch I. The detection of bone metastases in patients with high-risk prostate cancer: 99mTc-MDP Planar bone scintigraphy, single- and multi-field-of-view SPECT, 18F-fluoride PET, and 18F-fluoride PET/CT. *Journal of Nuclear Medicine: Official Publication, Society of Nuclear Medicine.* 2006;47(2):287–297.

56. Poulsen MH, Petersen H, Hoilund-Carlsen PF, et al. Spine metastases in prostate cancer: comparison of technetium-99m-MDP whole-body bone scintigraphy, [(18) F] choline positron emission tomography(PET)/computed tomography (CT) and [(18) F]NaF PET/CT. *BJU International.* 2014;114(6):818–823.

57. Wade AA, Scott JA, Kuter I, Fischman AJ. Flare response in 18F-fluoride ion PET bone scanning. *American Journal of Roentgenology.* 2006;186(6):1783–1786.

58. Scher HI, Morris MJ, Stadler WM, et al. Trial design and objectives for castration-resistant prostate cancer: updated recommendations from the Prostate Cancer Clinical Trials Working Group 3. *Journal of Clinical Oncology.* 2016;34(12):1402–1418.

59. Beheshti M, Vali R, Waldenberger P, et al. Detection of bone metastases in patients with prostate cancer by 18F fluorocholine and 18F fluoride PET-CT: a comparative study. *European Journal of Nuclear Medicine and Molecular Imaging.* 2008;35(10):1766–1774.

CHAPTER 11

Melanoma

ALIREZA REZAEE • ANDREAS BUCK • NIKLAUS SCHÄFER •
WERNER LANGSTEGER • MOHSEN BEHESHTI

BACKGROUND

General[1–3]

- Melanoma constitutes less than 2% of all skin cancer cases but is the most common leading cause of death from skin malignancies.
- It is the fifth and sixth most common cancer in Northern America among females and males.
- The most common site of involvement is the back in males and legs in females.
- There has been a rapid increase in the incidence rate in the last three decades.
- The incidence rate is higher in females before the age of 50 years but is twice and triple in males by the age of 65 and 80 years, respectively.
- Metastatic disease is the first presentation in 4% of newly diagnosed patients.

Early Clinical Symptoms[1–3]

- Mole-like lesion on the skin, growing in size with possible color change
- Nonhealing cutaneous sore lesion
- **ABCD** alarm signs: **A**symmetry, irregular **B**order, change in **C**olor, **D**iameter of >6 mm

Primary Diagnostic Procedure[1–3]

- Regular physical examination of the skin
- Biopsy of suspicious lesions
- Mutational analysis (BRAF, NRAS/C-KIT if BRAF wild type)

Standard Treatments[4–7]

- Full-thickness excisional biopsy to determine histology and Breslow thickness
- Wide excision (0.5 cm) for in situ melanoma, 1 cm for Breslow 2 mm, 2 cm for Breslow >2 mm
- Sentinel node for Breslow >1 mm (>0.75 mm if risk factors are present)
- Interferon adjuvant treatment (if micrometastases are present in the sentinel node)
- Chemotherapy and immunotherapy in cases of unresectable locoregional disease or systemic disease
- Tyrosine kinase inhibitors according to mutation analysis/checkpoint inhibitors
- Radiation therapy

Treatment Approach Based on Disease Stage

- Stage IA/B: Surgical resection of tumor (stage IB, if T1b > 0.75 mm, consider sentinel node)
- Stage IIA: Surgical resection of tumor (consider sentinel node)
- Stage IIB/C: Surgical resection of tumor (+sentinel node, ±adjuvant treatment)
- Stage IIIA/B/C: Surgical resection of tumor and involved lymph nodes (if feasible) + adjuvant therapy (also consider local radiation therapy to lymph node)
- Stage IV (or nonresectable stage III): Consider surgical resection of tumor and involved lymph nodes if needed, targeted therapy according to mutation analysis, checkpoint inhibitor treatment

Favorable Prognostic Factors[8,9]

- Depth of invasion <1 mm
- Clark level I
- No ulceration
- No lymph node metastasis at diagnosis
- Age less than 65 years
- Absent distant metastasis
- Female sex
- Origin in extremities
- No tumor vascularity and vascular invasion
- Low rate of mitosis and no regression
- Presence of tumor-infiltrating lymphocytes
- Normal serum lactate dehydrogenase level

Five-Year Survival[10]

- Stage 0: In situ melanoma (Clark level I): 99.9%
- Stage I: Invasive melanoma: 89%–95%
- Stage II: High-risk melanoma: 45%–79%
- Stage III: Locoregional metastasis: 24%–70%
- Stage IV: Distant metastasis: 7%–19%

TUMOR CHARACTERISTICS AND TYPICAL BEHAVIOR

Histopathology[11]

- Superficial spreading: 70%
- Nodular: 10%–15%
- Lentigo maligna: 5%–15%
- Acral lentiginous: 5%

Distribution and Localization[12]

The distribution and localization of primary tumors in males (M) and females (F) are given in Table 11.1.

N-lymph nodes

- Regional lymph nodes

M-distant metastases

- Skin: 50%–75%
- Lung: 70%–87%
- Liver: 54%–77%
- Brain: 36%–54%
- Bone: 23%–49%

TNM CLASSIFICATION[13,14]

The TNM classification is given in Tables 11.2 and 11.3.

TABLE 11.1
T-Primary Melanoma Localization and Distribution

	M (%)	F (%)
Head and neck	22	14
Trunk	38	17
Arm	17	21
Leg	15	42
Unspecified	8	6

GUIDELINES[13,15]

The European Society for Medical Oncology (ESMO) and National Comprehensive Cancer Network (NCCN) guidelines are given in Table 11.4.

EVIDENCE-BASED VIEWPOINTS[14,16–19]

- Fludeoxyglucose (FDG) PET/CT scan can play a role in more accurate diagnosis of metastatic melanoma.
- Evaluation of patients with advanced-stage malignant melanoma is recommended with chest radiography, CT scan of the abdomen, and FDG PET/CT if the screening tests or physical examinations are abnormal.
- FDG PET/CT is recommended for the pretreatment evaluation of patients with metastatic melanoma and in patients for whom radical dissection of involved lymph nodes or distant metastasectomy is planned. However, it is not recommended for patients with early-stage melanoma who are scheduled for sentinel lymph node biopsy.
- In advanced metastatic melanoma, FDG PET/CT is equally sensitive, but more specific, compared with CT and MRI for the detection of metastatic disease for both staging and restaging. It can also assess the response to treatment.
- FDG PET/CT is promising for the staging of advanced stage III and IV malignant melanoma and detection of soft tissue, lymph node, and visceral metastatic disease.

Cost-Effectiveness[20–22]

- The evaluation of high-risk malignant melanoma patients with FDG PET/CT saves money in patients' management by prevention of unnecessary thoracotomies in 20% of patients with pulmonary metastases.

TABLE 11.2
Melanoma TNM Classification

TNM	T1a	T1b	T2a	T2b	T3a	T3b	T4a	T4b
N0	IA	IB	IB	IIA	IIA	IIB	IIB	IIC
N1a	IIIA	IIIB	IIIA	IIIB	IIIA	IIIB	IIIA	IIIB
N1b	IIIB	IIIC	IIIB	IIIC	IIIB	IIIC	IIIB	IIIC
N2a	IIIA	IIIB	IIIA	IIIB	IIIA	IIIB	IIIA	IIIB
N2b	IIIB	IIIC	IIIB	IIIC	IIIB	IIIC	IIIB	IIIC
N2c	IIIB	IIIC	IIIB	IIIC	IIIB	IIIC	IIIB	IIIC
N3	IIIC	IIIC	IIIC	IIIC	IIIC	IIIC	IIIC	IIIC
M1abc	IV	IV	IV	IV	IV	IV	IV	IV

- FDG PET/CT resulted in a saving of $4400 per melanoma patient.
- Malignant melanoma with a saving to cost ratio of 1.95 is the third most cost-effective malignancy for overall saving after prostate and lung cancers, if evaluated with FDG PET/CT.
- Further prospective randomized clinical trials with a large number of patients are required to assess the cost-effectiveness of FDG PET/CT in malignancies such as malignant melanoma.

CLINICAL POINT OF VIEW

In recent years, the treatment of nonresectable or systemic malignant melanoma gained many new options. Tyrosine kinase inhibitors (TKIs), such as vemurafenib, have previously unseen high response rates in the subset of BRAF-mutated melanoma.[23]

More recently, new compounds, such as dabrafenib, used alone or in combination with other TKIs such as mitogen-activated protein kinase (MEK) inhibitors, have further improved patient outcomes. Also, immunotherapy, mainly checkpoint inhibitor treatment, was introduced successfully in patients with nonresectable or systemic melanoma. Especially CTLA4 blockade and more recently PD1/PD-L1 blockade showed important results. Therefore, TKI and checkpoint inhibitor of T-cell activation treatments are the current backbone to treat systemic malignant melanoma. Simplified, currently TKI, e.g., BRAF inhibition, is seen as standard in BRAF-mutated melanoma and checkpoint inhibition (e.g., PD1 blockade) is seen as standard in the BRAF wild type.

With the introduction of targeted therapy, imaging, and mainly molecular imaging, will need to adjust. Molecular imaging and early response will especially

TABLE 11.3
Melanoma TNM Classification

Primary Tumor (T)	Lymph Nodes (N)	Distant Metastasis (M)
T1 a,b: ≤1.0 mm T2 a,b: 1.01 to 2.0 mm T3 a,b: 2.01 to 4.0 mm T4 a,b: <4.0 mm a: Without ulceration b: With ulceration	N1: 1 lymph node a: Micrometastasis (clinically occult) b: Macrometastasis (clinically apparent) N2: 2 to 3 lymph nodes a: Micrometastasis b: Macrometastasis c: In transit met(s), satellite(s), without metastatic lymph nodes N3: 4 or more metastatic nodes or matted nodes or in-transit metastases or satellite(s) with metastatic node(s)	M1a: Distant skin, subcutaneous, or nodal metastases, normal lactate dehydrogenase (LDH) level M1b: Lung metastases, normal LDH level M1c: All other visceral metastases or any distant metastases with an elevated LDH level

TABLE 11.4
Melanoma ESMO and NCCN Guidelines

Clinical Guidelines	Initial Diagnosis (Primary Tumor)	N-Staging	M-Staging
ESMO	Recommended in • initial staging for tumors with T>T3a before surgery or SLNB	Recommended in • high-risk patients (thick primary tumor or after treatment of metastases)	Recommended in • high-risk patients (thick primary tumor or after treatment of metastases)
NCCN	Recommended in • stage III and IV initial staging • stage IIB-IV routine follow-up	Recommended in • stage III and IV initial staging and follow-up • evaluation of indeterminate lesions on CT scan	Recommended in • stage III and IV initial staging and follow-up • evaluation of specific signs and symptoms • evaluation of indeterminate lesions on CT scan • image areas not routinely studied in body CT scan (arms and legs)

ESMO, European Society for Medical Oncology; *NCCN,* National Comprehensive Cancer Network; *SLNB,* sentinel lymph node biopsy.

play a role in assessing active therapies at the earliest time point. Progressive metabolic disease in FDG PET/CT after two cycles of ipilimumab (YERVOY, Bristol Myers Squibb, NJ, USA) is highly predictive for further outcome.[24] Furthermore, functional imaging might be of use to assess either the mutational status or the local immune landscape in the tumor microenvironment.[25] The measurement of PD-L1 expression by PET using radiolabeled fragments might be of great interest in the future because these antigens are highly variable and successful treatment relies on the expression of PD1/PD-L1. Overall, melanoma serves as a great model for how to successfully implement functional imaging in the clinical routine to stage, restage, and monitor disease and FDG PET/CT has become a standard tool to assess malignant, high-risk melanoma in recent years. With the introduction of targeted therapies and the cessation of chemotherapy as standard treatment, many new challenges and opportunities for functional imaging arise.

PITFALLS[26]
False Positive

- Inflammation, such as postsurgical changes, granulomatous or infectious disease
- Physiologic uptake in brown fat tissue, skeletal muscles, or myocardium
- Physiologic activity in the bowel and urinary system
- Artifacts
- Pseudoprogression after checkpoint inhibitor treatment

False Negative

- Bone metastases that are obscured secondary to high bone marrow uptake from granulocyte-macrophage colony-stimulating factor stimulation
- Involved lymph nodes at the vicinity of brown fat tissue
- Bowel or peritoneal and mesenteric metastases that are obscured with physiologic bowel uptake
- Early-stage malignancy, hyperglycemic state, small lesions (<8 mm)

DISCUSSION

Based on the literature, the incidence of cutaneous malignant melanoma has been increasing during the past 30 years, specifically in Oceania. Therefore, early detection and appropriate management of the disease are warranted because the prognosis for patients with extensive metastatic disease is poor.

The primary diagnosis is made by careful physical examination of the skin and excisional full-depth biopsy of the suspicious lesions. However, multimodal imaging techniques are needed to evaluate possible regional or remote lymph node involvement or distant metastases.

Among the diagnostic imaging procedures, FDG PET/CT has been introduced as an eminent modality for staging in high-risk patients (>4 mm), evaluation of response to therapy, and follow-up in melanoma.

FDG PET/CT has the best sensitivity and specificity (approximately 90%) in the detection of metastatic lesions greater than 10 mm among imaging tools, including CT scan. In studies by Rodriguez Rivera, Wieder, and Xing, the sensitivity was calculated as 89%, 87%, and 86%, respectively. The specificity was calculated as 89%, 93%, and 91%, respectively. Also, Gellen and colleagues demonstrated an accuracy of 96% for FDG PET/CT in detecting melanoma metastases.[19,27–29]

A review of the major guidelines, such as NCCN and ESMO, reveals that utilization of FDG PET/CT is recommended in the initial staging and follow-up of patients with melanoma stage III and IV. It is also suitable for the exclusion of metastatic disease in patients with suspicious signs and symptoms, as well as clarification of concerning findings with other imaging modalities or laboratory data.

However, FDG PET/CT seems not to be the first-line diagnostic modality for staging and follow-up of patients with stage I and II melanoma.[13,15]

On the other hand, FDG PET/CT has limited sensitivity in the detection of metastases to the brain, one of the most common sites of cancer spread in melanoma. This is mainly because of the physiologic uptake of FDG by cerebral tissue. Therefore, contrast-enhanced MRI is suggested as the gold standard for the evaluation of cerebral metastases in melanoma. However, with the development of hybrid PET/MRI systems, this modality may offer an excellent diagnostic performance in the assessment of clinically advanced melanoma.[30,31]

To evaluate metastatic melanoma, whole-body (skull vertex to toes) FDG PET/CT instead of the usual limited skull base to midthigh scanning is the standard imaging protocol in most institutions. This protocol is expectedly more time consuming, and the patients receive more radiation dose from the additional CT scan. Some retrospective studies demonstrated that imaging the lower extremities provides no significant incremental information and does not change the patients' management, specifically when melanoma did not originate from the lower extremities. However, further studies are required to prove the hypothesis.[32]

Therapy Management

FDG PET/CT is also competent in upstaging of patients and management alteration, which prevents futile procedures or surgical interventions. A prospective multicenter study revealed that FDG PET/CT findings led to an upstaging to M1 status, with change of surgical management in about 18% of patients.[33]

These data were confirmed in a systematic review and meta-analysis of nine studies and a total of 623 patients with stage III malignant melanoma, showing that in about 22% of patients the stage and/or treatment approach was altered based on FDG PET/CT.[28]

Overall, the published prospective multicenter studies reported that FDG PET/CT is able to more accurately stage the disease in patients with melanoma compared with conventional imaging modalities, leading to change in therapeutic procedure in about 20% of the patients, particularly in advanced clinical stages.[34]

Prognostic Value

Many researchers assign a prognostic role to FDG PET/CT in the assessment of cutaneous malignant melanoma. A prospective study in patients with metastatic melanoma assessed the response to ipilimumab and found that FDG PET/CT can predict the therapy outcome in patients with stable and progressive disease.[35] The prognostic value of FDG PET/CT in patients with melanoma was assessed in some investigations. The researchers reported that those patients with melanoma with negative FDG PET/CT in follow-up imaging had a significantly lower risk of cancer-related mortality.[29]

In addition, they showed that the greater the maximum standardized uptake value (SUV_{max}) of the primary lesion, the poorer the prognosis for patients with melanoma. Furthermore, the SUV_{mean} in patients with nodal melanoma involvement was correlated with a shorter disease-free survival.[35–37]

Radiopharmaceuticals Beyond ^{18}F-FDG

With the development of radiopharmaceuticals beyond FDG, researchers are trying more specific radiotracers to image patients with melanoma, using PET/CT scanners. ^{18}F-dihydroxyphenylalanine (DOPA) PET/CT showed promising results with desirable sensitivity and specificity in the assessment of neuroendocrine tumors and melanoma, demonstrating that ^{18}F-DOPA avidity is caused mainly by the enhanced activity of L-DOPA decarboxylase. However, there are only a few studies reported in the literature.[38] ^{18}F-5-fluoropicolinamide has been introduced as a melanin-avid tracer that might be useful for melanoma staging.[39] Another melanin-specific probe, ^{18}F-MEL050, was introduced with the potential to evaluate metastatic melanoma.[40] Also, ^{18}F-fluorothymidine (FLT) showed potential impact in restaging metastatic melanoma.[41] However, further investigations are necessary to determine the role of new radiotracers in the clinical evaluation of cutaneous malignant melanoma.

TEACHING CASES

Case 1: Staging, Distant Metastases

Findings

A 50-year-old female with vulvar melanoma. FDG PET/CT shows a tracer-avid primary cancer in the vulvar region (A,B; arrow) with a large metabolically active right inguinal lymph node (C, arrow) and small metastatic lesion in the left liver lobe (E, arrow) and right lung (F, arrow). Sentinel node biopsy revealed lymph node micrometastases on the left inguinal region, which were negative on FDG PET/CT. Of incidental note is an FDG-avid benign uterine myoma (D, arrow) (Fig. 11.1).

Teaching points

- FDG PET/CT is an accurate modality for the evaluation of equivocal lesions on stand-alone CT.
- Lymphoscintigraphy and sentinel node biopsy are superior to FDG PET/CT in the detection of occult regional metastases, with a sensitivity of 94% and specificity of 100%.
- Although the 5-year survival of in situ melanoma is near 100%, it significantly diminishes in stage IV disease to <20%.
- The lung is the most common site of metastasis from melanoma.

Pitfalls

- Benign gynecologic neoplasms, such as myoma, could be FDG avid and result in false-positive reports.

Case 2: Restaging and Follow-Up

Findings

A 60-year-old female with history of right medial leg cutaneous melanoma. FDG PET/CT shows a faint tracer uptake in the right leg (A–C), corresponding to the primary tumor resection bed. There are FDG-avid metastatic lesions in the right thigh (A,D; arrow), gallbladder (A,E; arrow), and right lung (A,F; arrow). Follow-up images demonstrate an excellent metabolic response to therapy (B) but progressive disease with development of new small FDG-avid metastatic lesion in the left lung (C, arrow) (Fig. 11.2).

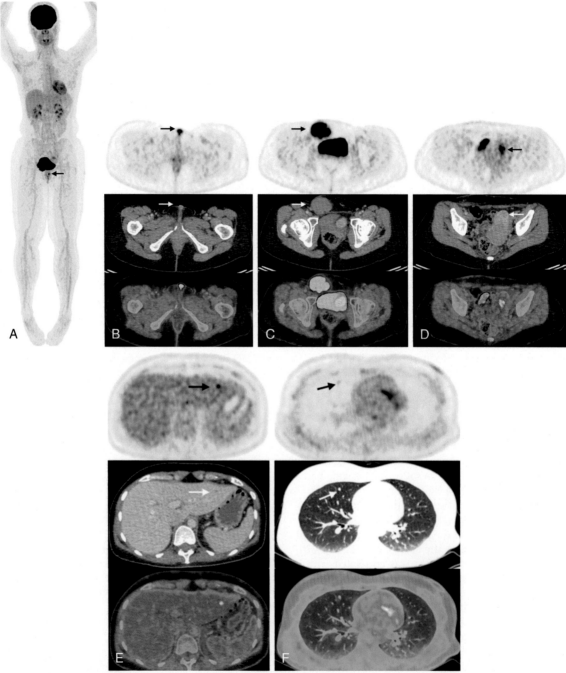

FIG. 11.1 FDG PET/CT showing a tracer-avid primary cancer in the vulvar region (A,B; *arrows*) with a large metabolically active right inguinal lymph node (C, *arrows*). Of incidental note is an FDG-avid benign uterine myoma (D, *arrows*). A small metastatic lesion in the left liver lobe (E, *arrows*) and right lung (F, *arrows*) is also seen.

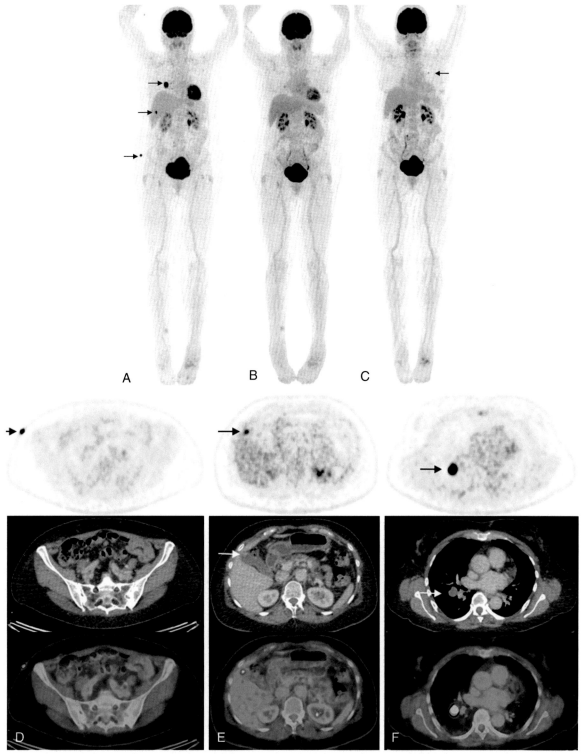

FIG. 11.2 A 60-year-old female with history of right medial leg cutaneous melanoma. FDG PET/CT shows faint tracer uptake in the right leg (A–C), corresponding to primary tumor resection bed. There are FDG-avid metastatic lesions in the right thigh (A and D, *arrow*), gallbladder (A and E, *arrow*) and the right lung (A and F, *arrow*). Follow-up images demonstrate excellent metabolic response to therapy (B) but progressive disease with development of new small FDG-avid metastatic lesion in the left lung (C, *arrow*).

Teaching points

- Melanoma presents with metastases in 4% of newly diagnosed patients.
- FDG PET/CT is currently used for extranodal staging, restaging, and recurrent melanoma.
- Although melanoma rarely metastasizes to the gallbladder, focal uptakes even in atypical localizations should be considered for further evaluation to exclude malignancy.
- The detection of small atypical metastasis to the gallbladder emphasizes again the superiority of FDG PET/CT to stand-alone CT in staging of melanoma.
- In addition to Breslow thickness, FDG PET/CT could be predictive of recurrence and prognosis.

Case 3: Treatment Evaluation

Findings

A 65-year-old male with remote history of cutaneous melanoma of the left back and several episodes of

recurrence. FDG PET/CT shows widespread tracer-avid lymph node metastases in the cervical, mediastinal, axillary, and abdominal regions (A). A posttherapy follow-up scan (B) demonstrates a favorable metabolic response in the axillary region; however, progressive disease is evident in the follow-up examination (C) with multiple new FDG-avid metastatic lesions (Fig. 11.3).

Teaching points

- FDG PET/CT is a promising modality for the assessment of treatment in melanoma.
- Male gender and lymph node involvement are among the poor prognostic factors in melanoma.

Case 4: Restaging

Findings

A 69-year-old male with remote history of melanoma, referred for further evaluation of an equivocal lesion in the head of the pancreas, incidentally detected on

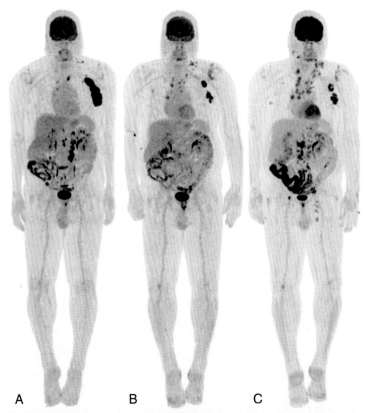

A   B   C

FIG. 11.3 FDG PET/CT showing widespread tracer-avid lymph node metastases in the cervical, mediastinal, axillary, and abdominal regions (A). A posttherapy follow-up scan (B) demonstrates a favorable metabolic response in the axillary region; however, progressive disease is evident in the follow-up examination (C), with multiple new FDG-avid metastatic lesions.

abdominal CT. The lesion was positive on FDG PET/CT (C, arrow) but negative on ^{68}Ga-DOTANOC PET/CT (D). FDG-avid lesions are noted in both adrenal glands (E, arrow) and the lungs (A), consistent with metastases. Of incidental note is a focal ^{68}Ga-DOTANOC uptake in the prostate gland, most likely benign in nature (Fig. 11.4).

Teaching points
- ^{68}Ga-DOTANOC PET/CT is a promising modality for the assessment of neuroendocrine tumors.
- Melanoma can show different behavior with atypical sites of metastases.
- FDG PET/CT is useful for the clarification of equivocal findings on conventional imaging modalities.

Pitfalls
- ^{68}Ga-DOTANOC uptake in the prostate gland could be physiologic or caused by a benign lesion and should not be interpreted as malignancy.

Case 5: Equivocal Findings on Conventional Imaging
Findings
A 54-year-old female with a history of melanoma, referred for further evaluation of an equivocal finding on stand-alone CT. There is a hypodense lesion in segment V of the liver on CT (B, arrow), which is not tracer avid on FDG PET/CT (Fig. 11.5).

Teaching points
- One of the indications of FDG PET/CT is for the assessment of equivocal lesions on conventional imaging modalities in patients with cancer.
- Age <65 years and female gender are among the favorable prognostic factors for melanoma.

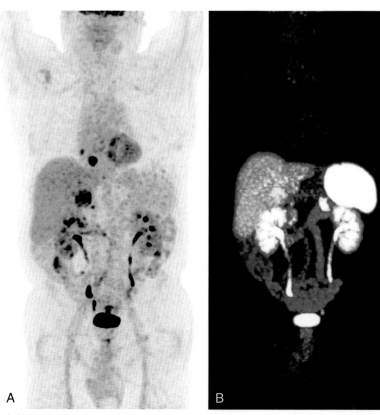

A   B

FIG. 11.4 A 69-year-old male with remote history of melanoma, referred for further evaluation of an equivocal lesion in the head of pancreas, incidentally detected on abdominal CT. The lesion was positive on FDG PET/CT (A and C, *arrow*) but negative on ^{68}Ga-DOTANOC PET/CT (B and D). FDG avid lesions are noted in both adrenal glands (E, *arrow*) as well as the lungs (A, *arrow*), but negative on ^{68}Ga-DOTANOC PET/CT (B, D, and F), consistent with metastases. Of incidental note is focal ^{68}Ga-DOTANOC uptake in the prostate gland, most likely benign in nature.

Continued

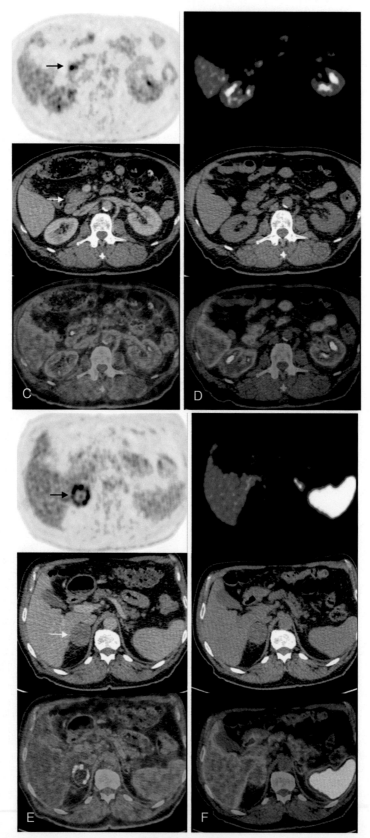

FIG. 11.4, cont'd

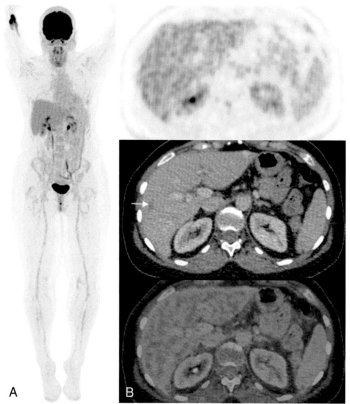

FIG. 11.5 A 54-year-old female with a history of melanoma, referred for further evaluation of an equivocal finding on stand-alone CT. There is a hypodense lesion in segment V of the liver on CT (B, *arrow*), which is not tracer avid on FDG PET/CT (A and upper B).

REFERENCES

1. American Cancer Society. *Cancer Facts & Figures*; 2016.
2. Siegel R, Naishadham D, Jemal A. Cancer statistics. *CA: A Cancer Journal for Clinicians*. January 2013;63(1):11–30.
3. James w, Berger T, Elston D, eds. *Andrews' Disease of the Skin: Clinical Dermatology*. 10th ed. Saunders Elsevier; 2009.
4. Bajetta E, Del Vecchio M, Bernard-Marty C, et al. Metastatic melanoma: chemotherapy. *Seminars in Oncology*. October 2002;29(5):427–445.
5. Chakraborty R, Wieland CN, Comfere NI. Molecular targeted therapies in metastatic melanoma. *Pharmacogenomics and Personalized Medicine*. 2013;6:49–56.
6. Kirkwood JM, Strawderman MH, Ernstoff MS, Smith TJ, Borden EC, Blum RH. Interferon alfa-2b adjuvant therapy of high-risk resected cutaneous melanoma: The Eastern Cooperative Oncology Group Trial EST 1684. *Journal of Clinical Oncology: Official Journal of the American Society of Clinical Oncology*. January 1996;14(1):7–17.
7. Swanson NA, Lee KK, Gorman A, Lee HN. Biopsy techniques. Diagnosis of melanoma. *Dermatologic Clinics*. October 2002;20(4):677–680.
8. Homsi J, Kashani-Sabet M, Messina JL, Daud A. Cutaneous melanoma: prognostic factors. *Cancer Control: Journal of the Moffitt Cancer Center*. October 2005;12(4): 223–229.
9. Murali R, Desilva C, Thompson JF, Scolyer RA. Factors predicting recurrence and survival in sentinel lymph node-positive melanoma patients. *Annals of Surgery*. June 2011;253(6):1155–1164.
10. Balch CM, Buzaid AC, Soong SJ, et al. Final version of the American Joint Committee on Cancer staging system for cutaneous melanoma. *Journal of Clinical Oncology: Official Journal of the American Society of Clinical Oncology*. August 15, 2001;19(16):3635–3648.
11. Liu V, Mihm MC. Pathology of malignant melanoma. *The Surgical Clinics of North America*. February 2003;83(1): 31–60. v.
12. Petrella T, Ernst S, Spatz A, Claveau J, Wong R, Smylie M. Canadian perspective on the clinical management of metastatic melanoma. *New Evidence in Oncology*. 2012:108–120.
13. *NCCN Clinical Practice Guidelines in Oncology. Melanoma*. 2016. Version 2. www.NCCN.org.

14. Melanoma of skin. In: Edge S, Byrd D, Compton C, eds. *AJCC Cancer Staging Manual.* 7th ed. Springer; 2009: 325–344.

15. Dummer R, Hauschild A, Lindenblatt N, Pentheroudakis G, Keilholz U, Committee EG. Cutaneous melanoma: ESMO clinical practice guidelines for diagnosis, treatment and follow-up. *Annals of Oncology: Official Journal of the European Society for Medical Oncology.* September 2015;26(suppl 5):v126–v132.

16. Krug B, Crott R, Lonneux M, Baurain JF, Pirson AS, Vander Borght T. Role of PET in the initial staging of cutaneous malignant melanoma: systematic review. *Radiology.* December 2008;249(3):836–844.

17. Sabel MS, Wong SL. Review of evidence-based support for pretreatment imaging in melanoma. *Journal of the National Comprehensive Cancer Network.* March 2009;7(3):281–289.

18. Stadelmann WK, McMasters K, Digenis AG, Reintgen DS. Cutaneous melanoma of the head and neck: advances in evaluation and treatment. *Plastic and Reconstructive Surgery.* May 2000;105(6):2105–2126.

19. Xing Y, Bronstein Y, Ross MI, et al. Contemporary diagnostic imaging modalities for the staging and surveillance of melanoma patients: a meta-analysis. *Journal of the National Cancer Institute.* January 19, 2011;103(2): 129–142.

20. Buck AK, Herrmann K, Stargardt T, Dechow T, Krause BJ, Schreyogg J. Economic evaluation of PET and PET/CT in oncology: evidence and methodologic approaches. *Journal of Nuclear Medicine: Official Publication, Society of Nuclear Medicine.* March 2010;51(3):401–412.

21. Krug B, Crott R, Roch I, et al. Cost-effectiveness analysis of FDG PET-CT in the management of pulmonary metastases from malignant melanoma. *Acta oncologica.* 2010;49(2):192–200.

22. Rohren EM, Turkington TG, Coleman RE. Clinical applications of PET in oncology. *Radiology.* May 2004;231(2):305–332.

23. Chapman PB, Hauschild A, Robert C, et al. Improved survival with vemurafenib in melanoma with BRAF V600E mutation. *The New England Journal of Medicine.* June 30, 2011;364(26):2507–2516.

24. Sachpekidis C, Larribere L, Pan L, Haberkorn U, Dimitrakopoulou-Strauss A, Hassel JC. Predictive value of early 18F-FDG PET/CT studies for treatment response evaluation to ipilimumab in metastatic melanoma: preliminary results of an ongoing study. *European Journal of Nuclear Medicine and Molecular Imaging.* March 2015;42(3):386–396.

25. Heskamp S, Hobo W, Molkenboer-Kuenen JD, et al. Noninvasive imaging of tumor PD-L1 expression using radiolabeled anti-PD-L1 antibodies. *Cancer Research.* July 15, 2015;75(14):2928–2936.

26. Tyler DS, Onaitis M, Kherani A, et al. Positron emission tomography scanning in malignant melanoma. *Cancer.* September 1, 2000;89(5):1019–1025.

27. Gellen E, Santha O, Janka E, et al. Diagnostic accuracy of (18)F-FDG-PET/CT in early and late stages of high-risk cutaneous malignant melanoma. *Journal of the European Academy of Dermatology and Venereology.* October 2015;29(10):1938–1944.

28. Rodriguez Rivera AM, Alabbas H, Ramjaun A, Meguerditchian AN. Value of positron emission tomography scan in stage III cutaneous melanoma: a systematic review and meta-analysis. *Surgical Oncology.* March 2014;23(1):11–16.

29. Wieder HA, Tekin G, Rosenbaum-Krumme S, et al. 18FDG-PET to assess recurrence and long term survival in patients with malignant melanoma. *Nuklearmedizin. Nuclear Medicine.* 2013;52(5):198–203.

30. Kruger S, Mottaghy FM, Buck AK, et al. Brain metastasis in lung cancer. Comparison of cerebral MRI and 18F-FDG-PET/CT for diagnosis in the initial staging. *Nuklearmedizin. Nuclear Medicine.* 2011;50(3):101–106.

31. Schwenzer NF, Pfannenberg AC. PET/CT, MR, and PET/MR in lymphoma and melanoma. *Seminars in Nuclear Medicine.* July 2015;45(4):322–331.

32. Lazaga FJ, Oz OK, Adams-Huet B, Anderson J, Mathews D. Comparison of whole-body versus limited whole-body 18F-FDG PET/CT scan in malignant cutaneous melanoma. *Clinical Nuclear Medicine.* November 2013;38(11):882–884.

33. Singnurkar A, Wang J, Joshua AM, Langer DL, Metser U. 18F-FDG-PET/CT in the staging and management of melanoma: a prospective Multicenter Ontario PET registry study. *Clinical Nuclear Medicine.* March 2016;41(3):189–193.

34. Bastiaannet E, Wobbes T, Hoekstra OS, et al. Prospective comparison of [18F]fluorodeoxyglucose positron emission tomography and computed tomography in patients with melanoma with palpable lymph node metastases: diagnostic accuracy and impact on treatment. *Journal of Clinical Oncology: Official Journal of the American Society of Clinical Oncology.* October 1, 2009;27(28):4774–4780.

35. Bastiaannet E, Hoekstra OS, de Jong JR, Brouwers AH, Suurmeijer AJ, Hoekstra HJ. Prognostic value of the standardized uptake value for (18)F-fluorodeoxyglucose in patients with stage IIIB melanoma. *European Journal of Nuclear Medicine and Molecular Imaging.* October 2012;39(10):1592–1598.

36. Hwang JP, Lim I, Na II, et al. Prognostic value of SUV-max measured by fluorine-18 fluorodeoxyglucose positron emission tomography with computed tomography in patients with gallbladder cancer. *Nuclear Medicine and Molecular Imaging.* June 2014;48(2):114–120.

37. Kang S, Ahn BC, Hong CM, et al. Can (18)F-FDG PET/CT predict recurrence in patients with cutaneous malignant melanoma? *Nuklearmedizin. Nuclear medicine.* 2011;50(3):116–121.

38. Caroli P, Nanni C, Rubello D, Alavi A, Fanti S. Non-FDG PET in the practice of oncology. *Indian Journal of Cancer.* April–June 2010;47(2):120–125.

39. Feng H, Xia X, Li C, et al. Imaging malignant melanoma with (18)F-5-FPN. *European Journal of Nuclear Medicine and Molecular Imaging*. January 2016;43(1):113–122.

40. Denoyer D, Greguric I, Roselt P, et al. High-contrast PET of melanoma using (18)F-MEL050, a selective probe for melanin with predominantly renal clearance. *Journal of Nuclear Medicine: Official Publication, Society of Nuclear Medicine*. March 2010;51(3):441–447.

41. Cobben DC, Jager PL, Elsinga PH, Maas B, Suurmeijer AJ, Hoekstra HJ. 3′-18F-fluoro-3′-deoxy-L-thymidine: a new tracer for staging metastatic melanoma? *Journal of Nuclear Medicine: Official Publication, Society of Nuclear Medicine*. December 2003;44(12):1927–1932.

CHAPTER 12

Brain Tumors

KARL-JOSEF LANGEN • ALEXANDER DRZEZGA • NORBERT GALLDIKS

BACKGROUND

General[1]

- Primary central nervous system (CNS) tumors account for about 1% to 2% of all malignancies.
- Gliomas are the second most common primary brain tumors, with an incidence of 4 to 5/100,000 individuals.
- Gliomas are the second leading cause of cancer mortality in adults under the age of 35 years and the fourth leading cause in those under the age of 54 years.
- Risk factors: Ionizing radiation and genetic predisposition account for only a small fraction of brain tumors.
- Brain metastases are the most frequent brain tumors, with an incidence of 8 to 14/100,000 individuals.[2]

Clinical Signs/Symptoms[3]

Common general signs and symptoms of brain tumors include the following:

- Hemiparesis
- Aphasia
- Seizures
- Visual changes
- Symptoms related to increased intracranial pressure, such as headaches, nausea, and vomiting
- Changes in personality, mood, mental capacity, and concentration

Diagnostic Procedures

Brain tumors have to be differentiated from other space-occupying lesions with similar appearance, such as demyelination, abscesses, and infarctions. Contrast-enhanced MRI is the method of first choice because of its superior soft tissue resolution, but contrast-enhanced CT is faster and therefore often used in clinically unstable patients for immediate management.

PET provides additional insight beyond conventional MRI into the biology of gliomas. The most widely used PET tracer, 2-18F-fluorodeoxyglucose (FDG), has only a limited use in brain tumors because of the high tracer uptake in the normal brain tissue. In contrast to FDG, the uptake of radiolabeled amino acids is low in the normal brain tissue but high in most brain tumors; thus, viable brain tumors can be depicted with a high tumor-to-background contrast. A key feature of amino acid tracers is the property to pass the intact blood–brain barrier (BBB), which allows depiction of the tumor mass beyond contrast enhancement in MRI[4] and differentiation of tumor progression from nonspecific treatment-related changes.[5] [11C-methyl]-methionine (MET) represents the longest established amino acid PET tracer, but tracers labeled with the longer lived fluorine-18 (half-life, 109.8 min), such as O-(2-[18F]-fluoroethyl)-L-tyrosine (FET) or 3,4-dihydroxy-6-[18F]-fluoro-L-phenylalanine (FDOPA), provide logistic advantages. Radiolabeled amino acids have become the preferred PET tracers in neurooncology, and the Response Assessment in Neuro-Oncology (RANO) group recommends the use of amino acid PET at all stages of patient management.[6] In Europe, [18F] FET is currently considered the tracer of choice at many centers active in brain tumor imaging (Table 12.1).

Prognostic Factors[7,10]

In addition to general prognostic factors, several genetic alterations have been associated with the prognosis of diffuse glioma (astrocytoma, oligodendroglioma, and glioblastoma). Knowledge of these alterations may also guide patient management (Tables 12.2 and 12.3). Generally accepted prognostic and, in part, predictive factors are the following:

- Age
- Karnofsky Performance Score
- DNA methylation of the O6-methylguanine-DNA methyltransferase (MGMT) gene promoter
- Mutation of isocitrate dehydrogenase (IDH) 1 and/or 2 genes
- Codeletion of chromosomes 1p and 19q
- Loss of ATRX expression

Survival[11]

- Glioblastoma: 15 months
- Anaplastic astrocytoma World Health Organization (WHO) grade III: 3.5 years

TABLE 12.1
Treatment Recommendations for Newly Diagnosed Gliomas[7–9]

Tumor Type	Suggested Treatment
ASTROCYTIC TUMORS	
• Diffuse astrocytomas (WHO grade II)	• Surgery followed by "Watch and Wait" strategy (low-risk patients) • Surgery plus radiation therapy followed by adjuvant procarbazine, lomustine, vincristine chemotherapy (high-risk patients)
• Anaplastic astrocytomas (WHO grade III)	• Surgery plus radiation therapy followed by adjuvant temozolomide chemotherapy
• Glioblastomas (WHO grade IV)	• Surgery plus radiation therapy with concurrent and adjuvant temozolomide chemotherapy
OLIGODENDROGLIAL TUMORS	
• Diffuse oligodendrogliomas (WHO grade II)	• Surgery followed by "Watch and Wait" strategy (low-risk patients) • Surgery plus radiation therapy followed by adjuvant procarbazine, lomustine, vincristine chemotherapy (high-risk patients)
• Anaplastic oligodendrogliomas with 1p/19q codeletion (WHO grade III)	• Surgery plus radiation therapy followed by adjuvant procarbazine, lomustine, vincristine chemotherapy

WHO, World Health Organization.

TABLE 12.2
Grading of Selected CNS Tumors According to the WHO Classification 2016 for Brain Tumors[10]

WHO Grade	
I	• Pilocytic astrocytoma • Subependymal giant cell astrocytoma
II	• Diffuse astrocytoma, IDH mutant • Oligodendroglioma, IDH mutant and 1p/19q codeleted • Pleomorphic xanthoastrocytoma • Ependymoma
III	• Anaplastic astrocytoma, IDH mutant • Anaplastic oligodendroglioma, IDH mutant and 1p/19q codeleted • Anaplastic pleomorphic xanthoastrocytoma
IV	• Glioblastoma, IDH wild type • Glioblastoma, IDH mutant • Diffuse midline glioma, H3 K27M mutant

CNS, central nervous system; *IDH*, isocitrate dehydrogenase; *WHO*, World Health Organization.

- Astrocytoma WHO grade II: 7 to 10 years
- Anaplastic oligodendroglioma WHO grade III: >10 years
- Oligodendroglioma WHO grade II: 10 to 15 years
- Pilocytic astrocytoma: 95% cure

TABLE 12.3
Guidelines of Amino Acid PET

EANM	European Association of Nuclear Medicine procedure guidelines for brain tumor imaging using labeled amino acid analogues	Vander Borght et al.[13]
RANO	Response Assessment in Neuro-Oncology (RANO) working group and European Association for Neuro-Oncology recommendations for the clinical use of PET imaging in gliomas	Albert et al.[6]
Deutsche Gesellschaft für Nuklearmedizin	German guidelines for brain tumor imaging by PET and SPECT using labeled amino acids	Langen et al.[14]

SPECT, single-photon emission computed tomography.

Histopathology[12]

Primary brain tumors include the following in decreasing order of frequency:
- Anaplastic astrocytomas and glioblastomas (38% of primary brain tumors)
- Meningiomas and other mesenchymal tumors (27% of primary brain tumors)

- Pituitary tumors
- Schwannomas
- CNS lymphomas
- Oligodendrogliomas
- Ependymomas
- Low-grade astrocytomas
- Medulloblastomas

Evidence-based Recommendations

- Amino acid PET in brain tumors is recommended in the evidence-based medical literature.[6,15]
- PET using radiolabeled amino acids provides substantial additional information on the tumor size of gliomas compared with CT or MRI.[16-19]
- Dynamic FET PET[20] and the "biologic tumor volume" (BTV) as assessed by amino acid PET at primary diagnosis are important predictors of prognosis.[21-23]
- Amino acid PET, especially FET PET, is a valuable tool in differentiating recurrent tumor from nonneoplastic changes in gliomas and brain metastasis.[5,24,25]
- Amino acid PET is helpful for therapy monitoring and provides an early assessment of therapy efficacy.[26-28]
- Amino acid PET avoids the cost and side effects of unnecessary invasive procedures.[29-31]

Cost-effectiveness

The cost-effectiveness of amino acid PET in the management of brain tumors has been analyzed with respect to amino acid PET-guided target selection for the diagnosis of gliomas, with respect to amino acid PET-guided surgery and therapy monitoring of antiangiogenic therapy.[29-31] The data suggest that the additional use of amino acid PET in the management of patients with cerebral gliomas has the potential to avoid overtreatment and corresponding costs, as well as unnecessary side effects to the patient.

CLINICAL POINT OF VIEW
Suspected Disease

- An increased amino acid uptake is highly predictive of a malignant brain lesion requiring rapid histologic clarification.
- A low amino acid uptake excludes a malignant brain lesion with high probability.
- A low amino acid uptake does not exclude a low-grade glioma (LGG) because 30% of LGGs exhibit only a low amino acid uptake.
- A moderately increased amino acid uptake can also be seen in acute inflammatory lesions, such as brain abscesses or demyelinating processes.

Imaging Tumor Extent and Biopsy Guidance

- Amino acid PET detects focal metabolic maxima for biopsy guidance, which is helpful in avoiding nondiagnostic biopsies.
- Amino acid PET can provide additional information on the extent of a brain tumor for planning of surgery and radiotherapy, especially in nonenhancing gliomas in MRI and CT.

Tumor Grading and Prognosis

- FDG PET is considered a relatively accurate predictor of tumor grade and prognosis of cerebral gliomas.
- Amino acid uptake shows a wide overlap between gliomas of different WHO grades, but dynamic FET can also differentiate between high-grade and low-grade gliomas with high accuracy.
- The BTV in amino acid PET is an independent predictor of prognosis.

The Diagnosis of Tumor Recurrence/ Progression

- Amino acid PET has high accuracy to differentiate progressive or recurrent tumor from treatment-related changes, such as pseudoprogression or radionecrosis.
- Amino acid PET has high accuracy to differentiate recurrent brain metastasis from radionecrosis after stereotactic radiosurgery.

Treatment Monitoring

- Amino acid PET is a sensitive method to detect response to therapy at an early stage of therapy and to predict survival.
- Amino acid PET has a high accuracy to differentiate tumor response from pseudoresponse during antiangiogenic therapy (Table 12.4).

DISCUSSION
Radiopharmaceuticals

PET using FDG is an established diagnostic method in most peripheral tumors. In cerebral gliomas, FDG uptake is correlated with the degree of malignancy of the tumor (WHO grading) and with the patient's outcome,[39-41] but the delineation of brain tumors is rather difficult because of the high rate of glucose metabolism in normal brain tissue. Another problem with FDG is the high tracer uptake in inflammatory cells. The most promising alternative for PET imaging of brain tumors can be found in markers of amino acid metabolism.

At present, the best established PET tracers for the investigation of brain tumors are radiolabeled amino acids of the class of large neutral amino acids, such as

MET, FET, and FDOPA.[42] The utilization of amino acids by both the white and gray matter of normal brain tissue is relatively low because of the limited demand for amino acids in neural tissue, which meets its energetic needs almost exclusively by metabolism of glucose and exhibits generally low cell division rates. On the other hand, most malignant brain lesions demonstrate significantly elevated amino acid utilization because of unspecific metabolism and high cell division rates. In consequence, most brain tumors can be distinguished from the surrounding normal tissue with high contrast, using amino acid PET imaging. Because large neutral amino acids are able to cross the BBB in healthy brain tissue, a disruption of the BBB, i.e., enhancement of contrast media on MRI scans, is not a prerequisite for intratumoral accumulation of MET, FET, and FDOPA. Consequently, the uptake of these tracers has been reported in many LGGs without BBB leakage.[4,20,43,44] The increased uptake of amino acids such as MET, FET, and FDOPA by cerebral glioma tissue and brain metastases seems to be caused predominantly by increased transport via the transport system L for large neutral amino acids, namely, the subtypes LAT1 and LAT2.[45–48] One study suggested that the trapping of FET within the cells is caused by the asymmetry of its intracellular and extracellular recognition by LAT1.[49] Some studies have shown that imaging of cerebral gliomas with MET, FET, and FDOPA is rather similar.[50–53] Nevertheless, there appear to be some differences in transport characteristics of MET, FET, and FDOPA. FET shows different patterns of time–activity curves in low-grade and high-grade gliomas (HGGs),[54–56] which were not observed with MET or FDOPA.[52,57] Because FDOPA is a precursor of dopamine, it also shows an uptake in the striatum and can be used to trace the dopaminergic pathway in the nigrostriatal region to evaluate the presynaptic function in patients with neurodegenerative and movement disorders.[58] This property may cause problems in the delineation of gliomas affecting the striatum.[42,59]

Most PET studies of cerebral gliomas have been performed with the amino acid MET,[60] although the short half-life of [11]C (20 min) limits the use of this technique to the few centers that are equipped with an in-house cyclotron facility. In contrast to MET, ^{18}F-labeled amino acids (half-life, 109 min), such as FET and FDOPA, can be transported from a cyclotron unit to multiple external PET centers. This enables a wider application of amino acid PET in clinical diagnosis. One of the best established ^{18}F-labeled amino acids is FET, which can be produced in large amounts for clinical purposes like the widely used FDG.[61–63]

Switzerland is the first country that has approved FET PET as a medical drug in 2014.[64]

Animal experiments have shown that, in contrast to MET, FET exhibits no uptake in inflammatory cells and in inflammatory lymph nodes, but some false-positive uptake has been observed for MET, FET, and FDOPA in brain abscesses and demyelinating processes and near cerebral ischemia and hematomas in animal experiments and in humans.[32–35,37,65,66] Therefore, an increased uptake of the tracers is not entirely specific for cerebral gliomas, although an increased amino acid uptake has a high positive predictive value for cerebral gliomas.[34,67] Furthermore, a low amino acid uptake does not exclude a brain tumor because approximately one-third of LGGs exhibit only a low amino acid uptake.[4,44,68,69] According to one meta-analysis, amino acid PET is considerably more sensitive than FDG PET to detect brain tumors and thus the PET tracers of choice for the initial assessment of brain tumors.[70] Radiolabeled amino acids have become the preferred PET tracers in neurooncology, and the RANO group recommends the use of amino acid PET at all stages of patient management.[6] Therefore, this chapter is focused on brain tumor imaging with MET, FET, and FDOPA, which are at present the best validated amino acid tracers for PET.

Imaging Tumor Extent and Biopsy Guidance

One of the most important aspects in the initial diagnosis of gliomas is the identification of tumor extension and the metabolically most active areas of the tumor.

TABLE 12.4
Pitfalls in Amino Acid PET

Condition	Comment	References
Brain abscess, inflammation	Rarely	Floeth et al.,[32] Hutterer et al.,[33] and Pichler et al.[34]
Hematoma	Increased uptake up to 45 d after bleeding	Salber et al.[35] and Ogawa et al.[36]
Infarction	Increased uptake up to 7 d after ischemia	Hutterer et al.[33] and Salber et al.[37]
Demyelination	Rarely	Floeth et al.[32] and Hutterer et al.[33]
Radionecrosis	Rarely	Hutterer et al.[38]
Epileptic seizures	Very rare	Hutterer et al.[146]

Representative tissue samples are vitally important for histologic tumor diagnosis, prognostication, and treatment planning. The diagnostic capacity of conventional MRI to depict the most aggressive areas in inhomogeneous gliomas is generally restricted and largely impossible in nonenhancing tumors. Local maxima of FDG uptake in heterogeneous gliomas are usually colocalized with the maximum amino acid uptake, but MET and FET PET have been shown to be considerably more sensitive than FDG PET for biopsy guidance.[71-73] The definition of an optimal biopsy site is especially difficult in gliomas showing no contrast enhancement on MRI. In a patient series of 22 histologically confirmed LGGs, FET PET identified a local maximum for biopsy guidance in 16 of the tumors (72%), whereas FDG identified a metabolic hot spot in only 2 (9%) of the LGGs.[71] In another study including 72 histologically confirmed diffuse LGGs, FET PET identified a local maximum in 79% of the tumors.[4] Other studies emphasize the role of kinetic analyses of FET uptake in gliomas: areas with an early peak in FET uptake followed by a descending time–activity curve are associated with areas of malignant transformation and poor prognosis.[20,69,74-77] These data suggest that amino acid PET is a useful tool for identifying metabolically suspicious areas in brain tumors to target biopsies. Nevertheless, it is not yet proven beyond doubt that the maximum concentration of amino acid uptake in gliomas corresponds to the most aggressive part of the tumor and further studies are needed to investigate this aspect.

Multiple studies in which the radiologic findings were compared with the histologic findings in tissue samples obtained by biopsy or open surgery have provided evidence that PET using radiolabeled amino acids detects the solid mass of gliomas and metabolically active tumor areas more reliably than either CT or MRI.[17,18,78,79] Furthermore, it has been demonstrated that integrating MET PET for resection guidance of HGGs provided a final target contour different from that obtained with MRI alone in about 80% of the procedures.[80] Complete resection of the tumor area with an increased amino acid uptake resulted in a significantly longer survival of patients, whereas the degree of contrast enhancement on the postoperative MRI scan did not have an impact on survival. Similar results have been observed with FET PET.[22,23,81] These data indicate that resection of malignant gliomas guided by amino acid PET may increase the amount of anaplastic tissue removed and thus patients' survival.

The improved imaging of glioma tissue using amino acid PET has also attracted interest for radiation treatment planning.[82-84] A number of centers have started to integrate amino acid imaging into CT- and MRI-based radiotherapy planning, particularly when high-precision radiotherapy is planned or in the setting of dose escalation studies or for the reirradiation of recurrent tumors.[83,85-90] An improved outcome of the patients with radiotherapy planning using amino acid imaging compared with conventional radiation therapy planning, however, has not yet been proven. A prospective study indicated that an integrated-boost intensity-modulated radiation dose escalation concept, which was based on FET PET-guided target volume delineation, showed no survival benefit for the patients.[84] The explanation for this may be found in the unfortunately overall low survival benefit of radiation therapy, with many recurrences occurring even within the radiated volume. This naturally limits the effects of an optimized definition of tumor borders.

Tumor Grading and Prognosis

FDG PET is considered a relatively accurate predictor of tumor grade and prognosis of cerebral gliomas.[39,40,91] However, in these studies the rate of correct identification of an HGG varied considerably. Furthermore, some studies observed no significant differences of FDG uptake in LGG and HGG.[92,93] Most PET studies employing amino acids have shown that gliomas of different WHO grades overlap in their degree of amino acid uptake, so that the tumor grade cannot be reliably predicted with this technique.[15] The use of amino acid tracers for glioma grading is limited by the relatively high uptake of amino acids in gliomas with oligodendroglial components[55,78,94] in spite of their better prognosis when compared with astrocytomas of the same grade. Most probably, these findings may reflect higher cell density, a different transport rate of the L-system of amino acid transporters, and higher microvessel density in oligodendroglial as compared with astrocytic gliomas.[78,95,96] The accuracy of static amino acid PET for the differentiation between LGG and HGG ranges between 70% and 80%.[4,55,60,70]

A number of studies have demonstrated that the evaluation of FET kinetics in the tumors may be more reliable to differentiate between HGG and LGG. HGGs are characterized by an early peak of the time–activity curve around 10 to 15 min after tracer injection followed by a decrease of FET uptake. In contrast, time–activity curves slightly and steadily increase in LGG of WHO grade II. By using dynamic evaluation of selected regions of the tumor, HGG and LGG could be distinguished with an accuracy of 70% to 90% in primary tumors and in recurrent tumors.[20,54-56,76,97] Furthermore, one study suggested that early static scans of FET uptake have a higher diagnostic accuracy for grading of gliomas than the standard 20 to 40 min scans, but this approach did not reach the accuracy of dynamic FET imaging.[98]

Although the prognostic value of ratios of amino acid uptake is controversial, some studies have reported that the BTV as assessed by amino acid PET at primary diagnosis is an independent prognostic factor.[21-23] Furthermore, textural parameters considering tumor heterogeneity might be an interesting approach to predict survival.[99]

More data on the prognostic value of amino acid PET are available for the subgroup of patients with LGG. In patients with LGG, longer survival has been reported for patients with a lower MET uptake in the tumors compared with those with a higher uptake.[100-103] Furthermore, the patients had a benefit from a surgical procedure only when an increased MET uptake was present.[100] By using FET PET, the combination with magnetic resonance (MR) morphology has also been found to be a significant prognostic predictor for patients with newly diagnosed LGG.[44] A baseline FET uptake and a circumscribed versus a diffuse growth pattern on MRI were highly significant predictors for the patients' clinical course and outcome. Thus, in patients with LGG, longer survival has been reported for patients with a lower amino acid uptake in the tumors compared with those with a higher uptake.[21-23,100-104]

Furthermore, as mentioned earlier, kinetic analyses of FET uptake in LGGs may be helpful in identifying areas of malignant transformation and poor prognosis.[20-23,69,74-77,100-104]

The Diagnosis of Tumor Recurrence/Progression

Conventional MRI has serious limitations in distinguishing recurrent glioma or metastases from nonspecific posttherapeutic changes, because pathologic contrast enhancement may reflect either regrowth of tumor or reactive changes after radiotherapy and/or chemotherapy.[105] The role of FDG PET in such cases is limited because of the frequency of nonspecific uptake.[106,107] Studies suggest that the specificity of FDG PET may be higher when PET CT is used.[108,109] Furthermore, contrast enhancement may be missing in recurrent LGGs and MRI cannot differentiate between tumor, edema, and nonspecific treatment-related changes. Multiple studies have shown that MET PET is highly sensitive in detecting recurrent gliomas but the specificity for the differentiation of vital tumor tissue from nonneoplastic changes is not optimal and in the range of 70% to 75%.[110-116] The accuracy of FET PET for the differentiation of tumor recurrence/progression from

nonneoplastic changes seems to be higher than that of MET PET. The lower specificity of MET may be explained by its higher affinity for macrophages compared with FET as demonstrated in animal experiments.[37,66] A sensitivity and specificity of FET PET for the detection of tumor recurrence/progression of 100% and 93%, respectively, have been reported compared with 93% and 50% for MRI alone.[117,118] Similar results have been reported for FDOPA.[119] A study of 124 patients with glioma demonstrated that the combined use of static and dynamic FET PET parameters differentiates progressive or recurrent glioma from treatment-related nonneoplastic changes with an accuracy of 93%.[5]

The role of amino acid PET has also been investigated in brain metastases because the differentiation of local recurrent brain metastasis from radiation-induced changes after radiotherapy using contrast-enhanced MRI alone is difficult. Similar to the results in recurrent gliomas, PET using MET has a moderate accuracy in differentiating recurrent metastatic brain tumor from radiation-induced changes, with a sensitivity and specificity of 70% to 80%.[113,120] The clinical usefulness of FET PET for the differentiation of local recurrent brain metastasis from radiation necrosis could be demonstrated in 31 patients with 40 metastases.[25] By using the tumor/brain ratios and the evaluation of FET kinetic studies, FET PET could differentiate local recurrent brain metastasis from radiation-induced changes with a high sensitivity (95%) and specificity (91%). By using FDOPA PET, a semiquantitative regions-of-interest analysis allowed the differentiation of recurrent or progressive brain metastasis from late or delayed radiation injury with a high sensitivity (81%) and specificity (84%).[121] One study reported on a sensitivity and specificity of FDOPA PET of more than 90% for differentiating radiation-induced changes from progressive disease in patients with brain metastases after stereotactic radiosurgery. In that study, FDOPA PET performed better than perfusion-weighted MRI.[59]

Treatment Monitoring

Imaging for radiologic response assessment in gliomas is based on serial measurements of T1- and T2-weighted MRI. Changes in apparent tumor size that are seen in MRI are taken as indicators of the response to therapy, but this approach is limited by the difficulty in distinguishing vital tumor tissue and unspecific treatment effects. FDG PET is considered not to be ideal to evaluate treatment response because of the high accumulation in nonspecific reactive changes in the tissue.[107] The feasibility and usefulness of MET, FDOPA, and FET PET for treatment assessment and follow-up after surgery, chemotherapy, and radiotherapy have been demonstrated in several studies. The currently available data suggest that a reduction of amino acid uptake of a glioma is a sign of a response to treatment. A prospective study investigating the prognostic value of early changes of FET uptake after postoperative radiochemotherapy (RCX) in patients with glioblastoma demonstrated that PET responders with a decrease of the tumor/brain ratio of more than 10% had a significantly longer disease-free survival and overall survival than patients with a stable or an increasing tracer uptake after RCX.[22,26] A reliable monitoring of temozolomide chemotherapy could also be demonstrated with MET in patients with recurrent HGG[42] and also in some experimental therapeutic approaches, such as radioimmunotherapy or convection-enhanced delivery of paclitaxel.[122,123] Furthermore, it has been shown that amino acid PET using FET is useful to assess failure of antiangiogenic treatment with bevacizumab earlier than MRI based on RANO criteria and to predict a favorable outcome of responders to bevacizumab.[28,124] A study including 30 patients reported that responders based on FDOPA PET data survived 3.5 times longer than nonresponders. In comparison, responders based on MRI data lived only 1.5 times longer than nonresponders.[125]

Alternative PET Tracers

The uptake of the proliferation marker [^{18}F]3′-deoxy-3′-fluorothymidine (FLT) is also correlated to the grade of malignancy and prognosis of cerebral gliomas,[126,127] but FLT is unable to identify the margin of gliomas because it is not able to pass the intact BBB and usually accumulates in areas with contrast enhancement on MRI only.[126,128–130] Furthermore, ^{11}C-choline or ^{18}F-fluorocholine has been used as a marker of cell membrane phospholipids in brain tumors and the uptake of these tracers correlates with the degree of malignancy in gliomas, but similar to FLT, choline derivatives are not able to pass the intact BBB.[131,132] Another interesting approach is to investigate the presence of intratumoral hypoxia using ^{18}F-fluoromisonidazole.[133–136] Hypoxia in tumors is a pathophysiologic consequence of structurally and functionally disturbed angiogenesis along with deterioration in the inability of oxygen to diffuse through tissues. A PET study in patients with cerebral gliomas demonstrated areas of hypoxia can differentiate glioblastomas from less malignant tumors.[137]

A promising target for brain tumor imaging is the mitochondrial translocator protein (TSPO), which is a component of the mitochondrial permeability transition pore and is strongly expressed by glioma cell lines.[138]

Formerly, TSPO ligands, such as ^{11}C-(R)PK11195, have been used mainly for PET imaging of inflammatory brain diseases as an indicator of microglial activation, but studies suggest a role of this method in the assessment of brain tumors as well.[139,140] One study has shown that TSPO expression may extend beyond the tumor margins in MRI and amino acid PET, indicating an infiltration zone that exhibited tumor progression in the further follow-up of the patients.[141] However, none of the PET methods mentioned earlier have found entry into clinical routine so far or proved superiority to amino acid PET imaging in brain tumor diagnosis.

Alternative MRI Approaches

Besides PET, functional or molecular MRI methods, such as perfusion-weighted imaging (PWI), diffusion-weighted imaging, and proton MR spectroscopy, can provide physiologic information beyond conventional MRI but have little molecular specificity.[142] It has been shown that PWI parameters correlated with the degree of malignancy of gliomas and seem to be useful in biopsy planning.[143] Proton MR spectroscopy (^{1}H-MRS) has been used for many years for the differential diagnosis of cerebral lesions of unknown type. Like amino acid imaging, ^{1}H-MRS yields metabolic information that is markedly more specific than that obtainable by conventional MRI for the differentiation of tumor tissue from nonspecific changes. The quality of the study can be impaired by susceptibility artifacts, a property that hampers the use of this method in patients with tumors in subcranial, frontobasal, or temporal locations or in patients who underwent surgery.[144] Although these advanced MRI methods are established and have been widely available for a long time, they are still not an integral part of the general guidelines. The fact that amino acid PET is widely used in centers that also have full access to the spectrum of functional and molecular MR methods emphasizes the additional value of amino acid PET beyond alternative MRI methods for brain tumor imaging.

TEACHING CASES

Case 1: Anaplastic Astrocytoma WHO Grade III

Findings

A 46-year-old female with a suspicious brain lesion. T1-weighted MRI (Fig. 12.1A) shows no pathologic contrast enhancement. T2-weighted MRI (Fig. 12.1B) shows widespread abnormalities in the frontal lobe. FET PET (Fig. 12.1C) identifies a tumor with a high tracer uptake in the right lower frontal lobe. Biopsy confirmed an anaplastic astrocytoma of the WHO grade III (Fig. 12.1).

Teaching points
- Amino acid PET can provide relevant additional information on the tumor extent of cerebral gliomas for therapy planning and biopsy guidance.
- Amino acids can pass the intact BBB and depict gliomas in brain areas showing no contrast enhancement in T1-weighted MRI.

Case 2: Diffuse Astrocytoma WHO Grade II
Findings
A 46-year-old female with suspicion of an LGG in the left frontal lobe. The lesion shows no contrast enhancement on T1-weighted MRI (Fig. 12.2A), widespread abnormalities in the T2-weighted MRI (Fig. 12.2B), and a low FDG uptake (Fig. 12.2C). FET PET (Fig. 12.2D) reveals an increased uptake and identifies a local maximum for biopsy guidance. A diffuse astrocytoma of the WHO grade II was confirmed by biopsy (Fig. 12.2).

Teaching points
- Amino acid PET is positive in 60% to 70% of LGGs and can improve biopsy guidance, whereas FDG PET is generally negative.
- Amino acids can pass the intact BBB and depict gliomas in brain areas showing no contrast enhancement in T1-weighted MRI.

Case 3: Radionecrosis
Findings
A patient with an anaplastic astrocytoma of the WHO grade III after brachytherapy with I-125 seeds, boost irradiation, and chemotherapy. Three years after the initiation of therapy the patient shows a ring-enhancing lesion in T1-weighted MRI (Fig. 12.3A), indicating tumor progression. FET PET (Fig. 12.3C) shows a low uptake in the lesion and increasing FET kinetics (Fig. 12.3D), which is consistent with treatment-related changes. A biopsy confirmed radionecrosis (Fig. 12.3).

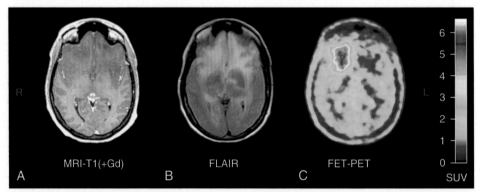

FIG. 12.1 T1-weighted MRI (A) showing no pathologic contrast enhancement. T2-weighted MRI FLAIR (B) shows widespread abnormalities in the frontal lobe. FET-PET (C) identifies a tumor with a high tracer uptake in the right lower frontal lobe.

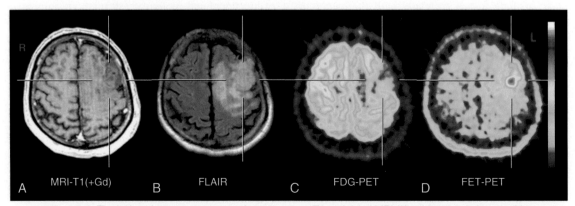

FIG. 12.2 The lesion shows no contrast enhancement on T1-weighted MRI (A), widespread abnormalities in the FLAIR MRI (B), and low FDG uptake (C). FET PET (D) reveals an increased uptake and identifies a local maximum for biopsy guidance.

Teaching points

- Amino acid PET has 90% accuracy in differentiating between recurrent tumor and treatment-related changes, such as radionecrosis. Dynamic FET PET helps to increase accuracy.
- A disruption of the BBB per se as indicated by contrast enhancement in T1-weighted MRI does not lead to an increased amino acid uptake.

Case 4: Glioblastoma (FDOPA PET)
Findings
A patient with a glioblastoma (WHO grade IV). T1-weighted MRI (Fig. 12.4A) shows a small area with contrast enhancement, and the T2-weighted MRI (Fig. 12.4B) shows diffuse signal abnormalities in the right hemisphere. FDOPA PET (Fig. 12.4C) identifies the tumor mass but differentiation from physiologic uptake in the striatum is difficult.

Teaching points

- FDOPA shows properties similar to those of MET or FET to depict brain tumors, but physiologic uptake in the striatum may disturb the proper delineation of brain tumors in the area of the striatum.
- FDOPA uptake in this glioblastoma demonstrates a considerably larger tumor extent as expected from the area of contrast enhancement in T1-weighted MRI.

Case 5: Glioblastoma (WHO Grade IV)
Findings
A patient with glioblastoma before and after RCX with concomitant temozolomide. One month after RCX (middle row), MRI (Fig. 12.5A and B) shows no major changes, whereas FET PET (Fig. 12.5C) indicates tumor response. Three months after the completion of RCX, MRI shows a ring-enhancing lesion (lower row), suggesting tumor progression, whereas FET PET indicates a responder with a decreasing amino acid uptake (Fig. 12.5).

Teaching points

- Amino acid PET can predict response to therapy earlier than MRI.
- Amino acid PET can help differentiate pseudoprogression from early tumor progression.

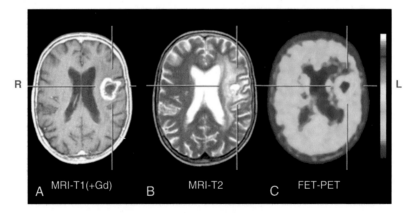

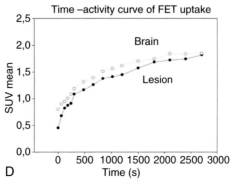

FIG. 12.3 Three years after the initiation of therapy the patient shows a ring-enhancing lesion in T1-weighted MRI (A), indicating tumor progression. FET PET (C) shows a low uptake in the lesion and increasing FET kinetics (D), which is consistent with treatment-related changes.

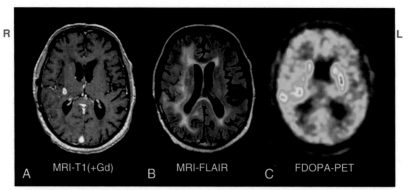

R ⎯ L

A MRI-T1(+Gd) B MRI-FLAIR C FDOPA-PET

FIG. 12.4 T1-weighted MRI (A) showing a small area with contrast enhancement and T2-weighted MRI (B) diffuse signal abnormalities in the right hemisphere. FDOPA PET (C) identifies the tumor mass but differentiation from physiologic uptake in the striatum is difficult.

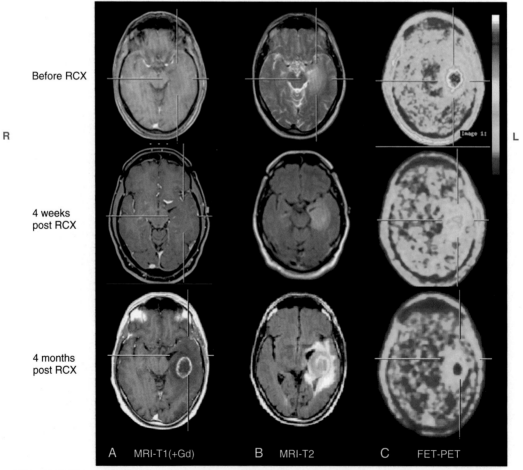

Before RCX

R ⎯ L

4 weeks post RCX

4 months post RCX

A MRI-T1(+Gd) B MRI-T2 C FET-PET

FIG. 12.5 One month after radiochemotherapy (RCX) (*middle row*), MRI (A and B) shows no major changes, whereas FET PET (C) indicates tumor response. Three months after the completion of RCX, MRI shows a ring-enhancing lesion (*bottom row*) suggesting tumor progression, whereas FET PET indicates a responder with decreasing amino acid uptake.

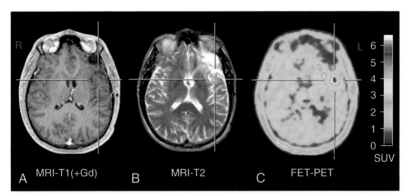

FIG. 12.6 T1-weighted MRI (A) shows no pathologic contrast enhancement. T2-weighted MRI shows widespread abnormalities (B) and is equivocal. FET PET (C) identifies an increased tracer uptake in the left temporal lobe. Tumor recurrence was confirmed histologically after resection.

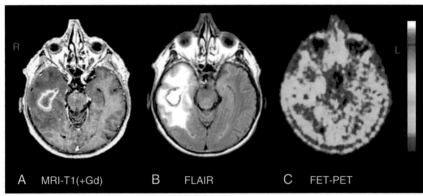

FIG. 12.7 A patient with a ring-enhancing lesion in the T1-weighted MRI (A) in the right temporal lobe and widespread abnormalities in the FLAIR MRI (B), which is highly suspicious for a glioblastoma or a brain metastasis. FET PET (C) shows a low tracer uptake, indicating a benign lesion. Biopsy yielded a brain abscess.

Case 6: Recurrent Anaplastic Oligoastrocytoma (WHO Grade III)

Findings

A patient with an anaplastic oligoastrocytoma (WHO grade III) after surgery followed by 10 cycles of chemotherapy with temozolomide. T1-weighted MRI (Fig. 12.6A) shows no pathologic contrast enhancement. T2-weighted MRI shows widespread abnormalities (Fig. 12.6B) and is equivocal. FET PET (Fig. 12.6C) identifies an increased tracer uptake in the left temporal lobe. Tumor recurrence was confirmed histologically after resection (Fig. 12.6).

Teaching points

- Amino acid PET has a high accuracy to differentiate recurrent tumor and treatment-related changes.
- Amino acid PET is especially helpful in recurrent tumors, showing no contrast enhancement in MRI.

Case 7: Brain Abscess

Findings

A patient with a ring-enhancing lesion in the T1-weighted MRI (Fig. 12.7A) and widespread abnormalities in the FLAIR MRI (B) in the right temporal lobe, which is highly suspicious for a glioblastoma or a brain metastasis. FET PET (Fig. 12.7C) shows a low tracer uptake, indicating a benign lesion. Biopsy yielded a brain abscess (Fig. 12.7).

Teaching points

- Amino acids usually exhibit a low uptake in brain abscesses and other inflammatory lesions, but false-positive cases with a moderately increased uptake have been reported.
- Again, a disruption of the BBB per se as indicated by contrast enhancement in T1-weighted MRI does not lead to an increased amino acid uptake.

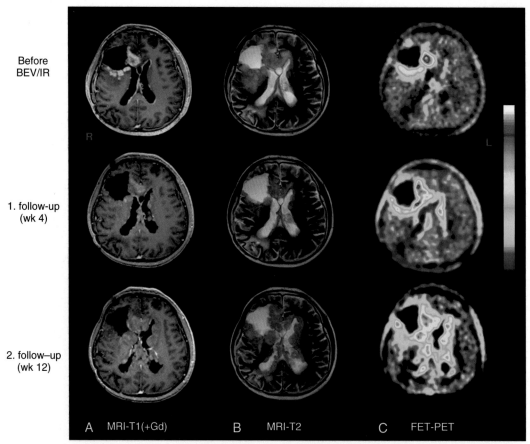

FIG. 12.8 The contrast-enhancing tumor (A) with an increased FET uptake (C) before therapy is shown in the upper row. After 4 weeks, bevacizumab and irinotecan (BEV/IR) MRI indicates partial response but FET PET indicates tumor progression, which is confirmed at the second follow-up.

Case 8: Pseudoresponse During Antiangiogenic Therapy

Findings

A patient with recurrent glioblastoma during antiangiogenic therapy with bevacizumab and irinotecan (BEV/IR). The contrast-enhancing tumor (Fig. 12.8A) with an increased FET uptake (Fig. 12.8C) before therapy is shown in the upper row. After 4 weeks, BEV/IR MRI indicates a partial response but FET PET indicates tumor progression, which is confirmed at the second follow-up (Fig. 12.8).

Teaching points

- Amino acid PET can detect pseudoresponse during antiangiogenic therapy, which is a frequent problem for conventional MRI.

- Treatment failure during antiangiogenic therapy can be detected up to 10 weeks earlier than with MRI and can help avoid ineffective treatment and side effects.

Case 9: Recurrent Brain Metastasis

Findings

A 50-year-old patient 16 months after stereotactic radiosurgery of a brain metastasis of malignant melanoma. T1-weighted MRI shows a contrast-enhancing lesion, which is equivocal for recurrent tumor or radionecrosis. FET uptake is increased, and the time–activity curve (early peak followed by a descent) is consistent with recurrent metastasis, which was confirmed by clinical course (Fig. 12.9).

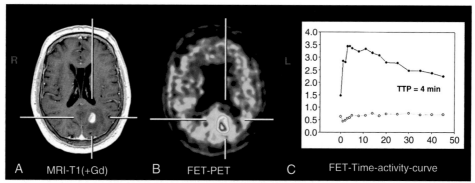

FIG. 12.9 T1-weighted MRI shows a contrast-enhancing lesion, which is equivocal for recurrent tumor or radionecrosis. FET uptake is increased, and the time–activity curve (early peak followed by a descent) is consistent with showing metastasis, which was confirmed by clinical course.

Status epilepticus with prolonged postictal left hemiparesis for 4 weeks

Nine weeks after seizure onset FET uptake has normalized

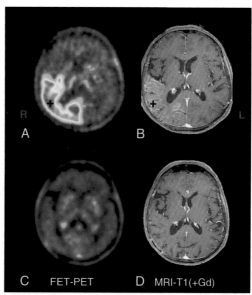

FIG. 12.10 FET PET (A) showed an increased uptake in the right temporoparietal cortex and contrast enhancement on T1-weighted MRI (B). Nine weeks after seizure onset and antiepileptic treatment, FET PET signal alterations completely resolved.

Teaching point

- Amino acid PET has a high accuracy in differentiating between recurrent metastasis and radiation injury after stereotactic radiosurgery.

Case 10: Pitfall Epilepsy
Findings

A 64-year-old female without residual tumor after treatment of a right frontal anaplastic astrocytoma WHO grade III developed a series of treatment-refractory motor partial seizures and a focal status epilepticus of the left arm and leg, followed by a severe and prolonged postictal left hemiparesis for 4 weeks. FET PET (Fig. 12.10A) showed an increased uptake in the right temporoparietal cortex and contrast enhancement on T1-weighted MRI (Fig. 12.10B). Nine weeks after seizure onset and antiepileptic treatment, FET PET signal alterations completely resolved (Fig. 12.10).

Teaching point

- An increased amino acid uptake caused by epileptic activity is a rare condition but needs to be considered in patients with treatment-refractory epilepsy.

CONCLUSION

Although FDG PET provides excellent results in imaging extracranial tumors, its use for brain tumor imaging is limited because of the poor tumor-to-background contrast. Meanwhile, a plethora of studies demonstrates that amino acid PET using established tracers, such as MET, FET, or FDOPA, may have substantial advantages over FDG and other tracers and adds valuable diagnostic information to that of conventional MRI in the assessment of patients with gliomas and other intracranial neoplasms. The benefits of amino acid PET over MRI for glioma imaging are manifold: better differentiation of equivocal lesions detected with MRI, prevention of inconclusive biopsies, improved targeting of surgery and radiotherapy to the true extent of the tumor so that healthy tissue is spared, differentiation between tumor progression and treatment-related changes so that overtreatment can be avoided, and early identification of tumor responses to therapy so that unnecessary adverse effects are avoided.[145] The RANO group recommends the use of amino acid PET at all stages of patient management: primary diagnosis, especially when MRI shows equivocal brain lesions; after diagnosis for defining the extent of the tumor to plan surgery and radiotherapy; in early treatment to differentiate between pseudoprogression and early tumor progression; at later stages of treatment for the identification of radionecrosis and treatment-related changes; and for monitoring of therapy.[6] The resulting improvement in diagnostic accuracy is expected to have patient-relevant benefits, particularly with respect to treatment planning and disease monitoring.

REFERENCES

1. Ostrom QT, Gittleman H, Liao P, et al. CBTRUS statistical report: primary brain and central nervous system tumors diagnosed in the United States in 2007–2011. *Neuro-oncology.* October 2014;16(suppl 4):iv1–iv63.
2. Nayak L, Lee EQ, Wen PY. Epidemiology of brain metastases. *Current Oncology Reports.* February 2012;14(1):48–54.
3. Alentorn A, Hoang-Xuan K, Mikkelsen T. Presenting signs and symptoms in brain tumors. *Handbook of Clinical Neurology.* 2016;134:19–26.
4. Rapp M, Heinzel A, Galldiks N, et al. Diagnostic performance of 18F-FET PET in newly diagnosed cerebral lesions suggestive of glioma. *Journal of Nuclear Medicine: Official Publication, Society of Nuclear Medicine.* February 2013;54(2):229–235.
5. Galldiks N, Stoffels G, Filss C, et al. The use of dynamic O-(2-18F-fluoroethyl)-L-tyrosine PET in the diagnosis of patients with progressive and recurrent glioma. *Neuro-oncology.* 2015;17:1293–1300.
6. Albert NL, Weller M, Suchorska B, et al. Response Assessment in Neuro-Oncology working group and European Association for Neuro-Oncology recommendations for the clinical use of PET imaging in gliomas. *Neuro-oncology.* 2016;18:1199–1208.
7. Weller M, van den Bent M, Hopkins K, et al. EANO guideline for the diagnosis and treatment of anaplastic gliomas and glioblastoma. *The Lancet Oncology.* August 2014;15(9):e395–e403.
8. Buckner JC, Shaw EG, Pugh SL, et al. Radiation plus Procarbazine, CCNU, and Vincristine in Low-Grade Glioma. *New England Journal of Medicine.* April 7, 2016;374(14):1344–1355.
9. van den Bent MJ, Brandes AA, Taphoorn MJ, et al. Adjuvant procarbazine, lomustine, and vincristine chemotherapy in newly diagnosed anaplastic oligodendroglioma: long-term follow-up of EORTC brain tumor group study 26951. *Journal of Clinical Oncology.* January 20, 2013;31(3):344–350.
10. Louis DN, Perry A, Reifenberger G, et al. The 2016 World Health Organization Classification of Tumors of the Central Nervous System: a summary. *Acta Neuropathologica.* June 2016;131(6):803–820.
11. Stupp R, Brada M, van den Bent MJ, Tonn JC, Pentheroudakis G. High-grade glioma: ESMO Clinical Practice Guidelines for diagnosis, treatment and follow-up. *Annals of Oncology.* September 2014;25(suppl 3):iii93–iii101.
12. Travis W, Colby T, Corrin B, Shimosato Y, Brambilla E. *WHO Histological Classification of Tumors: Histological Typing of Lung and Pleural Tumours.* 3rd ed. Berlin: Springer-Verlag; 1999.
13. Vander Borght T, Asenbaum S, Bartenstein P, et al. EANM procedure guidelines for brain tumour imaging using labelled amino acid analogues. *European Journal of Nuclear Medicine and Molecular Imaging.* November 2006;33(11):1374–1380.
14. Langen KJ, Bartenstein P, Boecker H, et al. German guidelines for brain tumour imaging by PET and SPECT using labelled amino acids. *Nuklearmedizin. Nuclear Medicine.* 2011;50(4):167–173.
15. Dunet V, Prior JO. Response to: performance of 18F-FET-PET versus 18F-FDG-PET for the diagnosis and grading of brain tumors: inherent bias in meta-analysis not revealed by quality metrics. *Neuro-oncology.* July 2016;18(7):1029–1030.
16. Kracht LW, Miletic H, Busch S, et al. Delineation of brain tumor extent with [11C]L-methionine positron emission tomography: local comparison with stereotactic histopathology. *Clinical Cancer Research: An Official Journal of the American Association for Cancer Research.* November 1, 2004;10(21):7163–7170.
17. Lopez WO, Cordeiro JG, Albicker U, et al. Correlation of 18F-fluoroethyl tyrosine positron-emission tomography uptake values and histomorphological findings by stereotactic serial biopsy in newly diagnosed brain tumors using a refined software tool. *OncoTargets and Therapy.* 2015;8:3803–3815.

18. Mosskin M, Ericson K, Hindmarsh T, et al. Positron emission tomography compared with magnetic resonance imaging and computed tomography in supratentorial gliomas using multiple stereotactic biopsies as reference. *Acta Radiology.* May-June 1989;30(3):225–232.

19. Pauleit D, Floeth F, Hamacher K, et al. O-(2-[18F] fluoroethyl)-L-tyrosine PET combined with MRI improves the diagnostic assessment of cerebral gliomas. *Brain: A Journal of Neurology.* March 2005;128(pt 3):678–687.

20. Jansen NL, Suchorska B, Wenter V, et al. Prognostic significance of dynamic 18F-FET PET in newly diagnosed astrocytic high-grade glioma. *Journal of Nuclear Medicine: Official Publication, Society of Nuclear Medicine.* January 2015;56(1):9–15.

21. Galldiks N, Dunkl V, Kracht LW, et al. Volumetry of [11C]-methionine positron emission tomographic uptake as a prognostic marker before treatment of patients with malignant glioma. *Molecular Imaging.* November-December 2012;11(6):516–527.

22. Piroth MD, Pinkawa M, Holy R, et al. Prognostic value of early [18F]fluoroethyltyrosine positron emission tomography after radiochemotherapy in glioblastoma multiforme. *International Journal of Radiation Oncology, Biology, Physics.* May 1, 2011;80(1):176–184.

23. Suchorska B, Jansen NL, Linn J, et al. Biological tumor volume in 18FET-PET before radiochemotherapy correlates with survival in GBM. *Neurology.* February 17, 2015;84(7):710–719.

24. Galldiks N, Dunkl V, Stoffels G, et al. Diagnosis of pseudoprogression in patients with glioblastoma using O-(2-[18F]fluoroethyl)-L-tyrosine PET. *European Journal of Nuclear Medicine and Molecular Imaging.* April 2015;42(5):685–695.

25. Galldiks N, Stoffels G, Filss CP, et al. Role of O-(2-18F-fluoroethyl)-L-tyrosine PET for differentiation of local recurrent brain metastasis from radiation necrosis. *Journal of Nuclear Medicine: Official Publication, Society of Nuclear Medicine.* 2012;53:1367–1374.

26. Galldiks N, Langen K, Holy R, et al. Assessment of treatment response in patients with glioblastoma using [18F] Fluoroethyl-L-Tyrosine PET in comparison to MRI. *Journal of Nuclear Medicine: Official Publication, Society of Nuclear Medicine.* 2012;53:1048–1057.

27. Galldiks N, Rapp M, Stoffels G, et al. Response assessment of bevacizumab in patients with recurrent malignant glioma using [18F]Fluoroethyl-L-tyrosine PET in comparison to MRI. *European Journal of Nuclear Medicine and Molecular Imaging.* January 2013;40(1): 22–33.

28. Hutterer M, Nowosielski M, Putzer D, et al. O-(2-18F-fluoroethyl)-L-tyrosine PET predicts failure of antiangiogenic treatment in patients with recurrent high-grade glioma. *Journal of Nuclear Medicine: Official Publication, Society of Nuclear Medicine.* June 2011;52(6):856–864.

29. Heinzel A, Muller D, Langen KJ, et al. The use of O-(2-18F-fluoroethyl)-L-tyrosine PET for treatment management of bevacizumab and irinotecan in patients with recurrent high-grade glioma: a cost-effectiveness analysis. *Journal of Nuclear Medicine: Official Publication, Society of Nuclear Medicine.* August 2013;54(8):1217–1222.

30. Heinzel A, Stock S, Langen KJ, Muller D. Cost-effectiveness analysis of FET PET-guided target selection for the diagnosis of gliomas. *European Journal of Nuclear Medicine and Molecular Imaging.* July 2012;39(7):1089–1096.

31. Heinzel A, Stock S, Langen KJ, Muller D. Cost-effectiveness analysis of amino acid PET-guided surgery for supratentorial high-grade gliomas. *Journal of Nuclear Medicine: Official Publication, Society of Nuclear Medicine.* April 2012;53(4):552–558.

32. Floeth FW, Pauleit D, Sabel M, et al. 18F-FET PET differentiation of ring-enhancing brain lesions. *Journal of Nuclear Medicine: Official Publication, Society of Nuclear Medicine.* May 2006;47(5):776–782.

33. Hutterer M, Nowosielski M, Putzer D, et al. [F-18]-fluoro-ethyl-L-tyrosine PET: a valuable diagnostic tool in neuro-oncology, but not all that glitters is glioma. *Neuro-oncology.* March 2013;15(3):341–351.

34. Pichler R, Dunzinger A, Wurm G, et al. Is there a place for FET PET in the initial evaluation of brain lesions with unknown significance? *European Journal of Nuclear Medicine and Molecular Imaging.* August 2010;37(8):1521–1528.

35. Salber D, Stoffels G, Oros-Peusquens AM, et al. Comparison of O-(2-18F-fluoroethyl)-L-tyrosine and L-3H-methionine uptake in cerebral hematomas. *Journal of Nuclear Medicine: Official Publication, Society of Nuclear Medicine.* May 2010;51(5):790–797.

36. Ogawa T, Hatazawa J, Inugami A, et al. Carbon-11-methionine PET evaluation of intracerebral hematoma: distinguishing neoplastic from non-neoplastic hematoma. *Journal of Nuclear Medicine: Official Publication, Society of Nuclear Medicine.* December 1995;36(12): 2175–2179.

37. Salber D, Stoffels G, Pauleit D, et al. Differential uptake of [18F]FET and [3H]L-methionine in focal cortical ischemia. *Nuclear Medicine and Biology.* November 2006;33(8):1029–1035.

38. Hutterer MGN, Hau P, Langen KJ. Pitfalls of [F18]-FET PET in the diagnostics of brain tumors. *Der Nuklearmediziner.* 2015;38:1–9.

39. Chen W. Clinical applications of PET in brain tumors. *Journal of Nuclear Medicine: Official Publication, Society of Nuclear Medicine.* September 2007;48(9):1468–1481.

40. Padma MV, Said S, Jacobs M, et al. Prediction of pathology and survival by FDG PET in gliomas. *Journal of Neuro-oncology.* September 2003;64(3):227–237.

41. Yoon JH, Kim JH, Kang WJ, et al. Grading of cerebral glioma with multiparametric MR imaging and 18F-FDG-PET: concordance and accuracy. *European Radiology.* February 2014;24(2):380–389.

42. Galldiks N, Langen KJ. Applications of PET imaging of neurological tumors with radiolabeled amino acids. *The Quarterly Journal of Nuclear Medicine and Molecular Imaging.* March 2015;59(1):70–82.

43. Bette S, Gempt J, Delbridge C, et al. Prognostic Value of O-[2-[18F]-Fluoroethyl]-L-Tyrosine-Positron Emission Tomography Imaging for Histopathologic Characteristics and Progression-Free Survival in Patients with Low-Grade Glioma. *World Neurosurgery.* May 2016;89:230–239.

44. Floeth FW, Pauleit D, Sabel M, et al. Prognostic value of O-(2-18F-fluoroethyl)-L-tyrosine PET and MRI in low-grade glioma. *Journal of Nuclear Medicine: Official Publication, Society of Nuclear Medicine.* April 2007;48(4):519–527.

45. Okubo S, Zhen HN, Kawai N, Nishiyama Y, Haba R, Tamiya T. Correlation of L-methyl-11C-methionine (MET) uptake with L-type amino acid transporter 1 in human gliomas. *Journal of Neuro-oncology.* September 2010;99(2):217–225.

46. Wiriyasermkul P, Nagamori S, Tominaga H, et al. Transport of 3-fluoro-L-alpha-methyl-tyrosine by tumor-upregulated L-type amino acid transporter 1: a cause of the tumor uptake in PET. *Journal of Nuclear Medicine: Official Publication, Society of Nuclear Medicine.* August 2012;53(8):1253–1261.

47. Youland RS, Kitange GJ, Peterson TE, et al. The role of LAT1 in 18F-DOPA uptake in malignant gliomas. *Journal of Neuro-oncology.* January 2013;111(1):11–18.

48. Papin-Michault C, Bonnetaud C, Dufour M, et al. Study of LAT1 Expression in Brain Metastases: Towards a Better Understanding of the Results of Positron Emission Tomography Using Amino Acid Tracers. *PLoS One.* 2016;11(6):e0157139.

49. Habermeier A, Graf J, Sandhofer BF, Boissel JP, Roesch F, Closs EI. System L amino acid transporter LAT1 accumulates O-(2-fluoroethyl)-L-tyrosine (FET). *Amino Acids.* February 2015;47(2):335–344.

50. Grosu AL, Astner ST, Riedel E, et al. An interindividual comparison of O-(2- [18F]fluoroethyl)-L-tyrosine (FET)- and L-[methyl-11C]methionine (MET)-PET in patients with brain gliomas and metastases. *International Journal of Radiation Oncology, Biology, Physics.* November 15, 2011;81(4):1049–1058.

51. Becherer A, Karanikas G, Szabo M, et al. Brain tumour imaging with PET: a comparison between [18F]fluorodopa and [11C]methionine. *European Journal of Nuclear Medicine and Molecular Imaging.* November 2003;30(11):1561–1567.

52. Kratochwil C, Combs SE, Leotta K, et al. Intra-individual comparison of 18F-FET and 18F-DOPA in PET imaging of recurrent brain tumors. *Neuro-oncology.* March 2014;16(3):434–440.

53. Weber WA, Wester HJ, Grosu AL, et al. O-(2-[18F]fluoroethyl)-L-tyrosine and L-[methyl-11C]methionine uptake in brain tumours: initial results of a comparative study. *European Journal of Nuclear Medicine.* May 2000;27(5):542–549.

54. Calcagni ML, Galli G, Giordano A, et al. Dynamic O-(2-[18F]fluoroethyl)-L-tyrosine (F-18 FET) PET for glioma grading: assessment of individual probability of malignancy. *Clinical Nuclear Medicine.* October 2011;36(10):841–847.

55. Popperl G, Kreth FW, Mehrkens JH, et al. FET PET for the evaluation of untreated gliomas: correlation of FET uptake and uptake kinetics with tumour grading. *European Journal of Nuclear Medicine and Molecular Imaging.* December 2007;34(12):1933–1942.

56. Weckesser M, Langen KJ, Rickert CH, et al. O-(2-[18F]fluoroethyl)-L-tyrosine PET in the clinical evaluation of primary brain tumours. *European Journal of Nuclear Medicine and Molecular Imaging.* April 2005;32(4):422–429.

57. Moulin-Romsee G, D'Hondt E, de Groot T, et al. Non-invasive grading of brain tumours using dynamic amino acid PET imaging: does it work for 11C-methionine? *European Journal of Nuclear Medicine and Molecular Imaging.* December 2007;34(12):2082–2087.

58. Sioka C, Fotopoulos A, Kyritsis AP. Recent advances in PET imaging for evaluation of Parkinson's disease. *European Journal of Nuclear Medicine and Molecular Imaging.* August 2010;37(8):1594–1603.

59. Cicone F, Filss CP, Minniti G, et al. Volumetric assessment of recurrent or progressive gliomas: comparison between F-DOPA PET and perfusion-weighted MRI. *European Journal of Nuclear Medicine and Molecular Imaging.* May 2015;42(6):905–915.

60. Singhal T, Narayanan TK, Jain V, Mukherjee J, Mantil J. 11C-L-methionine positron emission tomography in the clinical management of cerebral gliomas. *Molecular Imaging and Biology: MIB: The Official Publication of the Academy of Molecular Imaging.* January-February 2008;10(1):1–18.

61. Langen KJ, Hamacher K, Weckesser M, et al. O-(2-[18F]fluoroethyl)-L-tyrosine: uptake mechanisms and clinical applications. *Nuclear Medicine and Biology.* April 2006;33(3):287–294.

62. Wester HJ, Herz M, Weber W, et al. Synthesis and radiopharmacology of O-(2-[18F]fluoroethyl)-L-tyrosine for tumor imaging. *Journal of Nuclear Medicine: Official Publication, Society of Nuclear Medicine.* January 1999;40(1):205–212.

63. Hamacher K, Coenen HH. Efficient routine production of the 18F-labelled amino acid O-2-18F fluoroethyl-L-tyrosine. *Applied Radiation and Isotopes: Including Data, Instrumentation and Methods for Use in Agriculture, Industry and Medicine.* December 2002;57(6):853–856.

64. Swiss Agency for Therapeutic Products (Swissmedic). *Journal Swissmedic.* 2014;13:651.

65. Sala Q, Metellus P, Taieb D, Kaphan E, Figarella-Branger D, Guedj E. 18F-DOPA, a clinically available PET tracer to study brain inflammation? *Clinical Nuclear Medicine.* April 2014;39(4):e283–e285.

66. Salber D, Stoffels G, Pauleit D, et al. Differential uptake of O-(2-^{18}F-fluoroethyl)-L-tyrosine, L-^{3}H-methionine, and ^{3}H-deoxyglucose in brain abscesses. *Journal of Nuclear Medicine: Official Publication, Society of Nuclear Medicine*. December 2007;48(12):2056–2062.

67. Dunet V, Rossier C, Buck A, Stupp R, Prior JO. Performance of ^{18}F-fluoro-ethyl-tyrosine (^{18}F-FET) PET for the differential diagnosis of primary brain tumor: a systematic review and meta-analysis. *Journal of Nuclear Medicine: Official Publication, Society of Nuclear Medicine*. February 2012;53(2):207–214.

68. Herholz K, Holzer T, Bauer B, et al. ^{11}C-methionine PET for differential diagnosis of low-grade gliomas. *Neurology*. May 1998;50(5):1316–1322.

69. Unterrainer M, Schweisthal F, Suchorska B, et al. Serial ^{18}F-FET PET imaging of primarily ^{18}F-FET-negative glioma - does it make sense? *Journal of Nuclear Medicine: Official Publication, Society of Nuclear Medicine*. March 31, 2016.

70. Dunet V, Pomoni A, Hottinger A, Nicod-Lalonde M, Prior JO. Performance of ^{18}F-FET versus ^{18}F-FDG-PET for the diagnosis and grading of brain tumors: systematic review and meta-analysis. *Neuro-oncology*. March 2016;18(3):426–434.

71. Pauleit D, Stoffels G, Bachofner A, et al. Comparison of ^{18}F-FET and ^{18}F-FDG PET in brain tumors. *Nuclear Medicine and Biology*. October 2009;36(7):779–787.

72. Pirotte B, Goldman S, Massager N, et al. Combined use of ^{18}F-fluorodeoxyglucose and ^{11}C-methionine in 45 positron emission tomography-guided stereotactic brain biopsies. *Journal of Neurosurgery*. September 2004;101(3):476–483.

73. Plotkin M, Blechschmidt C, Auf G, et al. Comparison of F-18 FET-PET with F-18 FDG-PET for biopsy planning of non-contrast-enhancing gliomas. *European Radiology*. October 2010;20(10):2496–2502.

74. Galldiks N, Stoffels G, Ruge MI, et al. Role of O-(2-^{18}F-fluoroethyl)-L-tyrosine PET as a diagnostic tool for detection of malignant progression in patients with low-grade glioma. *Journal of Nuclear Medicine: Official Publication, Society of Nuclear Medicine*. December 2013;54(12):2046–2054.

75. Jansen NL, Suchorska B, Wenter V, et al. Dynamic ^{18}F-FET PET in newly diagnosed astrocytic low-grade glioma identifies high-risk patients. *Journal of Nuclear Medicine: Official Publication, Society of Nuclear Medicine*. February 2014;55(2):198–203.

76. Kunz M, Thon N, Eigenbrod S, et al. Hot spots in dynamic [18]FET-PET delineate malignant tumor parts within suspected WHO grade II gliomas. *Neuro-oncology*. March 2011;13(3):307–316.

77. Thon N, Kunz M, Lemke L, et al. Dynamic F-FET PET in suspected WHO grade II gliomas defines distinct biological subgroups with different clinical courses. *International Journal of Cancer*. May 2015;136:2132–2145.

78. Kracht LW, Friese M, Herholz K, et al. Methyl-[^{11}C]-l-methionine uptake as measured by positron emission tomography correlates to microvessel density in patients with glioma. *European Journal of Nuclear Medicine and Molecular Imaging*. June 2003;30(6):868–873.

79. Pauleit D, Stoffels G, Schaden W, et al. PET with O-(2-^{18}F-fluoroethyl)-L-tyrosine in peripheral tumors: first clinical results. *Journal of Nuclear Medicine: Official Publication, Society of Nuclear Medicine*. 2005;46:411–416.

80. Pirotte BJ, Levivier M, Goldman S, et al. Positron emission tomography-guided volumetric resection of supratentorial high-grade gliomas: a survival analysis in 66 consecutive patients. *Neurosurgery*. March 2009;64(3):471–481. discussion 481.

81. Buchmann N, Klasner B, Gempt J, et al. ^{18}F-Fluoroethyl-l-Thyrosine Positron Emission Tomography to Delineate Tumor Residuals After Glioblastoma Resection: A Comparison with Standard Postoperative Magnetic Resonance Imaging. *World Neurosurgery*. May 2016;89:420–426.

82. Grosu AL, Weber WA. PET for radiation treatment planning of brain tumours. *Radiotherapy and Oncology: Journal of the European Society for Therapeutic Radiology and Oncology*. September 2010;96(3):325–327.

83. Munck Af Rosenschold P, Costa J, Engelholm SA, et al. Impact of [^{18}F]-fluoro-ethyl-tyrosine PET imaging on target definition for radiation therapy of high-grade glioma. *Neuro-oncology*. May 2015;17(5):757–763.

84. Piroth MD, Pinkawa M, Holy R, et al. Integrated boost IMRT with FET-PET-adapted local dose escalation in glioblastomas. Results of a prospective phase II study. *Strahlentherapie und Onkologie: Organ der Deutschen Rontgengesellschaft… [et al]*. 2012;188:334–339.

85. Grosu AL, Weber WA, Franz M, et al. Reirradiation of recurrent high-grade gliomas using amino acid PET (SPECT)/CT/MRI image fusion to determine gross tumor volume for stereotactic fractionated radiotherapy. *International Journal of Radiation Oncology, Biology, Physics*. October 1, 2005;63(2):511–519.

86. Levivier M, Massager N, Wikler D, et al. Use of stereotactic PET images in dosimetry planning of radiosurgery for brain tumors: clinical experience and proposed classification. *Journal of Nuclear Medicine: Official Publication, Society of Nuclear Medicine*. July 2004;45(7):1146–1154.

87. Piroth MD, Pinkawa M, Holy R, et al. Integrated-boost IMRT or 3-D-CRT using FET-PET based auto-contoured target volume delineation for glioblastoma multiforme– a dosimetric comparison. *Radiation Oncology*. 2009;4:57.

88. Rickhey M, Koelbl O, Eilles C, Bogner L. A biologically adapted dose-escalation approach, demonstrated for ^{18}F-FET-PET in brain tumors. *Strahlentherapie und Onkologie: Organ der Deutschen Rontgengesellschaft… [et al]*. October 2008;184(10):536–542.

89. Rieken S, Habermehl D, Giesel FL, et al. Analysis of FET-PET imaging for target volume definition in patients with gliomas treated with conformal radiotherapy. *Radiotherapy and Oncology: Journal of the European Society for Therapeutic Radiology and Oncology*. December 2013;109(3):487–492.

90. Weber DC, Zilli T, Buchegger F, et al. [^{18}F]Fluoroethyltyrosine-positron emission tomography-guided radiotherapy for high-grade glioma. *Radiation Oncology*. 2008;3:44.

91. Delbeke D, Meyerowitz C, Lapidus RL, et al. Optimal cutoff levels of F-18 fluorodeoxyglucose uptake in the differentiation of low-grade from high-grade brain tumors with PET. *Radiology.* April 1995;195(1):47–52.

92. Kim S, Chung JK, Im SH, et al. ^{11}C-methionine PET as a prognostic marker in patients with glioma: comparison with ^{18}F-FDG PET. *European Journal of Nuclear Medicine and Molecular Imaging.* January 2005;32(1):52–59.

93. Miyake K, Shinomiya A, Okada M, Hatakeyama T, Kawai N, Tamiya T. Usefulness of FDG, MET and FLT-PET studies for the management of human gliomas. *Journal of Biomedicine & Biotechnology.* 2012;2012:205818.

94. Manabe O, Hattori N, Yamaguchi S, et al. Oligodendroglial component complicates the prediction of tumour grading with metabolic imaging. *European Journal of Nuclear Medicine and Molecular Imaging.* May 2015;42(6): 896–904.

95. Stockhammer F, Plotkin M, Amthauer H, van Landeghem FK, Woiciechowsky C. Correlation of F-18-fluoro-ethyltyrosine uptake with vascular and cell density in non-contrast-enhancing gliomas. *Journal of Neuro-oncology.* June 2008;88(2):205–210.

96. Wyss MT, Hofer S, Hefti M, et al. Spatial heterogeneity of low-grade gliomas at the capillary level: a PET study on tumor blood flow and amino acid uptake. *Journal of Nuclear Medicine: Official Publication, Society of Nuclear Medicine.* July 2007;48(7):1047–1052.

97. Popperl G, Kreth FW, Herms J, et al. Analysis of ^{18}F-FET PET for grading of recurrent gliomas: is evaluation of uptake kinetics superior to standard methods? *Journal of Nuclear Medicine: Official Publication, Society of Nuclear Medicine.* March 2006;47(3):393–403.

98. Albert NL, Winkelmann I, Suchorska B, et al. Early static ^{18}F-FET-PET scans have a higher accuracy for glioma grading than the standard 20–40 min scans. *European Journal of Nuclear Medicine and Molecular Imaging.* June 2016;43(6):1105–1114.

99. Pyka T, Gempt J, Hiob D, et al. Textural analysis of pretherapeutic [^{18}F]-FET-PET and its correlation with tumor grade and patient survival in high-grade gliomas. *European Journal of Nuclear Medicine and Molecular Imaging.* January 2016;43:133–141.

100. Ribom D, Eriksson A, Hartman M, et al. Positron emission tomography ^{11}C-methionine and survival in patients with low-grade gliomas. *Cancer.* September 15, 2001;92(6):1541–1549.

101. Smits A, Baumert BG. The clinical value of PET with amino acid tracers for gliomas WHO grade II. *International Journal of Molecular Imaging.* 2011;2011:372509.

102. Smits A, Westerberg E, Ribom D. Adding ^{11}C-methionine PET to the EORTC prognostic factors in grade 2 gliomas. *European Journal of Nuclear Medicine and Molecular Imaging.* January 2008;35(1):65–71.

103. Arbizu J, Tejada S, Marti-Climent JM, et al. Quantitative volumetric analysis of gliomas with sequential MRI and ^{11}C-methionine PET assessment: patterns of integration in therapy planning. *European Journal of Nuclear Medicine and Molecular Imaging.* May 2012;39:771–781.

104. Villani V, Carapella CM, Chiaravalloti A, et al. The role of PET [^{18}F]FDOPA in evaluating low-grade glioma. *Anticancer Research.* September 2015;35(9):5117–5122.

105. Brandsma D, van den Bent MJ. Pseudoprogression and pseudoresponse in the treatment of gliomas. *Current Opinion in Neurology.* December 2009;22(6):633–638.

106. Ricci PE, Karis JP, Heiserman JE, Fram EK, Bice AN, Drayer BP. Differentiating recurrent tumor from radiation necrosis: time for re-evaluation of positron emission tomography? *AJNR. American Journal of Neuroradiology.* March 1998;19(3):407–413.

107. Basu S, Alavi A. Molecular imaging (PET) of brain tumors. *Neuroimaging Clinics of North America.* November 2009;19(4):625–646.

108. Tripathi M, Sharma R, Varshney R, et al. Comparison of F-18 FDG and C-11 methionine PET/CT for the evaluation of recurrent primary brain tumors. *Clinical Nuclear Medicine.* February 2012;37(2):158–163.

109. Santra A, Kumar R, Sharma P, et al. F-18 FDG PET-CT in patients with recurrent glioma: comparison with contrast enhanced MRI. *European Journal of Radiology.* March 2012;81(3):508–513.

110. Crippa F, Alessi A, Serafini GL. PET with radiolabeled aminoacid. *The Quarterly Journal of Nuclear Medicine and Molecular Imaging.* April 2012;56(2):151–162.

111. Minamimoto R, Saginoya T, Kondo C, et al. Differentiation of Brain Tumor Recurrence from Post-Radiotherapy Necrosis with ^{11}C-Methionine PET: Visual Assessment versus Quantitative Assessment. *PLoS One.* 2015;10(7):e0132515.

112. Nihashi T, Dahabreh IJ, Terasawa T. Diagnostic accuracy of PET for recurrent glioma diagnosis: a meta-analysis. *AJNR. American Journal of Neuroradiology.* May 2013;34(5):944–950. S941-S911.

113. Terakawa Y, Tsuyuguchi N, Iwai Y, et al. Diagnostic accuracy of ^{11}C-methionine PET for differentiation of recurrent brain tumors from radiation necrosis after radiotherapy. *Journal of Nuclear Medicine: Official Publication, Society of Nuclear Medicine.* May 2008;49(5):694–699.

114. Tsuyuguchi N, Takami T, Sunada I, et al. Methionine positron emission tomography for differentiation of recurrent brain tumor and radiation necrosis after stereotactic radiosurgery–in malignant glioma. *Annals of Nuclear Medicine.* June 2004;18(4):291–296.

115. Ullrich RT, Kracht L, Brunn A, et al. Methyl-L-^{11}C-methionine PET as a diagnostic marker for malignant progression in patients with glioma. *Journal of Nuclear Medicine: Official Publication, Society of Nuclear Medicine.* December 2009;50(12):1962–1968.

116. Van Laere K, Ceyssens S, Van Calenbergh F, et al. Direct comparison of ^{18}F-FDG and ^{11}C-methionine PET in suspected recurrence of glioma: sensitivity, inter-observer variability and prognostic value. *European Journal of Nuclear Medicine and Molecular Imaging.* January 2005;32(1):39–51.

117. Popperl G, Gotz C, Rachinger W, Gildehaus FJ, Tonn JC, Tatsch K. Value of O-(2-[^{18}F]fluoroethyl)-L-tyrosine PET for the diagnosis of recurrent glioma. *European Journal of Nuclear Medicine and Molecular Imaging.* November 2004;31(11):1464–1470.

118. Rachinger W, Goetz C, Popperl G, et al. Positron emission tomography with O-(2-[¹⁸F]fluoroethyl)-L-tyrosine versus magnetic resonance imaging in the diagnosis of recurrent gliomas. *Neurosurgery.* September 2005;57(3):505–511. discussion 505–511.

119. Karunanithi S, Sharma P, Kumar A, et al. ¹⁸F-FDOPA PET/CT for detection of recurrence in patients with glioma: prospective comparison with ¹⁸F-FDG PET/CT. *European Journal of Nuclear Medicine and Molecular Imaging.* July 2013;40(7):1025–1035.

120. Tsuyuguchi N, Sunada I, Iwai Y, et al. Methionine positron emission tomography of recurrent metastatic brain tumor and radiation necrosis after stereotactic radiosurgery: is a differential diagnosis possible? *Journal of Neurosurgery.* May 2003;98(5):1056–1064.

121. Lizarraga KJ, Allen-Auerbach M, Czernin J, et al. ¹⁸F-FDOPA PET for differentiating recurrent or progressive brain metastatic tumors from late or delayed radiation injury after radiation treatment. *Journal of Nuclear Medicine: Official Publication, Society of Nuclear Medicine.* January 2014;55(1):30–36.

122. Popperl G, Goldbrunner R, Gildehaus FJ, et al. O-(2-[¹⁸F]fluoroethyl)-L-tyrosine PET for monitoring the effects of convection-enhanced delivery of paclitaxel in patients with recurrent glioblastoma. *European Journal of Nuclear Medicine and Molecular Imaging.* September 2005;32(9):1018–1025.

123. Popperl G, Gotz C, Rachinger W, et al. Serial O-(2-[¹⁸F]fluoroethyl)-L- -tyrosine PET for monitoring the effects of intracavitary radioimmunotherapy in patients with malignant glioma. *European Journal of Nuclear Medicine and Molecular Imaging.* July 2006;33(7): 792–800.

124. Galldiks N, Rapp M, Stoffels G, Dunkl V, Sabel M, Langen KJ. Earlier diagnosis of progressive disease during bevacizumab treatment using O-(2-¹⁸F-fluorethyl)-L-tyrosine positron emission tomography in comparison with magnetic resonance imaging. *Molecular Imaging.* August 1, 2013;12(5):273–276.

125. Schwarzenberg J, Czernin J, Cloughesy TF, et al. Treatment response evaluation using ¹⁸F-FDOPA PET in patients with recurrent malignant glioma on bevacizumab therapy. *Clinical Cancer Research: An Official Journal of the American Association for Cancer Research.* July 1, 2014;20(13):3550–3559.

126. Chen W, Cloughesy T, Kamdar N, et al. Imaging proliferation in brain tumors with ¹⁸F-FLT PET: comparison with ¹⁸F-FDG. *Journal of Nuclear Medicine: Official Publication, Society of Nuclear Medicine.* June 2005;46(6):945–952.

127. Collet S, Valable S, Constans JM, et al. [¹⁸F]-fluoro-L-thymidine PET and advanced MRI for preoperative grading of gliomas. *NeuroImage. Clinical.* 2015;8:448–454.

128. Hatakeyama T, Kawai N, Nishiyama Y, et al. ¹¹C-methionine (MET) and ¹⁸F-fluorothymidine (FLT) PET in patients with newly diagnosed glioma. *European Journal of Nuclear Medicine and Molecular Imaging.* November 2008;35(11):2009–2017.

129. Jacobs AH, Thomas A, Kracht LW, et al. ¹⁸F-fluoro-L-thymidine and ¹¹C-methylmethionine as markers of increased transport and proliferation in brain tumors. *Journal of Nuclear Medicine: Official Publication, Society of Nuclear Medicine.* December 2005;46(12):1948–1958.

130. Nowosielski M, DiFranco MD, Putzer D, et al. An intra-individual comparison of MRI, [¹⁸F]-FET and [¹⁸F]-FLT PET in patients with high-grade gliomas. *PLoS One.* 2014;9(4):e95830.

131. Ohtani T, Kurihara H, Ishiuchi S, et al. Brain tumour imaging with carbon-11 choline: comparison with FDG PET and gadolinium-enhanced MR imaging. *European Journal of Nuclear Medicine.* November 2001;28(11):1664–1670.

132. Sollini M, Sghedoni R, Erba PA, et al. Diagnostic performances of [¹⁸F]fluorocholine positron emission tomography in brain tumors. *The Quarterly Journal of Nuclear Medicine and Molecular Imaging.* September 1, 2015.

133. Kobayashi H, Hirata K, Yamaguchi S, Terasaka S, Shiga T, Houkin K. Usefulness of FMISO-PET for glioma analysis. *Neurologia medico-chirurgica.* 2013;53(11):773–778.

134. Koh WJ, Rasey JS, Evans ML, et al. Imaging of hypoxia in human tumors with [F-18]fluoromisonidazole. *International Journal of Radiation Oncology, Biology, Physics.* 1992;22(1):199–212.

135. Gerstner E, Zhang Z, Fink J, et al. ACRIN 6684: assessment of tumor hypoxia in newly diagnosed GBM using ¹⁸F-FMISO PET and MRI. *Clinical Cancer Research: An Official Journal of the American Association for Cancer Research.* October 2016;22:5079–5086.

136. Toyonaga T, Hirata K, Yamaguchi S, et al. F-fluoromisonidazole positron emission tomography can predict pathological necrosis of brain tumors. *European Journal of Nuclear Medicine and Molecular Imaging.* July 2016;43:1469–1476.

137. Hirata K, Terasaka S, Shiga T, et al. ¹⁸F-Fluoromisonidazole positron emission tomography may differentiate glioblastoma multiforme from less malignant gliomas. *European Journal of Nuclear Medicine and Molecular Imaging.* May 2012;39(5):760–770.

138. Winkeler A, Boisgard R, Awde AR, et al. The translocator protein ligand [¹⁸F]DPA-714 images glioma and activated microglia in vivo. *European Journal of Nuclear Medicine and Molecular Imaging.* May 2012;39(5):811–823.

139. Roncaroli F, Su Z, Herholz K, Gerhard A, Turkheimer FE. TSPO expression in brain tumours: is TSPO a target for brain tumour imaging? *Clinical and Translational Imaging.* 2016;4:145–156.

140. Su Z, Roncaroli F, Durrenberger PF, et al. The 18-kDa mitochondrial translocator protein in human gliomas: an ¹¹C-(R)PK11195 PET imaging and neuropathology study. *Journal of Nuclear Medicine: Official Publication, Society of Nuclear Medicine.* April 2015;56(4):512–517.

141. Jensen P, Feng L, Law I, et al. TSPO Imaging in Glioblastoma Multiforme: A Direct Comparison Between ¹²³I-CLINDE SPECT, ¹⁸F-FET PET, and Gadolinium-Enhanced MR Imaging. *Journal of Nuclear Medicine: Official Publication, Society of Nuclear Medicine.* September 2015;56(9):1386–1390.

142. Herholz K, Coope D, Jackson A. Metabolic and molecular imaging in neuro-oncology. *Lancet Neurology*. August 2007;6(8):711–724.

143. Dhermain FG, Hau P, Lanfermann H, Jacobs AH, van den Bent MJ. Advanced MRI and PET imaging for assessment of treatment response in patients with gliomas. *Lancet Neurology*. 2010;9:906–920.

144. Stadlbauer A, Prante O, Nimsky C, et al. Metabolic imaging of cerebral gliomas: spatial correlation of changes in O-(2-^{18}F-fluoroethyl)-L-tyrosine PET and proton magnetic resonance spectroscopic imaging. *Journal of Nuclear Medicine: Official Publication, Society of Nuclear Medicine*. 2008;49:721–729.

145. Langen KJ, Watts C. Neuro-oncology: amino acid PET for brain tumours - ready for the clinic? *Nature Reviews. Neurology*. 2016;12:375–376.

146. Hutterer, et al. *Journal of Nuclear Medicine*. 2017;58: 129–137.

Index

Note: 'Page numbers followed by "f" indicate figures and "t" indicate tables.'